Home Visitation Programs

Lori Roggman • Nancy Cardia
Editors

Home Visitation Programs

Preventing Violence and Promoting Healthy Early Child Development

Springer

Editors
Lori Roggman
Dept. Family, Consumer, and Human Development
Utah State University
Logan
Utah
USA

Nancy Cardia
Center for the Study of Violence
University of São Paulo
São Paulo
Brazil

Translation from the Portuguese language edition: Visitação domiciliar: promovendo o desenvolvimento e prevenindo violência e acidentes by Lori Roggman and Nancy Cardia,

ISBN 978-3-319-17983-4 ISBN 978-3-319-17984-1 (eBook)
DOI 10.1007/978-3-319-17984-1

Library of Congress Control Number: 2015946568

Springer Cham Heidelberg New York Dordrecht London

Printed on acid-free paper

Springer International Publishing AG Switzerland is part of Science+Business Media (www.springer.com)

Preface

Home visitation is a rapidly expanding approach to service delivery for families of infants and young children at risk for maltreatment or poor developmental support. There is an emerging global consensus that targeting children in their early years is key to mitigating the risks associated with early aggression and developmental delay. Home visitation programs are increasingly used in high-risk populations—typically facing multiple challenges related to poverty, mental illness, or isolation—to provide individualized services in family homes to help parents provide appropriate care and developmental support to infants and young children. Research and program descriptions presented in this volume show how home visiting interventions can help mitigate parents' stress, guide parents toward more positive parenting interactions, and help families move out of poverty. Parents have benefited from home visitation programs that have helped them educate and care for their children and develop age-appropriate strategies for regulating their children's aggressive behavior.

The success of several empirically tested home visitation programs has prompted a recent expansion of funding for home visitation in the USA and in other countries worldwide. The research literature, however, is still quite limited regarding the specific strategies and components of home visitation. Several researchers working in this area were invited to share their evidence-informed expertise at the international seminar on *Home Visitation Programs: Preventing Violence and Promoting Healthy Early Child Development*, held in 2011, in São Paulo in Brazil. Based on their presentations, these experts have written the chapters in this volume.

The chapters summarize and report research on home visiting services as a means of preventing violence and promoting early child development. The chapters guide the planning, implementation, and improvement of home visitation to provide culturally adaptable individualized infancy and early childhood services that address the roots of violence and promote optimal development. Part I, which is a two-part introduction, provides the rationale and challenges for home visitation in a multicultural international context. Part II includes chapters about research on home visitation evidence, design, development, evaluation, and quality improvement. Part III includes chapters on the implementation of specific home visitation programs in different settings around the world.

Each of the chapters in this book is based on either the implications of a particular research study (e.g., Korfmacher on training paraprofessional home visitors), a review of the research literature (e.g., Innocenti on innovation in evidence-based home visiting programs), or a detailed description of tested home visiting programs (e.g., Branker and colleagues on a tested home visiting program in the Caribbean). This collection of expertise in home visitation will be especially useful not only for program designers, administrators, and policy-makers who design and implement home visiting programs but also for those in multiple disciplines—social work, psychology, special education, and early childhood—who are the researchers and evaluators studying this approach to serve families with infants and young children. It is also our hope that that this book on home visitation research and implementation in the Americas provides a strong research-based foundation for students pursuing professional careers in which they will strive to reduce community and family violence by helping vulnerable families support the early development and resilience of their infants and young children.

Acknowledgments

We are grateful to Alessandra Guedes from the Pan-American Health Organization (PAHO) for connecting us with the Open Society Institute that provided funding for the seminar on home visiting held in São Paulo in 2011. At this seminar, the authors shared their work on home visiting that has evolved into the chapters in this book. We also thank the São Paulo State Foundation for the Support of Research (FAPESP), Mercedes Hinton who was then a program officer at the Open Society Institute, and Alex Butchart from the World Health Organization (WHO) who gave tremendous support for the home visiting program developed in São Paulo, along with Joanne Klevens at the US Center for Disease Control and Prevention (CDC), the Center for the Study on Violence of the University of São Paulo (NEV/USP) which organized the seminar and the University of São Paulo (USP) which hosted the seminar. In addition, we thank the families, children, and people working in the home visiting programs who have taught us all so much about how home visiting can help families support their children's health and development in different communities and contexts.

Contents

About the Editors

Lori Roggman (USA): Professor in the Department of Family, Consumer, and Human Development at Utah State University. She studies parenting and early intervention in relation to children's early social, cognitive, and language development. Dr. Roggman's career began as a Head Start home visitor and continued as a trainer and consultant for practitioners in infant/toddler and early childhood programs. She has conducted research on early parenting and on home visiting interventions to support parenting in Early Head Start and similar programs, and she coauthored *Developmental Parenting: A Guide for Early Childhood Practitioners*. She codeveloped the PICCOLO scale using 4500 observations of parenting interactions to develop a valid, reliable, and easy-to-use measure for both researchers and practitioners that gauges affection, responsiveness, encouragement, and teaching. She also codeveloped the Home Visit Rating Scales of home visiting quality. She has served in several technical advisory groups developing methods and measures to study services for families of infants, toddlers, and young children.

Nancy Cardia (Brazil): Professor and deputy coordinator of the Center for the Study of Violence and coordinator of the activities of knowledge transfer. She represents the center as a Collaborating Centre of the World Health Organization (WHO) in the issue of prevention of violence at the Department of Prevention of Violence and Injuries. She has organized the series of books *Police and Society* and the series *Human Rights Education*. Dr. Cardia is a member of the editing committee of the World Report on Violence against Children (UN/UNICEF), author of a book about murders of children in Brazil (WHO/PAHO). She compiled the module of *Youth Violence: Causes and Prevention* for the WHO TEACH-VIP and produced, for the PAHO/GTZ, a study on how to prevent youth violence and promote healthy development. She is the general coordinator of the pilot deployment of the program of domestic visitation for adolescent mothers and their children, a program to promote healthy development and prevent violence, and is also the coordinator of research on exposure to violence and its impact on attitudes, values, norms regarding violence, human rights, justice, and democracy.

About the Authors

Renato Alves (Brazil): PhD and master's degree holder in Psychology from the University of São Paulo. He holds a degree in Psychology from the Methodist University of São Paulo and a degree in Social Sciences from the University of São Paulo. He is a researcher at the Center for the Study of Violence at the University of São Paulo (NEV/USP) and professor of Psychology at the Methodist University of São Paulo.

Susan Michelle Branker (Barbados): A development and evaluation specialist consultant and a former programme director of the Bernard Van Leer Foundation's (BvLF) Caribbean Child Support Initiative (CCSI) Programme Management Unit (2001–2011) based in Barbados. She holds a bachelor of science degree in Sociology and Political Science from the University of the West Indies, Cave Hill Campus, Barbados, and a master of science degree in International Relations from the University of Southampton, United Kingdom. She has over 15 years of multi-country and multi-sector program management and development evaluation experience with a strong track record of performance in the start-up and replication of non-formal, culturally relevant and effective and approaches to early childhood development and parenting support. She presented the importance of quality, non-formal approaches to early childhood development and family support service provision to regional and international audiences in the Caribbean context and is a strong advocate for mainstreaming such approaches into the existing government systems and services.

Alberto Concha-Eastman (Colombia): Currently advisor on violence prevention and public health for the Mayor of Cali, Colombia. He was consultant of the regional Pan American Health Organization (PAHO/WHO-Washington) for the areas of Injuries and Violence Prevention and Sustainable Development and Environmental Health. He holds a master's degree in Epidemiology from Universidad del Valle, Colombia and a master of science degree in Epidemiology from the London School of Hygiene and Tropical Medicine. He has also been a visiting scholar at David Rockefeller Center for Latin American Studies at Harvard University.

Martha Julia Garcia-Sellers (USA): Professor, Tufts University, Child Development Department Director, Home-School Connection Program and the Family Values Project. She began her professional career in Guatemala as a psychologist in a multidisciplinary team carrying out applied research with malnourished children at the Institute of Nutrition of Central America and Panamá (INCAP), a unit of the Pan American Health Organization. Since completing her doctoral training in Child Development at Harvard University, she has devoted her efforts to the study of child-family assessment and preventive intervention of infants and preschool children. She is the founder and director of the Home-School Connection Program (H-SCP), a home visiting program strengthening communication among teachers, parents and children from immigrant families from Latin America living in the USA and in rural communities in Guatemala. At present, in collaboration with the Cultural Change Institute, she directs the Family Values Project for Hispanic and Brazilian immigrant families living in Boston, rural families living in Costa Rica, and Brazilian families in São Paulo.

Breanna Gassner (USA): Graduate student with a master's degree in American Studies and a degree in Human Development and Family Studies. She has worked as a research assistant and data analyst on projects related to bias and racial prejudice and has presented her research at national conferences. She currently works as an administrative assistant and tutor in the Learning Center at the Pennsylvania State University, Shenango Campus.

Aline Mizutani Gomes (Brazil): Researcher at the Center for the Study of Violence at the University of São Paulo (NEV/USP). She collaborated in the development of a home visiting program for pregnant adolescents and their children to prevent violence and secure a healthy development, being a visitor herself as well as a supervisor for paraprofessional visitors. She has a master's and an MA degree in Psychology as well as a Psychologist degree (five-year degree). She was a home visitor and continued as a trainer in the Infância Saudável (a home visitation program). At the Center for the Study of Violence, her research interests include early child development, adolescent pregnancy, and violence prevention.

Mark S. Innocenti (USA): Associate professor of psychology at Utah State University and director of the Research and Evaluation Division of the Center for Persons with Disabilities, a university center of excellence for the development of people with disabilities. He has over 30 years of experience in multidisciplinary work with children at risk and with disabilities and their families and has coordinated a series of research projects, including a 10-year longitudinal study on the effects and costs of early intervention with children with disabilities and a study of early literacy and bilingual early language support. His current research focuses on developing strategies and evaluation assessments for home visitation programs and in evaluating preschool education as a means of preventing later special education.

Jon Korfmacher (USA): Associate professor at the Erikson Institute. His research focuses on differential responses of children and families to early childhood intervention programs. He is interested in understanding why families participate in these programs, what the experience is like for them, and what types of services work best for different families under different circumstances. He also studies the training and professional development of early childhood service providers. He is also a faculty associate with the Herr Research Center for Children and Social Policy and a graduate fellow of ZERO TO THREE.

Horis Lynch (Barbados): Former research assistant with the Caribbean Child Support Initiative Programme Management Unit in Barbados. He holds a bachelor of science degree in Political Science and Law from the University of the West Indies and is interested in Social Policy Research and the effects of early childhood intervention on children's development from school entry to early adulthood. He studies family, school, and other social influences on children's educational success and contextual factors that influence adolescent development, particularly for rural minorities.

William McGuigan (USA): Associate professor of Human Development and Family Studies at the Pennsylvania State University, Shenango Campus. He is a certified family life educator and a member of the American Professional Society on the Abuse of Children, the American Sociological Association, and the National Council on Family Relations. He has served on the review board of Child Abuse & Neglect: The International Journal. His research focuses on child abuse, family violence, and the effectiveness of home visitation programs.

Maristela G. Monteiro (USA): Senior advisor in alcohol and substance abuse at the Pan American Health Organization (PAHO). She joined PAHO in December 2003, after working for nearly 10 years in Geneva at the World Health Organization, coordinating the area of alcohol and substance abuse. She is a medical doctor with a PhD in Psychopharmacology from the Federal University of São Paulo, Brazil.

Alder Mourão (Brazil): Researcher at the Center for the Study of Violence at the University of São Paulo (NEV/USP). He collaborated in the development of a home visiting program to promote healthy early child development as well as to prevent violence for a high-risk group as a visitor and as a supervisor. He has a master's and an MSc in Nursing. His research focuses on public and family health, early child development, and violence prevention.

Clive Murray (Barbados): Communication for development specialist with over 10 years of progressive work experience in the nonprofit sector in the Caribbean region. He has developed and managed initiatives in the areas of communication and advocacy for early childhood development, community development, donor management, and media relations. He holds a master of arts degree in Social Development and Sustainable Livelihoods from the University of Reading, United Kingdom and a bachelor of arts in media and communication from the University of the West Indies (UWI) Mona, Kingston, Jamaica.

S. Darius Tandon (USA): Associate professor at Northwestern University Feinberg School of Medicine where he is also associate director of Center for Community Health. He is interested in understanding how to address psychosocial risk factors, particularly maternal depression, among women using early childhood intervention programs. Much of his recent work involves the integration of a cognitive-behavioral stress management intervention into early childhood programs with the aim of preventing the onset and worsening of depression.

Nick Wechsler (USA): Infant specialist and the director for Program Development for the Ounce of Prevention Fund in Illinois, USA. For the Ounce, he has developed, trained, and supported numerous program strategies and services to promote secure parent–child relationships in both home- and center-based programs. These activities include: video intervention, doula services, the Community-Based Family Administered Neonatal Activities (C-B FANA, a perinatal guide for home visitors), infant mental health services and consultation, reflective supervision, and Dr. T. Berry Brazelton's Touchpoints.

J. Leonardo Yánez (Bernard van Leer Foundation/Netherlands): Senior program officer for Latin America at the Bernard van Leer Foundation. He worked in academia, NGOs, and government in Venezuela on primary and preschool care and education before joining the foundation in 2000, initially coordinating the "Effectiveness Initiative" before moving onto developing and managing programs in the Latin America region. He was national director of Preschool Education and general director of Programme Coordination for Social Development in Venezuela and ex-chairman of Primary and Preschool Education Department at the Andrés Bello University. He has contributed to the design, implementation, and evaluation of programmes for Early Childhood Care and Development, and worked as consultant for UNICEF, Social Science Research Centre, Book's Bank, National Institute for Child and Youth, Ministries of Family and Social Development, Education and Planning, among others.

Part I
Introduction to Home Visiting and its Challenges

Chapter 1
Introduction: Home Visitation as a Primary Prevention Tool for Violence

Alberto Concha-Eastman

Primary prevention has been demonstrated as the most effective way to avoid the development of diseases or the risks of situations that jeopardize people's lives. Vaccines, applied early in life, are the single best example of primary prevention. Thanks to global efforts, smallpox was globally eradicated in 1978. Polio does not exist anymore in the Americas. New vaccines are under investigation to attack other preventable diseases. If people stop drinking when driving, then no alcohol-related traffic crashes would happen anymore.

In the case of violence and aggression, there might not be a "vaccine" available, but it is well known that a nonviolent intrafamily environment will significantly reduce the likelihood that children will become aggressors later on in their lives. Violence is a multicausal and multilevel phenomenon. Roots of violence have been identified at individual, family, and community interactions as well as at macro-societal level. This complexity makes it more difficult to have a unique tool to prevent or control its occurrence or prevalence. There is, however, a global consensus that targeting children in their early years is the key to mitigating the social and individual environmental risks associated with youth violence and aggression (Maggi et al., 2005). The earlier an intervention is put in place, the larger the likelihood it will result in positive outcomes. Just as vaccines that are applied to infants and toddlers, social and family programs that go to the roots of early aggression and violence can be named as primary violence prevention programs.

This primary violence prevention approach has gained more adherents since violence has been accepted as a public health issue, shifting from repression and control to prevention based on an intersectoral and multidisciplinary approach. Public health is not medicine, it is "…the collective intervention by the state and civil

We must address the roots of violence. Only then will we transform the past century's legacy from a crushing burden into a cautionary lesson. Nelson Mandela, foreword to the WHO World Report on Violence and Health, 2002

A. Concha-Eastman (✉)
Cali, Colombia
e-mail: alberto.conchaeastman@gmail.com

L. Roggman, N. Cardia (eds.), *Home Visitation Programs*,
DOI 10.1007/978-3-319-17984-1_1

society to protect and improve the health of the people. It is a social practice of an interdisciplinary nature" (Pan American Health Organization, 2002). Addressing the roots of violence is, however, a challenge. It requires working on the social determinants of aggression as close as possible to their origin. Social determinants of health, as defined by the World Health Organization (WHO) and Commission on Social Determinants of Health (CSDH), are "the circumstances in which people grow, live, work, and age" (Commission on Social Determinants of Health, 2008, p. 2), and consequently as the first of the commission's recommendations they state, "Improve the well-being of girls and women and the circumstances in which their children are born, put major emphasis on early child development (ECD) and education for girls and boys, improve living and working conditions and create social protection policy supportive of all, and create conditions for a flourishing older life" (Commission on Social Determinants of Health, 2008, p. 44). Strategies aimed at enhancing parents' capacity to raise their offspring and build a creative and bonding relationship are badly needed as part of a primary violence prevention effort.

Aggression develops early in life. ECD literature suggests that children are at risk for aggressive development if they live in a stressful family environment, if they are physically abused, or are poor and living in vulnerable neighborhoods. Neuroscience research on ECD shows that the brain of a child is very sensitive to external influences in early childhood. The conditions to which children are exposed, including the quality of relationships and language environment, literally "sculpt" the developing brain (Mustard, 2007). As the CSDH pointed out, "investments in ECD are one of the most powerful that countries can make—in terms of reducing the escalating chronic disease burden in adults, reducing costs for judicial and prison systems, and enabling more children to grow into healthy adults who can make a positive contribution to society, socially and economically." Interventions that mitigate parents' stress, keep parents from abusing their children, or help families move out of poverty may encourage parents to support their children's development of age-appropriate strategies for regulating aggressive behavior. Young children who manifest severe and pervasive forms of aggression demonstrate significant levels of social impairment in preschool and beyond and are therefore more likely to develop chronic antisocial behaviors and compounding mental health problems.

For the above reasons, a very powerful recommendation of the WHO CSDH clearly states, "5.1. WHO and UN Children's Fund (UNICEF) set up an interagency mechanism to ensure policy coherence for early child development such that, across agencies, a comprehensive approach to early child development is acted on" (Commission on Social Determinants of Health, 2008, p. 51).

In different environments, research has shown that by 17 months of age, the onset of physical aggression was reported for close to 80 % of the children (Tremblay et al., 2006). Fortunately, by preschool age most children have "unlearned" aggression, but for a small percentage (5–8 %) aggression persists in their life span (Farrington, 1995). Programs that demonstrate effectiveness in reducing aggression in children contribute to the reduction of risk behaviors, aggression, violence, and delinquency later on in the children's lives (Anderson et al., 2003; Bowles, Akpokodje, & Tigere, 2005). Nonetheless, there are also factors that reduce the likelihood of a child ever becoming involved in risky behaviors. Some of the identified protective factors are family ties, empowerment, strengthened communication, positive life expectations, constructive use of time, commitment to learning, and enhanced social skills.

Parents from low-income families in vulnerable and disfranchised conditions need support to educate and look after their children. Children who have been loved, guided, cared for, and properly supported have better school performance, enjoy better health, show improved socialization skills, and are better able, later in their adolescence and youth, to confront different risks and challenges. In the long term, they also have fewer rates of criminal and delinquent activities. Identifying the proper target group as early as possible in their social environment, that is, pregnant women and their partners as well as their children from birth up to age six living in deprived neighborhoods where intrafamily violence, insecurity, substance abuse, unsafe sex, and aggression are prevalent, is key for potential success.

Knowledge, skills, and access to ECD are scarce in developing countries. Besides, institutional services for children do not usually include ECD programs. An ECD program that integrates home visitation outreach as a tool to approach families linked to institutional services is seen as a primary prevention initiative. As aggression is the earliest detectable and preventable problem behavior in children, home visitation may be the most adequate tool as a primary aggression and violence prevention initiative to be developed jointly with communities and institutions through educating and supporting families. For instance, the Nurse–Family Partnership, developed in the USA by Olds, is an evidence-based nurse home visiting program designed to improve the health, well-being, and self-sufficiency of young first-time parents and their children. Findings suggest that the likelihood of child abuse and accidents is reduced, the likelihood of children having improved developmental outcomes as they reach school age is increased, and the likelihood of antisocial behavior in children when they reach their teens is reduced (Olds et al. 1997). In Brazil, another home visiting program has shown powerful impacts on children's developmental outcomes. The *Primeira Infancia Melhor* (PIM) Program (The Better Early Childhood Development Program), broadly implemented since 2003, has trained personnel in 367 municipalities (74 %) of the State of Rio Grande Do Sul on PIM, and 267 of these have been properly enabled for its implementation. In its 2010 evaluation, the program showed significant advantages in development for children participating in the intervention group, compared with those in the control group, in motor skills, language development, social interaction, and cognitive skills (PIM, 2011).

Specifically, this type of initiative focuses on developing parenting skills, encouraging parental improvement in education and empowerment, explaining the rights for adequate mental and physical health care for both the pregnant women and their unborn infants, and improving pregnant women and their partners' understanding of their parenting role. Training health-care personnel at different levels on the theories and practice of ECD and home visitation initiatives as well as advocating and promoting the integration of health and family services for children are required. The concept of an integral ECD program has to be promoted, emphasizing the need for wide local implementation and for a sustainability plan.

The home visitation programs described by Martha Garcia-Sellers (Chap. 11, this volume) are based on a home-school model in East Boston and Somerville (Massachusetts) in the USA, targeting playground toddlers or children from Latin American immigrant families and also implemented in Pastores, a rural community in Guatemala, targeting preschool to third-grade children. These programs show the possibility of success when the community needs are met to build an intrafamily bonding relationship that goes beyond the program itself. Outcomes can be perpetuated when involvement from participants is encouraged and maintained.

Complementary to these examples of good practice was the emphasis of Mark Innocenti (Chap. 9, also this volume) on the need to have a basis of research evidence for home visitation program models. In his presentation, he showed results of the home visiting evidence of effectiveness (HomVEE; Paulsell, Avellar, Martin, & Del Grosso, 2010) for a set of home visitation models targeting pregnant women and their children up to age 5. The results show various positive impacts on maternal and child health, child development, school readiness, reductions in child maltreatment, reductions in juvenile delinquency, positive parenting practices, and other impacts. Despite not reaching a full positive evaluation of each model in each impact, the HomVEE results clearly send the message that there are positive results based on properly designed and implemented home visitation programs, regardless of concerns on their cost, in particular in the USA, where evaluations are demanded.

Effective home visiting programs begin with a clear vision. For example, a home visitation program in the difficult conditions of the Khayelitsha neighborhood, Cape Town, South Africa, has a clearly predefined vision: "The Parent Centre strives to contribute to a society in which every parent/caregiver is able to raise resilient children in ways in which they can develop their full potential, protected from victimization and abuse in communities free from violence" (Barries, 2011, p. 5), meaning that change is possible even in very difficult circumstances. Barries pointed out some lessons learned that apply not only for her context but also to many others, such as the need to make supervision for all program staff because some clients, despite support and information, may continue to struggle with parenting and may need statutory intervention; need to network and partner; need to implement vital ongoing training; and the need to make a rigorous selection of staff. These recommendations are crucial to implementing a home visitation program in difficult settings.

It is important to stress that in many communities there is limited access for vulnerable families to health and family support services. In general, those that are currently offered in developing countries do not have the required knowledge about violence prevention and do not address parenting skills to identify and prevent aggression and deal with anger. Home visitation programs show promise at the earliest period of infancy. Positive, early preventive interventions through parent–child interactions and parenting skills can be a highly protective factor against adverse child outcomes. Through a well-planned ECD Home Visitation program, mothers, fathers, and other caregivers' skills can be enhanced, and access to health services for pregnant women and young mothers can be improved.

Much work is needed to have ECD Home Visitation programs fully installed and sustained. As a key approach to primary violence prevention for lowering the risk of aggression, delinquency, and crime, these home visitation approaches have to be expanded. Our obligation is to maintain our conviction and commitment to this work because the need to continue working to reduce violence and aggression is a must.

References

Anderson, L. M., Fielding, J. E., Fullilove, M. T., Scrimshaw, S. C., & Carande-Kulis, V. G. (2003). Methods for conducting systematic reviews of the evidence of effectiveness and economic efficiency of interventions to promote healthy social environments. *American Journal of Preventive Medicine, 24*(3), 25–31.

Barries, V. (2011, May). *Parent-infant intervention home visiting programme: An attachment-based parent-infant intervention provided by community counselors*. International Seminar on Home Visitation Programs: Preventing Violence and Promoting Healthy Early Child Development. São Paulo, Brazil.

Bowles, R., Akpokodje, J., & Tigere, E. (2005). Evidence-based approaches to crime prevention in developing countries. *European Journal on Criminal Policy and Research, 11*(3–4), 347–377.

Commission on Social Determinants of Health. (2008). *Closing the gap in a generation: Health equity through action on the social determinants of health*. Final Report of the Commission on Social Determinants of Health. Geneva, Switzerland: World Health Organization.

Farrington, D. P. (1995). The development of offending and antisocial behaviour from childhood: Key findings from the Cambridge Study in Delinquent Development. *Journal of Child Psychology and Psychiatry, 36*(6), 929–964.

Maggi, F., Irwin, G. L., Siddiqi, A., Poureslami, I., Hertzman, E., & Hertzman, C. (2005). *International perspectives one early child development*. Analytic and Strategic Review Paper prepared by the Knowledge Network for Early Child Development of the Commission on the Social Determinants of Health, Geneva, Switzerland: World Health Organization.

Mustard, J. F. (2007). Experience-based brain development: Scientific underpinnings of the importance of early child development in a global world. In M. E. Young & L. M. Richardson (Eds.), *Early child development: From measurement to action* (pp. 43–71). Washington, DC: World Bank.

Olds, D. L., Eckenrode, J., Henderson, C. R., Kitzman, H., Powers, J., Cole, R., Sidora, K., Morris, P., Pettitt, L. M., & Luckey, D. (1997). Long term effects of home visitation on maternal life course and child abuse and neglect: Fifteen year follow-up of a randomized control trial. *Journal of the American Medical Association, 278*, 637–643.

Pan American Health Organization. (2002). *Public health in the Americas. Conceptual renewal, performance assessment, and bases for action, scientific and technical publication No. 589*. Washington, DC: Pan American Health Organization.

Paulsell, D., Avellar, S., Martin, E. S., & Del Grosso, P. (2010). *Home visiting evidence of effectiveness review: Executive summary* (No. 6938). Mathematica Policy Research.

Programa Primeira Infância Melhor. (2011). *Segundo Corte Avaliativo*, Boletim Informativo. http://www.pim.saude.rs.gov.br/a_PIM/boletinsInformativos/Boletim-EdicaoEspecial-SegundoCorteAvaliativo.pdf. Accessed 7 Aug 2011.

Tremblay, R. E., Japel, C., Pérusse, D., Boivan, M., Zoccolillo, M., Montplaisir, J., & McDuff, P. (2006). The search for age of "onset" of physical aggression: Rousseau and Bandura revisited. *Criminal Behavior and Mental Health, 9*(1), 8–23.

Alberto Concha-Eastman MD, MSc (Colombia): Currently advisor on Violence Prevention and Public Health for the Mayor of Cali, Colombia. He was the consultant of the regional Pan American Health Organization (PAHO/WHO-Washington) for the areas of injuries and violence prevention and sustainable development and environmental health. He holds a master's degree in epidemiology from Universidad del Valle, Colombia, and a master of science in Epidemiology from the London School of Hygiene and Tropical Medicine. He has also been a visiting scholar at the David Rockefeller Center for Latin American Studies at Harvard University.

Chapter 2
The Four Challenges of Home Visitation Programs: Alcohol and Substance Abuse, Intrafamilial Violence, and Mental Disorders

Maristela G. Monteiro

The use of alcohol and other drugs is particularly serious in high-risk communities and is related to their availability and cost; therefore, consumption will be higher where they are widely available and have a low cost (Babor et al., 2010a, 2010b). The harms caused by alcohol are proportionally higher in low- and middle-income countries, partly, due to the lack of services and resources, including an absence of enforced policies, safe roads, electricity, health services, police presence, and safe leisure spaces (World Health Organization, 2011). The harms caused by alcohol increase where there are no policies in place, either at local or national levels to reduce access to alcoholic beverages, limit excessive drinking, sales to minors, sales to intoxicated people, or the marketing and promotion of alcohol products. One of the most important negative results of excessive drinking is violent and aggressive behavior, which can aggravate already existing violent situations in the family or in the community (Pan American Health Organization, 2010). The use of other drugs—especially stimulants, such as cocaine, crack, methamphetamines, and other related substances—is also associated with violence (World Health Organization, 2004). Home visitors may need training to recognize symptoms of alcohol and substance abuse and to convey clear messages about the dangers of excessive alcohol and drug use, and the available community services to reduce such problems.

Alcohol and stimulant drugs, in particular, are associated with violence, but intrafamilial violence occurs even when alcohol use or other substance use is not excessive (WHO/London School of Hygiene and Tropical Medicine, 2010). Often, this type of violence is prevalent in countries with more social and gender inequalities, where laws and policies are lacking for the prevention of violence and reduction of its impact on women and families, and in cultures in which violence is more accepted (WHO/Commission on Social Determinants of Health, 2008). As a result, in communities that do not offer equal access to education and employment for women and in which men have much more power than women, the risk of violence against women and children is greater and can be aggravated by the excessive

M. G. Monteiro (✉)
Alcohol and Substance Abuse, Pan American Health Organization, Washington, DC, USA
e-mail: monteirm@paho.org

L. Roggman, N. Cardia (eds.), *Home Visitation Programs*,
DOI 10.1007/978-3-319-17984-1_2

use of alcohol (Pan American Health Organization, 2008). Home visitors are often the only persons who may witness intrafamilial violence, and in some cases home visitors could be at risk of violence.

Finally, when not treated, mental disorders—such as depression, schizophrenia, and other conditions—can interfere with the acceptance of home visitation programs and adherence to them. In the majority of countries, there are significant gaps in the treatment of mental disorders due to a lack of specialized services, services integrated in primary health care, or trained professionals and access to essential medicines (World Health Organization, 2010a, 2005b). The stigma attached to mental disorders prevents people—both men and women—from seeking help or discussing their emotions with health professionals, specialized or not (World Health Organization, 2010b; Room, 2005). For example, postpartum depression can lead the mother to neglect the child, underestimating or not interacting with their babies, which may result in developmental delays that could be avoided (Murray & Cooper, 1997). Depression and problems with alcohol or other drugs can affect women, victims of violence, making it difficult to develop bonds with their children and provide care to them (Romito et al., 2009). It is also possible that violent men with untreated mental disorders have a compromised capacity to promote the healthy development of their children and care for them. Violence against children is also relatively common, varying from verbal abuse to maltreatment and extreme punishments, which are not reported to health professionals due to fears of separation, police involvement, or retaliation by the other parent (Pan American Health Organization, 2011).

These are issues with difficult solutions. These challenges constitute significant barriers to the inclusion of affected children and high-risk families in home visitation programs. At the same time, these are precisely the families which would most benefit from these programs. Therefore, it is urgent to do research and build the capacity of home visitation workers and others responsible for these programs. To build healthy and safe communities, it is fundamental that these issues be dealt with under the lens of social and human rights. This way, these problems can be minimized in the most efficient way so that families feel safe and comfortable to talk, confidentially, about the risks they are facing, receive information on how to reduce them, seek care and treatment for mental health issues, and obtain support to change their life conditions (MacArthur Foundation Network, 2010).

These challenges point to the association between social determinants of health and the efficacy and sustainability of home visitation programs. Social and gender equity—through the development of sustainable programs and policies to promote the healthy and safe development of individuals and communities, and at the same time to protect and promote human rights—can be the way to expand the utilization and impact of home visitation programs in other parts of the world (Room et al., 2006; Schmidt et al., 2010; WHO/Commission on Social Determinants of Health, 2008).

References

Babor, T., Caetano, R., Casswell, S., Edwards, G., Giesbrecht, N., Graham, K., et al. (2010a). *Alcohol: No ordinary commodity—Research and public policy* (2nd ed.). New York: Oxford University Press.
Babor, T. F., et al. (2010b). *Drug policy and the public good*. Oxford: Oxford University Press.
Kumpfer, K. L., Alvarado, R., Kendal, K., Beesley, S., Cavanass-Lee, C. (2002). *Strengthening America's families* (CSAP/OJJDP monograph). Salt Lake City: Department of Health Promotion and Education, College of Health, University of Utah.
MacArthur Foundation Network on SES and Health. (2010). The biology of disadvantage: Socioeconomic status and health. *Annals of the New York Academy of Sciences, 1186,* 1–275.
Murray, L., Cooper, P. J. (1997). Postpartum depression and child development. *Psychological Medicine, 27*(2), 253–260.
Pan American Health Organization. (2008). *Multicentric study on gender, alcohol, culture and harms; final report*. Washington, DC: PAHO.
Pan American Health Organization. (2010). Unhappy hours: Alcohol and partner aggression in the Americas. In K. Graham, S. Bernards, M. Munné, & S. C. Wilsnack (Eds.), *Scientific publication no. 631*. Washington, DC: PAHO.
Pan American Health Organization. (2011). Bibliografía sobre abuso o maltrato infantile. In A. Concha-Eastman, Y. Benguigui, & R. Salgado (Eds.), *Serie HCT/AIEPI-44.E.* Washington, DC: PAHO.
Romito, P., Pomicino, L., Lucchetta, C., Scrimin, F., Turan, J. M. (2009). The relationships between physical violence, verbal abuse and women's psychological distress during the postpartum period. *Journal of Psychosomatic Obstetrics Gynaecology, 30*(2), 115–121.
Room, R. (2005). Stigma, social inequality and alcohol and drug use. *Drug and Alcohol Review, 24*, 143–155.
Room, R., Mäkelä, P., Schmidt, L., & Rehm, J. (2006). *Alcohol, health disparities and development*. Geneva: World Health Organization. (Expert committee meeting document)
Schmidt, L., Mäkelä, P., Rehm, J., & Room, R. (2010). Alcohol: Equity and social determinants. In E. Blas, & A. Sivasankara Kurup (Eds.), *Equity, social determinants and public health programmes* (pp. 11–29). Geneva: World Health Organization. http://www.who.int/social_determinants/en/.
World Health Organization. (2004). *Neuroscience of psychoactive substance use and dependence*. Geneva: World Health Organization.
World Health Organization. (2005a). *Substance use among young people in urban environments*. Geneva: World Health Organization.
World Health Organization. (2005b). *Mental health atlas*. Geneva: World Health Organization.
World Health Organization. (2010a). *Atlas on substance use: Resources for the prevention and treatment of substance use disorders*. Geneva: World Health Organization.
World Health Organization. (2010b). *Mental health and development: Targeting people with mental health conditions as a vulnerable group*. Geneva: World Health Organization.
World Health Organization. (2011). *Global status report on alcohol and health*. Geneva: World Health Organization.
World Health Organization Commission on Social Determinants of Health. (2008). *Closing the gap in a generation: Health equity through action on the social determinants of health*. Geneva: World Health Organization.
World Health Organization London School of Hygiene and Tropical Medicine. (2010). *Preventing intimate partner and sexual violence against women: Taking action and generating evidence*. Geneva: World Health Organization.

Maristela G. Monteiro MD, PhD (USA): Senior advisor in alcohol and substance abuse at the Pan American Health Organization (PAHO). She joined PAHO in December 2003, after working for nearly 10 years in Geneva at the World Health Organization, coordinating the area of alcohol and substance abuse. She is a medical doctor with a PhD in Psychopharmacology, from the Federal University of São Paulo, Brazil.

Part II
Home Visiting Programs and Practices: Research and Evaluation

Chapter 3
Home Visiting to Enhance Child Development in the Context of Violence: Possibilities and Limitations

Jon Korfmacher and Lori Roggman

Children who are victims or witnesses of violence are more likely to show early and persistent aggressive behavior (Baldry, 2003; Cummings, Goeke-Morey, & Papp, 2004; Margolin & Gordis, 2000). Violence and aggression are sadly common in very poor communities, in which poverty creates additional stress that is associated with more childhood aggression (Guerra, Huesmann, Tolan, Van Acker, & Eron, 1995; Tremblay et al., 2004). Childhood aggression is also higher when parents are insensitive, harsh, or abusive (National Institute of Child Health and Development (NICHD) Early Child Care Research Network (ECCRN), 2004; Tremblay et al., 2004). These influences are rarely entirely separate and confined to a single generation. Children who live in poor families and communities are more likely to experience aggression at home and in their neighborhoods and are also more likely to become aggressive at a young age and remain aggressive in adolescence and adulthood, suggesting an intergenerational cycle of aggression and violence (Cappell & Heiner, 1990).

Home visiting programs may be able to help families interrupt this cycle by improving parenting, supporting children's positive development, and decreasing children's behavior problems (Avellar & Suplee, 2013; Moss et al., 2011). This chapter examines the links between violence exposure and children's early aggression, as well as the importance of children's early development for their resilience to stress and self-regulation of aggression. We explore aspects of early environments that support children's development and resilience, with a particular focus on the potential of home visiting to reduce the risk of violence and aggression. Without repeating what is explored in other chapters of this book (see, e.g., chapters in this volume by Innocenti, Korfmacher, and Roggman), we place this discussion in the context of evidence that supports the effectiveness of home visiting to improve parenting and

J. Korfmacher (✉)
Erikson Institute, Chicago, USA
e-mail: jkorfmacher@erikson.edu

L. Roggman
Utah State University, Logan, USA

L. Roggman, N. Cardia (eds.), *Home Visitation Programs*,
DOI 10.1007/978-3-319-17984-1_3

child development. We conclude by applying these findings to the expansion and improvement of home visiting in international contexts.

Violence Exposure and Aggression

Children in many families and communities are exposed to violence, either as victims or as witnesses. In 2012, in the USA, child protective service agencies identified 686,000 children, about 9 of every 1000 children and 22 of every 1000 infants under age 1, who were "found to be victims" of child maltreatment, either by abuse or by neglect (Children's Bureau, 2013). Most of these agency-confirmed maltreatment cases, three in four, were due to neglect, but rates of abuse may actually be higher than these data suggest. In a random sample of over 1400 US men and women, 1 in 5 adults, or 200 of every 1000, reported that they had been physically abused during their childhood (Briere & Elliott, 2003). Rates of violence exposure are similarly high: One in four US children witness family violence in their homes during childhood (Hamby, Finkelhor, Turner, & Ormrod, 2011). In other parts of the world, the situation is similar: An average of 23 % of adults report abuse during their childhood, and 25–50 % of children, across countries, report being abused (Pinheiro, 2006; Butchart et al., 2006). These direct experiences of violence in young children's communities and families have been clearly associated with childhood and adolescent aggression (Evans, Davies, & DiLillo, 2008; Lansford et al., 2007; Margolin & Gordis, 2000). Even indirect experiences, such as when children witness domestic violence at home, are linked with aggression (Baldry, 2003), and the combination of abuse and violence exposure is an especially powerful predictor of childhood aggression (Bourassa, 2007; Hughes, Parkinson, & Vargo, 1989). Children who are physically punished, even if not considered victims of abuse, are also more likely to show aggressive behavior (Afifi, Brownridge, Cox, & Sareen, 2006). Children with persistent aggressive behavior in early childhood are likely to show later aggression and violence (Brame, Nagin, & Tremblay, 2001; Duke, Pettingell, McMorris, & Borowsky, 2010; Nagin & Tremblay, 1999), including violence in their families and communities when they are adults (Cappell & Heiner, 1990; American Psychological Association, 1996).

To disrupt this cycle of violence, children need good care in healthy families. Safe, stable, nurturing family relationships are protective factors that can prevent the intergenerational transmission of abuse in families (Jaffee et al., 2013; Schofield, Lee, & Merrick, 2013). These relationships, however, are often fragile in conditions of poverty and violence, and given the high rates of maltreatment noted above, parents cannot always be counted on as protectors of their children. Parents living in these kinds of stressful conditions, often themselves victims and witnesses of violence, are more likely to show the kinds of harsh, punitive, and insensitive or uninvolved care that contributes to children's early and persistent aggression (Chang, Schwartz, Dodge, & McBride-Chang, 2003; Kimonis et al., 2006; Knutson, DeGarmo, Koeppl, & Reid, 2005; NICHD ECCRN, 2004; Olson, Bates,

Sandy, & Lanthier, 2000). Parenting styles certainly vary by culture, but even across ethnic and cultural groups, parents' harshness is associated with more child aggression in the home and more child emotional problems both at home and in school (Ho, Bluestein, & Jenkins 2008).

These aspects of harsh or unreliable parenting that underlay children's early aggression are associated not only with poverty but also with various other risk factors that come with poverty: chronic stress, traumatic experiences, poor education, and poor mental health (Banyard, Williams, & Siegel, 2003; Farrington & Loeber, 2000; Frias-Armenta & McCloskey, 1998; Lee, 2009; Martorell & Bugental, 2006; Romano, Tremblay, Boulerice, & Swisher, 2005). In the context of various combinations of these environmental and parenting factors, children's early development and lifelong health and functioning can be greatly compromised (Anda et al., 2006), and early and persistent aggression becomes far more likely (Putnam, 2006).

It is important to consider that there is variation in the path that emerges from early aggression. Aggressive behavior in children as young as age 2 or 3 is not uncommon and typically, in the context of safe, secure, nurturing relationships, decreases over time as children develop better self-regulation skills rather than persisting into later aggression (Eisenberg et al., 2001; Hill, Degnan, Calkins, & Keane, 2006; Alink et al., 2006; Tremblay et al., 2004; Tremblay, 2000). A risk factor for persistent aggression, however, is early insecure attachment (DeMulder, Denham, Schmidt, & Mitchell, 2000; Finzi, Ram, Har-Even, Shnit, & Weizman, 2001; Lyons-Ruth, Alpern, & Repacholi, 1993; NICHD ECCRN, 2004; Ooi, Ang, Fung, Wong, & Cai, 2006; Aguilar, Sroufe, Egeland, & Carlson, 2000). Children's attachment security depends on their experiences of sensitive and responsive care during infancy (De Wolff & Van IJzendoorn, 1997), but in the absence of that kind of parenting, especially when parenting is sometimes frightening, children develop insecure attachments that can be expressed in anger and aggression (Lyons-Ruth, 1996; Lyons-Ruth, Easterbrooks, & Davidson, 1997). An insecure parent–child relationship may be even more likely to lead to aggression if parents use physical punishment, which is associated with both insecure attachment and childhood aggression (Coyl, Roggman, & Newland, 2002; Posada & Pratt, 2008; Roggman & Cook, 2011; Weiss, Dodge, Bates, & Pettit, 1992).

As this brief review demonstrates, there are multiple causes of violence in early childhood and multiple impacts of this violence in children's later functioning. Clearly, however, parents exert a powerful influence on the experience of a young child, and the parent–child relationship can filter and buffer the impact of the larger sociocultural context. Parenting, then, offers an opening for early intervention efforts. Effective early interventions help parents to provide more sensitive parenting to support secure attachment and provide more developmentally supportive parenting to help children learn to communicate and regulate their emotions and behaviors. Parenting that is neither harsh nor indifferent, but instead responsive and engaged, can interrupt and moderate the effects of stressful, impoverished, or violent environments on aggression and other negative developmental outcomes (Schofield et al., 2013).

Longitudinal research demonstrates four core developmental principles that guide effective early interventions. First, development in the earliest years predicts lifelong outcomes in multiple developmental domains—physical, cognitive, language, social, and emotional development. Second, factors that put early development at risk are cumulative and include not only experiences with violence but also other adverse experiences associated with living in poverty—experiences that often occur before children can remember them, but that predict long-term negative outcomes in health, relationships, and all domains of development. Third, much of children's development occurs in the context of relationships, mostly with their parents, who are also likely to have experienced violence and adversity in their families and communities. Fourth, this grim situation can be offset by positive parent–child relationships that provide developmentally supportive early environments in which parents prevent violence, protect children's safety, and promote children's resilience and in which children can develop and thrive.

Using Family Interventions to Reduce Violence and Aggression

Interventions that increase the kind of parenting that supports children's early development have the potential to disrupt the intergenerational cycle of violence (Jaffee et al., 2013). The key question, of course, is: How do we promote positive and engaged parenting in the communities and families where it is arguably both most needed and where it is most at risk not to happen? At this intersection of early childhood and violence, various national and international policies and practices have been suggested to reduce both children's exposure to violence and children's development of early aggression. In the USA the Centers for Disease Control and Prevention (CDC) have described a series of steps to create safe, stable, nurturing relationships in children's lives, including implementing evidence-based programs for parents and caregivers (CDC, 2013). The CDC recommends programs that include components associated with effectiveness, such as teaching parents positive childrearing strategies and alternatives to physical punishment, emphasizing the importance of nurturing relationships with their children, and providing opportunities for parents to actively practice these skills with their children (c.f., Kaminski, Valle, Filene, & Boyle, 2008). These are common components of home visitation programs (see below) that aim to facilitate parents' safe, stable, and nurturing relationships with infants and young children.

Internationally, the World Health Organization (WHO) recommends programs to support parent–child relationships and notes the appropriateness of home visiting to provide these services (WHO, 2009). The United Nations Children's Fund (UNICEF), as well, has recently highlighted the possibility of home visitation to protect children from violence (UNICEF, 2014). WHO and UNICEF (2012) have also collaborated on a curriculum focused on enhancing early child development and parent–child interaction guidance provided by community health workers, home visitors, or other health-care providers, the *Care for Child Development* curriculum. By intervening in infancy and early childhood, the CDC, UNICEF, and WHO intend such programs to help parents protect their children from violence and exposure to violence, provide nurturance and support for their children's early development and resilience, and decrease the incidence of their children's aggressive behavior so it does not persist and escalate to abuse and violence in their adulthood.

The Potential of Home Visiting Effectiveness to Prevent Maltreatment

Home visiting is, in essence, a service-delivery mechanism, where support and guidance are provided in a home setting. A number of service systems in early childhood may use home visiting, including early intervention to children with identified delays and disabilities, preschool programming where the teacher may visit the child in the home to increase family connections to the classroom, or child welfare where there is immediate concern for child safety. In general, however, the term *home visiting* (in particular, early childhood home visiting) has come to define a particular type of preventive intervention, in which professionals (or trained paraprofessionals) regularly visit the home to provide information and guidance to families with young children, many of whom qualify for services based on various risk factors, such as poverty or teen parenthood.

Home visiting, as it is currently understood, has been around in the USA since at least the 1970s (see Halpern, 1999, for a history), emerging from multiple lines of intervention, including public health, family support, and education. From the beginning, there has been debate about its evidence and its effectiveness (e.g., Gomby, Culross, & Behrman, 1999), although a consensus is emerging that home visiting "works," but perhaps not as strongly as hoped or across as many areas of functioning as hoped.

One of the controversial areas of outcome is the ability of home visiting to prevent child maltreatment. As has been noted by others (MacMillan et al., 2009), home visiting is often "sold" or encouraged in policy and practice circles as a strategy to reduce child maltreatment. Generally, based on meta-analyses of studies using group comparison or pre–post designs, home visiting programs aiming to reduce child maltreatment have shown significant but small effects on reducing child maltreatment and improving parent functioning and parent–child interaction, (e.g., Geeraert, Van den Noortgate, Grietens, & Onghena, 2004). Rigorous randomized controlled trials have shown home visiting impacts on reduced child maltreatment, but only for a few program models. One of those models is Nurse Family Partnership (NFP), a model of home visiting developed initially in the USA that focuses on first-time, low-income mothers and, true to its name, uses nurses as home visitors. Results from multiple randomized trials have justifiably established NFP as an evidence-based home visiting intervention (see Olds, 2006). Child maltreatment rates have shown significant reductions in only one NFP trial (Elmira), although a second trial (Memphis) showed reductions in hospital emergency room visits for injuries and ingestions and recently reported reductions in long-term child mortality (Olds et al., 2014) .

As of 2014, the Home Visiting Evidence of Effectiveness (HomVEE) Review (Avellar, Paulsell, Sama-Miller, & Del Grosso, 2014), updated from previous reviews, identified six home visiting programs that showed evidence of reductions in child maltreatment, based on studies that met the review's methodological criteria. One of the programs was NFP. Studies of several other home visiting programs can be criticized as based only on parent report, such as Healthy Families New York (Dumont et al., 2008) or based on only a single trial, such as Even Start in New Zealand (Fergusson, Grant, Horwood, & Ridder, 2005), Child FIRST (Lowell, Carter, Godoy, Paulicin, & Briggs-Gowan, 2011), or Parents as Teachers (PAT; Drazen & Haust, 1993). SafeCare Augmented, in one trial, showed maltreatment reductions not only in parent-reported abuse but also in child welfare reports of child exposure to domestic violence (Silovsky et al., 2011). A recent study of Early Head Start (EHS) showed that school-age children who had been in EHS programs across multiple states had significantly fewer child welfare agency encounters regarding maltreatment, documented in state administrative data, compared with children in a randomly assigned control group (Green et al., 2014), but the study did not analyze home visiting programs separately from center-based programs.

What are the implications of these findings? One home visiting program (NFP) has shown some evidence of child maltreatment or mortality reduction in some, but not all, of its trials, and a few other home visiting programs have shown reductions in maltreatment in a single trial, but home visiting programs have not yet shown strong *consistent* evidence, based on rigorous research methodology, that they can be counted on to prevent maltreatment, despite their promise. Furthermore, only a few home visiting programs have shown any reductions in children's exposure to interpersonal violence (e.g., Silovsky et al., 2011), and little evidence suggests that home visiting directly prevents family interpersonal violence or the effects of violence exposure on children (see Feder et al., 2009), although a recent trial of the Domestic Violence Enhanced Home Visitation (DOVE) model suggests that it is possible to include interpersonal violence education in *prenatal* home visiting (see Decker et al., 2012).[1]

Established Home Visiting Programs That Promote Parenting and Child Development

Evidence is considerably stronger for home visiting programs to improve positive parenting and child development than to prevent experiences with violence. Most home visiting programs have focused on improving children's overall positive

[1] In addition, there are evidence-based interventions that can help children to cope with the impact of trauma and domestic violence once it occurs, such as child–parent psychotherapy (Lieberman & Van Horn, 2011; Moss et al., 2011).

development, the foundation of long-term positive life trajectories and the basis of resilience in the face of adversity, and most attempt to do this by encouraging positive parenting, the key to buffering the effects of other negative influences. Some of these home visiting programs have aimed to improve parenting and child development more generally, while others have targeted specific parenting or child development domains, such as improving maternal sensitivity or reducing child behavior problems. When parents are more positive and more sensitive, children have fewer behavior problems, and child maltreatment and childhood aggression are far less likely (Chang et al. 2003; Knutson et al., 2005; NICHD ECCRN, 2004). If home visiting programs demonstrate an impact in improved parenting and child development, outcomes that are likely to lead directly or indirectly to reductions in child maltreatment, they may offer important avenues for intervention as well as prevention.

Positive, sensitive parenting and child behavior and development outcomes have been tested in a number of home visitation programs. In the USA, the most widely implemented evidence-based home visiting programs serving families of infants have all shown scientific evidence of positive impacts on parenting and child development (Avellar et al., 2014): EHS-home visiting, Healthy Families America (HFA), NFP, and PAT. These well-established home visiting programs deliver health and education services through individualized home visits to parents. Each program model organization provides detailed guidance on implementation for new programs using their models. What they have in common is that each program is implemented through regularly scheduled home visits made to at-risk families by trained and supervised practitioners, who meet individually with a parent and child (and often additional family members) to promote safe, secure, nurturing environments beginning in the first year of infancy or sooner. Although they were all developed in the USA, these program models or similar replications of them are in use outside of the USA as well.

EHS home visiting programs, implemented according to established performance standards to increase parenting skills and improve the learning environment of the home, have demonstrated positive parenting impacts on the home environment and parenting interactions and child impacts of fewer social behavior problems and more engagement when playing with their parents (Jones Harden, Chazan-Cohen, Raikes, & Vogel, 2012; Love et al., 2005). HFA, in which home visitors promote bonding and attachment and link families to medical and other services, has shown evidence of higher quality of the home environment (Duggan et al., 2007), less harsh punitive parenting (Duggan et al., 2004; DuMont et al., 2008; LeCroy & Krysik, 2011), along with fewer child behavior problems—including aggression—and better academic achievement (Caldera et al., 2007, Kirkland & Mitchell-Herzfeld, 2012). NFP, in which visiting nurses build supportive relationships with new mothers to promote healthy pregnancy and early infancy, has shown positive parenting impacts on the quality of the home environment and parenting interactions (Kitzman et al., 1997; Olds et al., 2002), positive child impacts on fewer behavior problems and better academic achievement (Kitzman et al., 2010; Olds et al., 2004), and reductions in child maltreatment (Kitzman et al., 1997; Olds et al., 1997). Although PAT, in which home visitors use activities from an established curriculum to help parents support early development, shows more mixed results than other models, it has demonstrated an impact on better overall quality of the home environment (Wagner, Cameto, & Gerlach-Downie, 1996).

These programs have been used in a wide range of communities, from dangerous urban neighborhoods in which home visitors work in pairs to increase their personal safety to isolated rural homes that may require an hour or more of traveling time in each direction. Nevertheless, their effectiveness in international contexts, although expanding rapidly, needs rigorous testing to ensure that their effectiveness is generalizable to an even broader range of cultures and social systems.

One other US home visiting program that serves families with infants and has shown high-quality research evidence of both parenting and child outcomes is the Play and Learning Strategies (PALS) program, and only the infant part of the program shows adequate evidence of positive impacts (Avellar et al., 2014). The PALS infant program serves families with children 5 months to 1 year, in 10 home visiting sessions that last 90 min each, during which a parent educator facilitates parents' mastery of specific skills for interacting with their infants to strengthen their bond and stimulate early language, cognitive, and social development. This parenting skills program, using video examples and feedback, has produced positive changes in parenting measured through direct observation of mother–infant interaction. Mothers were video recorded while interacting with their infants, and trained observers noted a wide range of positive and negative parenting behaviors. Mothers in the PALS Infant program were substantially more responsive, warm, sensitive, encouraging, supportive, and verbally stimulating and less intrusive and harsh with their infants, compared with those randomly assigned to a comparison group (Landry, Smith, & Swank, 2006).

These impacts are important in parenting behavior, particularly for families in impoverished or violent communities because these are the kinds of key parenting behaviors that are associated with children's early development and that predict their later development (Cook, Roggman, & Boyce, 2011; Roggman, Cook, Innocenti, Jump Norman, & Christiansen, 2013; Tamis-LeMonda, Shannon, Cabrera, & Lamb, 2004). These outcomes are thereby likely to improve children's resilience to the effects of stressful, impoverished, or violent early environments (Schofield et al., 2013).

In New Zealand, the Early Start program serves at-risk families with newborn children up to age 5. Home visitors in this program create a collaborative, problem-solving partnership with the family to increase child and family health and well-being. Families with high needs may receive up to 3 hours of services per week that is gradually reduced through four levels, from 3 hours per 2 weeks to 1 hour per month to 1 hour per 3 months. The program has shown improvements in child development and positive parenting, along with reductions in child maltreatment.

Early Start also adapted their program to serve an indigenous population, consulting with representatives from that community, hiring and training home visitors from the indigenous community to serve the families, and establishing a board with half the members from the indigenous community to ensure a respectful and sensitive perspective of families. In this group as well as the mainstream group, parents served by Early Start reported more positive childrearing practices and fewer behavior problems in their children, and in the mainstream group, parents in Early Start also reported less punitive parenting beliefs (Avellar et al., 2014; Fergusson et al., 2005), compared with parents randomly assigned to a comparison group. Both the impacts on children's behavior problems and the improvements in parenting suggest that the collaborative, problem-solving partnership approach of this program may offer an important strategy to increase resilience and reduce aggression in children and families from diverse cultures.

Promising Research on Home Visiting to Improve Parenting and Child Development

Together, high-quality studies testing the impact of established home visiting program models have demonstrated that these models can improve various positive outcomes in parenting and child development across a range of communities, using a variety of approaches from a number of disciplinary perspectives. The evidence-based home visiting programs discussed so far provide ongoing comprehensive support over long periods of time in weekly or monthly home visits and are established programs that continue to operate. Other research has tested more brief and focused in-home parenting interventions that are much shorter term and not part of continuing standardized comprehensive service programs (see Juffer, Bakermans-Kranenburg, & Van IJzendoorn, 2014). Instead, these interventions have been implemented as part of experiments to test the effectiveness of theoretically guided interventions designed to cause specific effects in parenting behavior or child development.

In an experimental intervention in Holland, home visitors worked with low-income Dutch mothers in 2-hour home visits three times over 3 months (van den Boom, 1994), to promote secure infant attachment by encouraging maternal sensitivity during naturally occurring mother–infant interactions in the home, what the researcher referred to as "the most direct way to affect behavior" (p. 1459). To encourage sensitivity, home visitors guided mothers to imitate their babies, to be quiet when a baby looked away, and to sooth their babies when in distress. As a result, the mothers in this brief home visiting intervention, compared with those randomly assigned to a control group, became significantly more sensitive and stimulating with their infants, and even more importantly, the infants were less than half as likely to develop insecure attachments. Given the link between attachment insecurity and early aggression (NICHD ECCRN, 2004), the impacts of this quite brief home visiting intervention support the potential of focused home visiting approaches that last only a few weeks to improve parenting and children's development.

More recently in Canada (Moss et al., 2011), an 8-week home visiting intervention incorporated weekly video observation and feedback with mothers of children ages 12 and 71 months who were being monitored by a community or child welfare agency for maltreatment. The intervention showed strong evidence of better maternal sensitivity in the program group, and with it, less maltreatment and less early childhood aggression. In the USA, professional practitioners implemented a ten-session in-home intervention for foster children ages 4 to 60 months by successfully training foster parents to be more responsive and supportive of children's self-regulation (Dozier et al., 2006). Together, these kinds of brief in-home parenting interventions and others that have increased mothers' sensitive parenting suggest that home visiting has the potential to have powerful focused impacts on key aspects of parenting, even when the home visiting intervention is brief and the dosage rather small (6–12 h).

A meta-analysis of parenting interventions focused specifically on maternal sensitivity showed that across many of these interventions, those that were most effective lasted less than 16 weeks, used video feedback, and included fathers (Bakermans-Kranenburg, Van IJzendoorn, & Juffer, 2003). Most of the interventions were implemented in families' homes, but the few that were not did not show significantly less effectiveness at improving sensitivity. Also, the age of the child at the onset of the intervention did not seem to matter across parenting sensitivity interventions, even though most of us believe that earlier is better (e.g., Dozier et al., 2006), suggesting that evidence-based home visiting programs that begin after the first year, such as Family Check-Up (beginning at age 2) and Home Instruction for Parents of Preschool Youngsters (HIPPY; beginning at age 3) may be appropriate in some communities. For very focused goals, such as improving maternal sensitivity, these brief home visiting interventions may be feasible when resources are scarce, when meeting in homes is challenging or dangerous, or when interventions begin at a wide range of child ages.

Most home visiting interventions that have shown scientifically tested impacts have a broad array of goals that are relevant to the overall aim of decreasing violence and aggression in families and communities: safe, secure, and nurturing relationships, of course, but also prenatal and neonatal health, strong language support in parent–child interactions, practical strategies for solving child and family problems, and family access to needed child and family services. Home visiting approaches that have been effective at increasing positive supportive parenting and improving children's developmental outcomes were tested in communities where infants and young children are at risk for poor outcomes because of poverty and violence in the family community.

Most of these programs have been in urban settings, but home visiting programs are also used in rural communities where social isolation and limited access to resources can increase the stress of poverty. Home visiting may ease the travel burden for families seeking services, but in some remote areas the travel burden on home visiting programs can be daunting if families live far from communities and far from each other. As an alternative, some programs have implemented home visits from a distance, "tele-visiting," in which families may "meet" with a home visitor by telephone or by Internet contact (e.g., Kelso, Fiechtl, Olsen, & Rule, 2009). One examination of this approach showed even higher quality of home visiting practices and stronger impacts than in a comparison group randomly assigned to face-to-face home visits (Blaiser, Behl, Callow-Heusser, & White, 2013).

Other interventions have incorporated text messaging into home visiting interventions as an attempt to keep families connected to their home visitor in-between visits (Carta, Lefever, Bigelow, Borkowski and Warren, 2013; Jabaley, Lutzker, Whitaker, & Self-Brown, 2011). This may also be helpful in rural programs where more frequent home visits may not be practical. A wide range of goals, disciplines, strategies, and technologies are incorporated into home visiting programs. Which home visiting program will best fit a particular community depends on the needs and the available resources of that community.

Ways to Expand and Improve Home Visiting in International Contexts

What are the implications of these findings for home visiting in parts of the world that are not North America, given that 90 % of the research on home visiting comes from the USA or Canada (Mikton & Butchart, 2009)? How can home visiting be adapted to more populations, cultures, and contexts to prevent violence or buffer its effects on young children? A full international review of home visiting is beyond the scope of this short chapter. Readers are referred to other chapters in this book that highlight initiatives in South America and the Carribean, regions that have seen a steady increase in interest in early childhood intervention, including home visiting (see, e.g., chapters in this volume by Branker et al. and Cárdia et al.; see also Araujo, López-Boo, & Puyana, 2013). Other areas of the world with attention to building up early childhood home visiting include Eastern Europe, where the UNICEF regional office is attempting to use existing visiting nurse infrastructures that were developed during the Cold War era to promote a more holistic approach to early child development and well-being (UNICEF, 2012); and Asia, where a number of home visiting models are being developed and tested, such as the Lady Health Worker Program in Pakistan (Yousafzai, Rasheed, Rizvi, Armstrong, & Bhutta, 2014)[2] and community-based maternal and newborn care programs with postnatal home visits in Bangladesh, Malawi, and Nepal (Sitrin et al., 2013).

The justification for the use of home visiting services in low- and middle-income countries is not too different from the rationale in higher-income countries such as the USA: Home visiting provides a service mechanism to support caregivers of children who may not otherwise seek out such services. In some programs in South America, such as in Peru's *Cuna Más*, a federal initiative to support at-risk families during the early childhood period, home visits are a primary service delivery mechanism to rural areas and happen in extremely isolated communities in the Andes Mountains or the Amazonian Rain Forest.

Home visiting services internationally also face similar issues as in the USA, such as the development of evidence-based practices, the adaption or adoption of

[2] See also the ongoing Lancet series on early childhood development in low- and middle-income countries (e.g., Engle et al., 2011).

these practices in new communities and settings, hiring and training of qualified staff, and the scaling-up of effective practices. These challenges, however, may be exacerbated in low- and middle-income countries, where there are more concentrated areas of poverty, malnutrition, and restricted learning opportunities for young children. For example, established international entities (such as WHO) that can leverage resources to fund programming strongly promote the use of evidence-based home visiting models as the best investment for preventing violence and promoting positive child development (e.g., MacMillan et al., 2009; MacMillan & Mikton, 2013). These models were often originally developed in the USA or Canada, where the programs have been most closely studied. But these models often have certain assumptions built into their implementation, such as the ready availability of nurses for home visitors or cultural universality in optimal parenting, which can make them difficult to use without substantial adaptations. These adaptations, in turn, often do not readily align with the practices in place when the program model was originally tested. These programs also may be expensive to purchase the rights to use and, even with adaptations, may be expensive to implement and especially expensive to sustain beyond demonstration projects. In light of these limitations, home visiting models originally developed in the Carribean, including Jamaica (Grantham McGregor et al., 1991) and Cuba (Tinajero, 2010), are being more widely disseminated and used in the Latin American region as well as other parts of the world.

Home visiting programs in low- and middle-income countries may also face challenges because of limited resources and infrastructure within their countries. *Cuna Más*, for example, provides home visits to families living in communities with limited cell phones, communication grids, or even electricity. Televisiting and text messages are not, at this point, feasible supplements or replacements for in-person contacts, despite their touting as innovative practices in home visiting programs in higher-income countries. Who to use as home visitors and how to support their work is also a challenge, particularly for countries that may not have a strong professional base of health and human service practice or that have few higher education institutions that can provide a large enough educated workforce.

Given all of these challenges, however, the home visiting initiatives that are beginning in these countries are noteworthy and provide examples of innovative practices that high-income countries could well learn from. Many countries (such as Brazil and Peru) are attempting ambitious inter-sectorial collaborations, where ministries of health, social welfare, and education work together to support early childhood programming across their departments. Integrating early childhood home visiting curricula into existing health practices, such as by using community health workers who already provide services to disadvantaged communities, is also a strategy increasingly being adopted.

Given this increase in home visiting activity, the need for careful examination and study of these practices is paramount. Unfortunately, many home visiting services in low- and middle-income countries exist in a "gray area," where programs undergo little evaluation, with few efforts to share findings or lessons learned from these initiatives. There is little international awareness of these programs, and few opportunities for these programs to share common experiences and challenges or measurement and evaluation strategies. Beyond the rare randomized trial, little information is available about program implementation or effectiveness. In short, there is a strong need for monitoring, evaluation, and research strategies that can be integrated into existing home visiting services to provide meaningful information about their conduct and their outcomes.

This also suggests the need for attention to be paid on the development and dissemination of measures that are efficient and reliable. Programs often struggle with finding linguistically appropriate and culturally valid measures for their cultural setting. Simple translations of tools that have been developed in other settings with WEIRD (Western, educated, industrialized, rich, and democratic) populations (Henrich, Heine, & Norenzayan, 2010) are often not sufficient to provide meaningful information to programs or the stakeholders who support them.

Conclusion

Although it may be a promising strategy, it is important to not oversell home visiting as *the* solution to childhood violence. Home visiting should be seen as only one mechanism within a comprehensive system of services devoted to preventing violence against children and promoting their health and well-being. Home visiting cannot do it all and will have only limited outcomes if it is the sole service available to families. Other interventions, such as conditional cash transfers or other poverty alleviation methods, preventive health services, and carefully implemented media content can and should be used as well (Engle et al., 2011). But as a part of a system that supports families in impoverished and often violent communities, effective, well-planned, and carefully monitored home visiting programs may be able to help families provide more support for children's positive development and decrease children's early aggression and behavior problems.

References

Afifi, T. O., Brownridge, D. A., Cox, B. J., & Sareen, J. (2006). Physical punishment, childhood abuse and psychiatric disorders. *Child Abuse & Neglect, 30*(10), 1093–1103.

Aguilar, B., Sroufe, L., Egeland, B., & Carlson, E. (2000). Distinguishing the early-onset/persistent and adolescence-onset antisocial behavior types: From birth to 16 years. *Development and Psychopathology, 12*(02), 109–132.

Alink, L. R., Mesman, J., Van Zeijl, J., Stolk, M. N., Juffer, F., Koot, H. M., & Van IJzendoorn, M. H. (2006). The early childhood aggression curve: Development of physical aggression in 10-to 50-month-old children. *Child Development, 77*(4), 954–966.

American Psychological Association. (1996). *Violence and the family: Report by the American Psychological Association Presidential Task Force on Violence and the Family*. Washington, DC: American Psychological Association.
Anda, R. F., Felitti, V. J., Bremner, J. D., Walker, J. D., Whitfield, C. H., Perry, B. D., & Giles, W. H. (2006). The enduring effects of abuse and related adverse experiences in childhood. *European Archives of Psychiatry and Clinical Neuroscience, 256*(3), 174–186.
Araujo, M. C., López-Boo, F., & Puyana, J. M. (2013). *Overview of early childhood development services in Latin America and the Caribbean*. Washington, DC: Inter-American Development Bank.
Avellar, S. A., & Supplee, L. H. (2013). Effectiveness of home visiting in improving child health and reducing child maltreatment. *Pediatrics, 132*(Supplement 2), S90–S99.
Avellar, S., Paulsell, D., Sama-Miller, E., & Del Grosso, P. (2014). *Home visiting evidence of effectiveness review: Executive summary*. Washington, DC: Office of Planning, Research, an Evaluation, Administration for Children and Families, U.S. Department of Health and Human Services.
Bakermans-Kranenburg, M. J., Van IJzendoorn, M. H., & Juffer, F. (2003). Less is more: Meta-analyses of sensitivity and attachment interventions in early childhood. *Psychological Bulletin, 129*(2), 195–215.
Baldry, A. C. (2003). Bullying in schools and exposure to domestic violence. *Child Abuse & Neglect, 27*(7), 713–732.
Banyard, V. L., Williams, L. M., & Siegel, J. A. (2003). The impact of complex trauma and depression on parenting: An exploration of mediating risk and protective factors. *Child Maltreatment, 8*(4), 334–349.
Blaiser, K. M., Behl, D., Callow-Heusser, C., & White, K. R. (2013). Measuring costs and outcomes of tele-intervention when serving families of children who are deaf/hard-of-hearing. *International Journal of Telerehabilitation, 5*(2), 3–10.
Bourassa, C. (2007). Co-occurrence of interparental violence and child physical abuse and its effect on the adolescents' behavior. *Journal of Family Violence, 22*(8), 691–701.
Brame, B., Nagin, D. S., & Tremblay, R. E. (2001). Developmental trajectories of physical aggression from school entry to late adolescence. *Journal of Child Psychology and Psychiatry, 42*(4), 503–512.
Briere, J., & Elliott, D. M. (2003). Prevalence and psychological sequelae of self-reported childhood physical and sexual abuse in a general population sample of men and women. *Child Abuse & Neglect, 27*(10), 1205–1222.
Butchart, A., Phinney Harvey, A., Mian, M., Fürniss, T., Kahane, T., & The World Health Organization Department of Injuries and Violence Prevention and the International Society for Prevention of Child Abuse and Neglect. (2006). *Preventing child maltreatment: A guide to taking action and generating evidence*. Geneva: World Health Organization.
Caldera, D., Burrell, L., Rodriguez, K., Crowne, S. S., Rohde, C., & Duggan, A. (2007). Impact of a statewide home visiting program on parenting and on child health and development. *Child Abuse & Neglect, 31*(8), 829–852. doi:10.1016/j.chiabu.2007.02.008.
Cappell, C., & Heiner, R. B. (1990). The intergenerational transmission of family aggression. *Journal of Family Violence, 5*(2), 135–152.
Carta, J. J., Lefever, J. B., Bigelow, K., Borkowski, J., & Warren, S. F. (2013). Randomized trial of a cellular phone-enhanced home visitation parenting intervention. *Pediatrics, 132*(Supplement 2), S167–S173.
Centers for Disease Control and Prevention. (2013). *Essentials for childhood: Steps to create safe, stable, and nurturing relationships*. Atlanta: Center for Disease Control.
Chang, L., Schwartz, D., Dodge, K. A., & McBride-Chang, C. (2003). Harsh parenting in relation to child emotion regulation and aggression. *Journal of Family Psychology, 17*(4), 598–606.
Children's Bureau (U.S. Department of Health and Human Services, Administration for Children and Families, Administration on Children, Youth and Families). (2013). *Child maltreatment 2012 [online]*. Washington, DC: Government Printing Office. http://www.acf.hhs.gov/sites/default/files/cb/cm2012.pdf. Accessed 25 Jan 2015.

Cook, G. A., Roggman, L. A., & Boyce, L. K. (2011). Fathers' and mothers' cognitive stimulation in early play with toddlers: Predictors of 5th grade reading and math. *Family Science, 2*(2), 131–145.
Coyl, D. D., Roggman, L. A., & Newland, L. (2002). Stress, maternal depression, and negative mother–infant interactions in relation to infant attachment. *Infant Mental Health Journal, 23,* 145–163.
Cummings, E. M., Goeke-Morey, M. C., & Papp, L. M. (2004). Everyday marital conflict and child aggression. *Journal of Abnormal Child Psychology, 32*(2), 191–202.
Decker, M. R., Frattaroli, S., McCaw, B., Coker, A. L., Miller, E., Sharps, P., & Gielen, A. (2012). Transforming the healthcare response to intimate partner violence and taking best practices to scale. *Journal of Women's Health, 21*(12), 1222–1229.
DeMulder, E. K., Denham, S., Schmidt, M., & Mitchell, J. (2000). Q-sort assessment of attachment security during the preschool years: Links from home to school. *Developmental Psychology, 36*(2), 274.
Dozier, M., Peloso, E., Lindhiem, O., Gordon, M. K., Manni, M., Sepulveda, S., & Levine, S. (2006). Developing evidence-based interventions for foster children: An example of a randomized clinical trial with infants and toddlers. *Journal of Social Issues, 62*(4), 767–785.
Drazen, S. M., & Haust, M. (1993, August). *Raising reading readiness in low-income children by parent education.* Paper presented at the annual meeting of the American Psychological Association.
Duggan, A., McFarlane, E., Fuddy, L., Burrell, L., Higman, S. M., Windham, A., & Sia, C. (2004). Randomized trial of a statewide home visiting program: Impact in preventing child abuse and neglect. *Child Abuse & Neglect, 28*(6), 597–622.
Duggan, A., Caldera, D., Rodriguez, K., Burrell, L., Rohde, C., & Crowne, S. S. (2007). Impact of a statewide home visiting program to prevent child abuse. *Child Abuse & Neglect, 31*(8), 801–827.
Duke, N. N., Pettingell, S. L., McMorris, B. J., & Borowsky, I. W. (2010). Adolescent violence perpetration: Associations with multiple types of adverse childhood experiences. *Pediatrics, 125*(4), e778–e786.
DuMont, K., Mitchell-Herzfeld, S., Greene, R., Lee, E., Lowenfels, A., Rodriguez, M., & Dorabawila, V. (2008). Healthy Families New York (HFNY) randomized trial: Effects on early child abuse and neglect. *Child Abuse & Neglect, 32*(3), 295–315.
Eisenberg, N., Cumberland, A., Spinrad, T. L., Fabes, R. A., Shepard, S. A., Reiser, M., & Guthrie, I. K. (2001). The relations of regulation and emotionality to children's externalizing and internalizing problem behavior. *Child Development, 72*(4), 1112–1134.
Engle, P. L., Fernald, L. C., Alderman, H., Behrman, J., O'Gara, C., Yousafzai, A., & Iltus, S. (2011). Strategies for reducing inequalities and improving developmental outcomes for young children in low-income and middle-income countries. *Lancet, 378*(9799), 1339–1353.
Evans, S. E., Davies, C., & DiLillo, D. (2008). Exposure to domestic violence: A meta-analysis of child and adolescent outcomes. *Aggression and Violent Behavior, 13*(2), 131–140.
Farrington, D. P., & Loeber, R. (2000). Epidemiology of juvenile violence. *Child and Adolescent Psychiatric Clinics of North America, 9*(4), 733–748.
Feder, G., Ramsay, J., Dunne, D., Rose, M., Arsene, C., Norman, R., & Taket, A. (2009). How far does screening women for domestic (partner) violence in different health-care settings meet criteria for a screening programme? Systematic reviews of nine UK national screening committee criteria. *Health Technology Assessment (Winchester, England), 13*(16), 1–91.
Fergusson, D. M., Grant, H., Horwood, L. J., & Ridder, E. M. (2005). Randomized trial of the Early Start program of home visitation. *Pediatrics, 116*(6), e803–e809.
Finzi, R., Ram, A., Har-Even, D., Shnit, D., & Weizman, A. (2001). Attachment styles and aggression in physically abused and neglected children. *Journal of Youth and Adolescence, 30*(6), 769–786.
Frias-Armenta, M., & McCloskey, L. A. (1998). Determinants of harsh parenting in Mexico. *Journal of Abnormal Child Psychology, 26*(2), 129–139.

Geeraert, L., Van den Noortgate, W., Grietens, H., & Onghena, P. (2004). The effects of early prevention programs for families with young children at risk for physical child abuse and neglect: A meta-analysis. *Child Maltreatment, 9*(3), 277–291.

Gomby, D. S., Culross, P. L., & Behrman, R. E. (1999). Home visiting: Recent program evaluations: Analysis and recommendations. *The Future of Children, 9*(1), 4–26.

Grantham-McGregor, S. M., Powell, C. A., Walker, S. P., & Himes, J. H. (1991). Nutritional supplementation, psychosocial stimulation, and mental development of stunted children: The Jamaican Study. *Lancet, 338,* 1–5.

Green, B. L., Ayoub, C., Bartlett, J. D., Von Ende, A., Furrer, C., Chazan-Cohen, R., Vallotton, C., & Klevens, J. (2014). The effect of Early Head Start on child welfare system involvement: A first look at longitudinal child maltreatment outcomes. *Children and Youth Services Review, 42,* 127–135.

Guerra, N. G., Huesmann, L. R., Tolan, P. H., Van Acker, R., & Eron, L. D. (1995). Stressful events and individual beliefs as correlates of economic disadvantage and aggression among urban children. *Journal of Consulting and Clinical Psychology, 63*(4), 518.

Halpern, R. (1999). *Fragile families, fragile solutions: A history of supportive services for families in poverty*. New York: Columbia University Press.

Hamby, S. L., Finkelhor, D., Turner, H. A., & Ormrod, R. (2011). *Children's exposure to intimate partner violence and other family violence*. Washington, DC: US Department of Justice, Office of Justice Programs. Office of Juvenile Justice and Delinquency Prevention.

Henrich, J., Heine, S. J., & Norenzayan, A. (2010). The weirdest people in the world? *Behavioral and Brain Sciences, 33*(2–3), 61–83.

Hill, A. L., Degnan, K. A., Calkins, S. D., & Keane, S. P. (2006). Profiles of externalizing behavior problems for boys and girls across preschool: The roles of emotion regulation and inattention. *Developmental Psychology, 42*(5), 913–928.

Ho, C., Bluestein, D. N., & Jenkins, J. M. (2008). Cultural differences in the relationship between parenting and children's behavior. *Developmental Psychology, 44*(2), 507–522. http://dx.doi.org/10.1037/0012-1649.44.2.507.

Hughes, H. M., Parkinson, D., & Vargo, M. (1989). Witnessing spouse abuse and experiencing physical abuse: A "double whammy"? *Journal of Family Violence, 4*(2), 197–209.

Jabaley, J. J., Lutzker, J. R., Whitaker, D. J., & Self-Brown, S. (2011). Using iPhones™ to enhance and reduce face-to-face home safety sessions within SafeCare®: An evidence-based child maltreatment prevention program. *Journal of Family Violence, 26*(5), 377–385.

Jaffee, S. R., Bowes, L., Ouellet-Morin, I., Fisher, H. L., Moffitt, T. E., Merrick, M. T., & Arseneault, L. (2013). Safe, stable, nurturing relationships break the intergenerational cycle of abuse: A prospective nationally representative cohort of children in the United Kingdom. *Journal of Adolescent Health, 53*(4), S4–S10.

Jones Harden, B., Chazan Cohen, R., Raikes, H., & Vogel, C. (2012). Early Head Start home visitation: The role of implementation in bolstering program benefits. *Journal of Community Psychology, 40*(4), 438–455.

Juffer, F., Bakermans-Kranenburg, M. J., & Van IJzendoorn, M. H. (2014). Attachment-based interventions. In P. Holmes & S. Farnfield (Eds.), *The Routledge handbook of attachment: Implications and interventions* (pp. 83–103). New York: Routledge.

Kaminski, J. W., Valle, L. A., Filene, J. H., & Boyle, C. L. (2008). A meta-analytic review of components associated with parent training program effectiveness. *Journal of Abnormal Child Psychology, 36,* 567–589.

Kelso, G. L., Fiechtl, B. J., Olsen, S. T., & Rule, S. (2009). The feasibility of virtual home visits to provide early intervention: A pilot study. *Infants and Young Children, 22*(4), 332–340.

Kimonis, E. R., Frick, P. J., Boris, N. W., Smyke, A. T., Cornell, A. H., Farrell, J. M., & Zeanah, C. H. (2006). Callous-unemotional features, behavioral inhibition, and parenting: Independent predictors of aggression in a high-risk preschool sample. *Journal of Child and Family Studies, 15*(6), 741–752.

Kirkland, K., & Mitchell-Herzfeld, S. (2012). *Evaluating the effectiveness of home visiting services in promoting children's adjustment in school: Final report to the Pew Center on the*

States. Rensselaer: New York State Office of Children and Family Services, Bureau of Evaluation and Research.
Kitzman, H., Olds, D. L., Henderson, C. R., Hanks, C., Cole, R., Tatelbaum, R., & Barnard, K. (1997). Effect of prenatal and infancy home visitation by nurses on pregnancy outcomes, childhood injuries, and repeated childbearing. A randomized controlled trial. *JAMA: The Journal of the American Medical Association, 278*(8), 644–652.
Kitzman, H. J., Olds, D. L., Cole, R. E., Hanks, C. A., Anson, E. A., Arcoleo, K. J., Luckey, D. W., Knudtson, M. D., Henderson, C. R., & Holmberg, J. R. (2010). Enduring effects of prenatal and infancy home visiting by nurses on children: Follow-up of a randomized trial among children at age 12 years. *Archives of Pediatrics and Adolescent Medicine, 164*(5), 412–418.
Klamer, A., Lando, A., Pinborg, A., & Greisen, G. (2005). Ages and Stages Questionnaire used to measure cognitive deficit in children born extremely preterm. *Acta Paediatrica, 94*(9), 1327–1329.
Knutson, J. F., DeGarmo, D., Koeppl, G., & Reid, J. B. (2005). Care neglect, supervisory neglect, and harsh parenting in the development of children's aggression: A replication and extension. *Child Maltreatment, 10*(2), 92–107.
Landry, S. H., Smith, K. E., & Swank, P. R. (2006). Responsive parenting: Establishing early foundations for social, communication, and independent problem-solving skills. *Developmental Psychology, 42*(4), 627–642.
Lansford, J. E., Miller-Johnson, S., Berlin, L. J., Dodge, K. A., Bates, J. E., & Pettit, G. S. (2007). Early physical abuse and later violent delinquency: A prospective longitudinal study. *Child Maltreatment, 12*(3), 233–245.
LeCroy, C. W., & Krysik, J. (2011). Randomized trial of the Healthy Families Arizona home visiting program. *Children and Youth Services Review, 33*(10), 1761–1766.
Lee, Y. (2009). Early motherhood and harsh parenting: The role of human, social, and cultural capital. *Child Abuse & Neglect, 33*(9), 625–637.
Lieberman, A. F., & Van Horn, P. (2011). *Psychotherapy with infants and young children: Repairing the effects of stress and trauma on early attachment*. New York: Guilford Press.
Love, J. M., Kisker, E. E., Ross, C., Raikes, H., Constantine, J., Boller, K., & Vogel, C. (2005). The effectiveness of Early Head Start for 3-year-old children and their parents: Lessons for policy and programs. *Developmental Psychology, 41*(6), 885–901.
Lowell, D. I., Carter, A. S., Godoy, L., Paulicin, B., & Briggs-Gowan, M. J. (2011). A randomized controlled trial of Child First: A comprehensive home-based intervention translating research into early childhood practice. *Child Development, 82*(1), 193–208.
Lyons-Ruth, K. (1996). Attachment relationships among children with aggressive behavior problems: The role of disorganized early attachment patterns. *Journal of Consulting and Clinical Psychology, 64*(1), 64–73.
Lyons-Ruth, K., Alpern, L., & Repacholi, B. (1993). Disorganized infant attachment classification and maternal psychosocial problems as predictors of hostile-aggressive behavior in the preschool classroom. *Child development, 64*(2), 572–585.
Lyons-Ruth, K., Easterbrooks, M. A., & Davidson, C. (1997). Infant attachment strategies, infant mental lag, and maternal depressive symptoms: Predictors of internalizing and externalizing problems at age 7. *Developmental Psychology, 33*(4), 681–692.
MacMillan, H., & Mikton, C. (2013). Prevention of child maltreatment and associated impairment: An evidence-based overview. WHO Violence and Injury Prevention Webinar. http://www.who.int/violence_injury_prevention/capacitybuilding/child_maltreatment_prevention_mikton_macmillan.ppt. Accessed 25 Jan 2015.
MacMillan, H. L., Wathen, C. N., Barlow, J., Fergusson, D. M., Leventhal, J. M., & Taussig, H. N. (2009). Interventions to prevent child maltreatment and associated impairment. *Lancet, 373*(9659), 250–266.
Margolin, G., & Gordis, E. B. (2000). The effects of family and community violence on children. *Annual Review of Psychology, 51*(1), 445–479.

Martorell, G. A., & Bugental, D. B. (2006). Maternal variations in stress reactivity: Implications for harsh parenting practices with very young children. *Journal of Family Psychology, 20*(4), 641.

Mikton, C., & Butchart, A. (2009). Child maltreatment prevention: A systematic review of reviews. *Bulletin of the World Health Organization, 87,* 353–361.

Moss, E., Dubois-Comtois, K., Cyr, C., Tarabulsy, G. M., St-Laurent, D., & Bernier, A. (2011). Efficacy of a home-visiting intervention aimed at improving maternal sensitivity, child attachment, and behavioral outcomes for maltreated children: A randomized control trial. *Development and Psychopathology, 23*(1), 195–210.

Nagin, D., & Tremblay, R. E. (1999). Trajectories of boys' physical aggression, opposition, and hyperactivity on the path to physically violent and nonviolent juvenile delinquency. *Child Development, 70*(5), 1181–1196.

National Institute of Child Health and Development (NICHD) Early Child Care Research Network (ECCRN). (2004). Trajectories of physical aggression from toddlerhood to middle childhood: Predictors, correlates, and outcomes. *Monographs of the Society for Research in Child Development, 69*(4), vii–1.

Olds, D. L. (2006). The nurse-family partnership: An evidence-based preventive intervention. *Infant Mental Health Journal, 27*(1), 5–25.

Olds, D. L., Eckenrode, J., Henderson, C. R., Kitzman, H., Powers, J., Cole, R., & Luckey, D. (1997). Long-term effects of home visitation on maternal life course and child abuse and neglect. Fifteen-year follow-up of a randomized trial. *JAMA: The Journal of the American Medical Association, 278*(8), 637–643.

Olds, D. L., Robinson, J., O'Brien, R., Luckey, D. W., Pettitt, L. M., Henderson, C. R., & Talmi, A. (2002). Home visiting by paraprofessionals and by nurses: A randomized, controlled trial. *Pediatrics, 110*(3), 486.

Olds, D. L., Kitzman, H., Cole, R., Robinson, J., Sidora, K., Luckey, D. W., & Holmberg, J. (2004). Effects of nurse home-visiting on maternal life course and child development: Age 6 follow-up results of a randomized trial. *Pediatrics, 114*(6), 1550–1559.

Olds, D. L., Kitzman, H., Knudtson, M. D., Anson, E., Smith, J. A., & Cole, R. (2014). Effect of home visiting by nurses on maternal and child mortality: Results of a 2-decade follow-up of a randomized clinical trial. *JAMA Pediatrics, 168*(9), 800–806.

Olson, S. L., Bates, J. E., Sandy, J. M., & Lanthier, R. (2000). Early developmental precursors of externalizing behavior in middle childhood and adolescence. *Journal of Abnormal Child Psychology, 28,* 119–133.

Ooi, Y. P., Ang, R. P., Fung, D. S., Wong, G., & Cai, Y. (2006). The impact of parent–child attachment on aggression, social stress and self-esteem. *School Psychology International, 27*(5), 552–566.

Pinheiro, P. S. (2006). *Rights of the child: Report of the independent expert for the United Nations study on violence against children.* New York: United Nations.

Posada, G., & Pratt, D. M. (2008). Physical aggression in the family and preschoolers' use of the mother as a secure base. *Journal of Marital and Family Therapy, 34*(1), 14–27.

Putnam, F. W. (2006). The impact of trauma on child development. *Juvenile and Family Court Journal, 57*(1), 1–11.

Roggman, L. A., & Cook, G. A. (2011). Attachment, aggression, and family risk in a low-income sample. *Family Science, 1*(3–4), 191–204.

Roggman, L. A., Cook, G. A., Innocenti, M. S., Jump Norman, V., & Christiansen, K. (2013). Parenting Interactions with Children: Checklist of Observations Linked to Outcomes (PICCOLO) in diverse ethnic groups. *Infant Mental Health Journal, 34*(4), 290–306.

Romano, E., Tremblay, R. E., Boulerice, B., & Swisher, R. (2005). Multilevel correlates of childhood physical aggression and prosocial behavior. *Journal of Abnormal Child Psychology, 33*(5), 565–578.

Schofield, T. J., Lee, R. D., & Merrick, M. T. (2013). Safe, stable, nurturing relationships as a moderator of intergenerational continuity of child maltreatment: A meta-analysis. *Journal of Adolescent Health, 53*(4), S32–S38.

Silovsky, J. F., Bard, D., Chaffin, M., Hecht, D., Burris, L., Owora, A., Beasley, L., Doughty, D., & Lutzker, J. (2011). Prevention of child maltreatment in high-risk rural families: A randomized clinical trial with child welfare outcomes. *Children and Youth Services Review, 33,* 1435–1444.

Sitrin, D., Guenther, T., Murray, J., Pilgrim, N., Rubayet, S., Ligowe, R., & Moran, A. (2013). Reaching mothers and babies with early postnatal home visits: The implementation realities of achieving high coverage in large-scale programs. *PLoS ONE, 8(7),* e68930. doi:10.1371/journal.pone.0068930.

Tamis-LeMonda, C. S., Shannon, J. D., Cabrera, N. J., & Lamb, M. E. (2004). Fathers and mothers at play with their 2-and 3-year-olds: Contributions to language and cognitive development. *Child development, 75*(6), 1806–1820.

Tinajero, A. R. (2010). Scaling-up early child development in Cuba: Cuba's Educate Your Child program: Strategies and lessons from the expansion process, working paper 16. Washington, DC: Wolfensohn Center for Development at Brookings.

Tremblay, R. E. (2000). The development of aggressive behaviour during childhood: What have we learned in the past century? *International Journal of Behavioral Development, 24*(2), 129–141.

Tremblay, R. E., Nagin, D. S., Séguin, J. R., Zoccolillo, M., Zelazo, P. D., Boivin, M., & Japel, C. (2004). Physical aggression during early childhood: Trajectories and predictors. *Pediatrics, 114*(1), e43–e50.

UNICEF. (2012). *Securing the foundations of human development: Policy brief for the Regional Office for Central & Eastern Europe, Commonwealth of Independent States*. Geneva: UNICEF. http://www.unicef.org/ceecis/ECD_Policy_Brief_-_Securing_the_Foundations_of_Human_Development_2012.pdf.Downloaded at Accessed 24 Jan 2015..

UNICEF. (2014). *Ending violence against children: Six strategies for action*. New York: UNICEF.

van den Boom, D. C. (1994). The influence of temperament and mothering on attachment and exploration: An experimental manipulation of sensitive responsiveness among lower-class mothers with irritable infants. *Child Development, 65*(5), 1457–1477.

Wagner, M., Cameto, R., & Gerlach-Downie, S. (1996). *Intervention in support of adolescent parents and their children: A final report on Teen Parents as Teachers demonstration*. Menlo Park: SRI International.

Weiss, B., Dodge, K. A., Bates, J. E., & Pettit, G. S. (1992). Some consequences of early harsh discipline: Child aggression and a maladaptive social information processing style. *Child Development, 63*(6), 1321–1335.

Wolff, M. S., & Van IJzendoorn, M. H. (1997). Sensitivity and attachment: A meta-analysis on parental antecedents of infant attachment. *Child Development, 68*(4), 571–591.

World Health Organization. (2009). *Preventing violence through the development of safe, stable and nurturing relationships between children and their parents and caregivers*. Geneva: World Health Organization.

World Health Organization, & UNICEF. (2012). *Care for Child Development: Improving the care of young children*. Geneva: World Health Organization.

Yousafzai, A. K., Rasheed, M. A., Rizvi, A., Armstrong, R., & Bhutta, Z. A. (2014). Effect of integrated responsive stimulation and nutrition interventions in the Lady Health Worker programme in Pakistan on child development, growth, and health outcomes: A cluster-randomised factorial effectiveness trial. *Lancet, 384*(9950), 1282–1293.

Jon Korfmacher PhD (USA): Associate professor at the Erikson Institute. His research focuses on differential responses of children and families to early childhood intervention programs. He is interested in understanding why families participate in these programs, what the experience is like for them, and what types of services work best for different families under different circumstances. He also studies the training and professional development of early childhood service providers. He is also a faculty associate with the Herr Research Center for Children and Social Policy and a graduate fellow of ZERO TO THREE.

Lori Roggman (USA): Professor in the Department of Family, Consumer, and Human Development at Utah State University. She studies parenting and early intervention in relation to children's early social, cognitive, and language development. Her career began as a Head Start home visitor and continued as a trainer and consultant for practitioners in infant/toddler and early childhood programs. She has conducted research on early parenting and on home visiting interventions to support parenting in Early Head Start and similar programs. She has also coauthored the book named *Developmental Parenting: A Guide for Early Childhood Practitioners*. She codeveloped the PICCOLO scale using 4500 observations of parenting interactions to develop a valid, reliable, easy-to-use measure for both researchers and practitioners that gauges affection, responsiveness, encouragement, and teaching. She also codeveloped the Home Visit Rating Scales of home visiting quality. She has served in several technical advisory groups developing methods and measures to study services for families of infants, toddlers, and young children.

Chapter 4
Developmental Parenting Home Visiting to Prevent Violence: Monitoring and Evaluating

Lori Roggman

Young children who experience abuse or exposure to violence are at high risk for long-term negative outcomes, in both poor development and increasingly aggressive behavior, if they do not have the buffering protection of stable supportive parenting (Olson, Lopez-Duran, Lunkenheimer, Chang, & Sameroff, 2011; Shonkoff, 2010; Tremblay et al., 2004). Without safe, stable, and nurturing relationships, young children with aggressive behavior problems are likely to remain aggressive and become adults who are abusive and violent (Jaffee et al., 2013; Nagin & Tremblay, 2001), thereby continuing an intergenerational cycle of violence (Cappell & Heiner, 1990). Nevertheless, most young children who show early aggression have parents who help them learn other ways to express and regulate their emotions and behaviors so that they do not maintain high levels of aggression (Tremblay, 2000). Parenting that supports children's early development can help children gain communication and self-regulation skills and thereby provide a foundation of resilience to environmental stress (Armstrong, Birnie-Lefcovitch, & Ungar, 2005; Masten, 2001), but many parents need help to provide that support. Home visiting programs designed to provide such support to parents have shown evidence of effectiveness in interrupting the cycle of violence by improving parenting and thereby reducing children's early aggressive behavior (Moss et al., 2011).

Home visiting that increases positive parenting behaviors can effectively promote children's early development (Chazen-Cohen et al., 2009). A *developmental parenting* approach to home visiting emphasizes parenting strengths, incorporates practices guided by observation and feedback regarding specific parenting behaviors, and is adaptable to each individual family in their culture. The approach focuses on parenting behaviors that support child development, that change as a child develops, and that can be developed. Parenting shown in research to support children's early development includes parenting behaviors in the domains of warmth, responsiveness, encouragement, and cognitive stimulation (Bernier, Whipple, &

L. Roggman (✉)
Utah State University, Logan, Utah, USA
e-mail: LoriRoggman@gmail.com

L. Roggman, N. Cardia (eds.), *Home Visitation Programs*,
DOI 10.1007/978-3-319-17984-1_4

Carlson, 2010; Farah et al., 2008; Kiernan & Mensah, 2011; Kim-Cohen, Moffitt, Caspi, & Taylor, 2004; Schore, 2001).

A developmental parenting approach to home visiting engages parents by using specific strategies that (1) build partnerships with families that focus on child development, (2) respond to family strengths as resources for supporting children's development, (3) facilitate developmentally supportive parenting interactions, and (4) work collaboratively and nonintrusively with parents to support children's development. Considered separately, these specific home visiting practices are supported by the research literature (Dunst, Bruder, Trivette, & Hamby, 2006; Heinicke, Rineman, Ponce, & Guthrie, 2001; Hebbeler & Gerlach-Downie, 2002; Roggman, Boyce, Cook, & Jump, 2001). Implemented in combination, this set of home visiting practices has shown experimental evidence of improving parenting, even in the stressful circumstances of poverty and with children with disabilities, by increasing developmentally supportive parenting and decreasing harsh parenting, thereby increasing child attachment security, reducing early childhood aggression, and improving other developmental outcomes (Boyce, Innocenti, Roggman, Jump Norman, & Ortiz, 2010; Boyce et al., 2010; Roggman, Boyce, & Cook, 2009; Roggman & Cook, 2011). This home visiting approach thus has the potential to disrupt the cycle of abuse and aggression.

These home visiting practices are similar to those implemented in many home visiting programs, including the US Early Head Start program for infants and toddlers who, because they are from low-income families experiencing high levels of stress, are considered at risk for negative developmental outcomes, including insecurity and aggression. Nevertheless, when these practices were assessed using an adaptation of our home visiting practices measure (*Home Visit Rating Scales-Adapted (HOVRS-A),* Roggman et al., 2010) in the Early Head Start Family and Child Experiences Study (Baby FACES), a national descriptive study of Early Head Start, the average home visitor showed only moderate use of these practices (Bryans, Cohen, & Raikes, 2011). Programs need to emphasize the use of these skills by home visitors. Home visitors typically require ongoing training and supervision focused directly on these practices in order to employ them effectively enough to help the highest-risk parents to support their children's early development. For these reasons, monitoring and evaluating home visiting programs is especially important to ensure home visiting effectiveness with high-risk families.

Logic Model of Developmental Parenting Home Visiting

A logic model of the developmental parenting approach can guide the process of monitoring and evaluating a home visiting program. From left to right, Fig. 4.1 shows a multicomponent logic model in which monitoring and evaluating a home visiting program can support effective home visiting practices to promote the kinds of parenting interactions that support children's early development. This model can guide the monitoring and evaluation of home visiting programs by identifying specific practices underlying developmental parenting home visiting fidelity and by suggesting ways of measuring home visiting outcomes. This model therefore has the potential to improve home visiting programs.

Home visiting programs may usefully adapt this model to include details that describe their own program. For a program to develop their own logic model, program staff members should address the following questions: (1) Which child outcomes are the most important? (2) How can parents support these child outcomes? (3) Which home visiting strategies can best help parents provide this support? (4) What can help or get in the way of these strategies being effective? To monitor or evaluate a home visiting program, the quality of each component of the program's logic model needs to be observed and/or measured regularly, compared across time, and used to improve home visiting quality.

The following sections of this chapter will review research evidence and knowledge about each component of the developmental parenting home visiting logic model, moving from right to left. First, child development will be considered in relation to key environmental stress factors that can lead to poor developmental outcomes and aggressive behavior. The parenting behaviors that can support positive child outcomes even in highly stressful environments will then be described, followed by a review of the home visiting practices that can promote these parenting behaviors. Finally, a process will be described for monitoring and evaluating home visiting practices and program outcomes for children and parents.

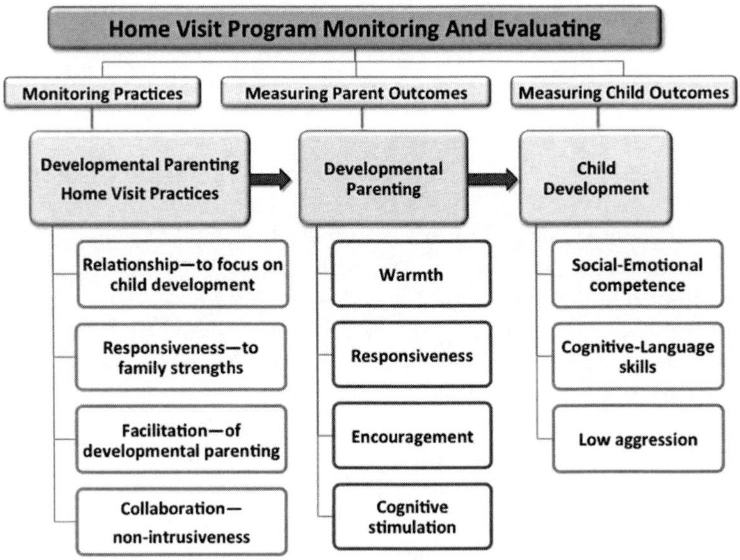

Fig. 4.1 Logic model for monitoring and evaluating developmental parenting home visiting

Environmental Stress and Aggression in Early Childhood

Chronic or severe environmental stress, often referred to as toxic stress, can interfere with children's early development and increase the risk of childhood aggression. The aim of developmental parenting home visiting is to improve outcomes for infants and young children at risk for developmental problems and aggressive behavior due to highly stressful environments. Improvements in children's social-emotional development can actually reverse children's reactions to highly stressful conditions by reducing their overall reactivity and vulnerability to stress (Schore, 2001). When young children are supported in their development in the context of consistent close relationships, they are more resilient to the risks of these multiple negative outcomes that may result from living in chronically stressful early environments (Garner, 2013; Johnson, Riley, Granger, & Riis, 2013; Shonkoff et al., 2012; Thompson, 2014). Without that support, children who live in environments with extended periods of high levels of stress are at risk for long-term chronic and often severe negative effects on their health, development, and psychological functioning (Middlebrooks & Audage, 2008; Shonkoff, 2010). Infants and young children are particularly vulnerable to chronic stress because their early brain development is likely to be adversely affected by high levels of stress, and they become more likely over time to experience increased reactivity to stress, often expressed in early aggression and observed in delayed development (Haller, Harold, Sandi, & Neumann, 2014; Lupien, McEwen, Gunnar, & Heim, 2009; O'Neal et al., 2010). Some of the most damaging sources of stress for young children include maltreatment, parent mental illness or substance abuse, and extreme poverty.

Maltreatment

Children's experiences of maltreatment, in the form of abuse or neglect or in the form of exposure to domestic violence, have negative impacts on their health and development. Such children show impairments in stress hormone regulation, sleep patterns, and coping abilities (Anda et al., 2006; Bugental, Martorell, & Barraza, 2003; Cicchetti, Rogosch, Howe, & Toth, 2010; Schore, 2001). They also show delayed and limited language abilities (Eigsti & Cicchetti, 2004), which are associated with physical aggression in young children (Séguin, Parent, Tremblay, & Zelazo, 2009). In addition, they are more likely to show signs of attachment insecurity (Lyons-Ruth, Easterbrooks, & Cibelli, 1997), which is also associated with early aggression (DeMulder, Denham, Schmidt, & Mitchell, 2000; Finzy, Anca, Har-Even, Shnit, & Weizman, 2001; Lyons-Ruth, Alpern, & Repacholi, 1993; NICHD ECCRN, 2004; Ooi, Ang, Fung, Wong, & Cai, 2006; Weinfield, Sroufe, Egeland, & Carlson, 1999). Childhood maltreatment is related to a variety of predictive factors, including parenting stress (Taylor, Guterman, Lee, & Rathouz, 2009), low levels of maternal education, and large family size (Dubowitz et al., 2011); but two of the most consistent predictors are parental depression and substance abuse problems

(Chemtob, Gudiño, & Laraque, 2013; Dubowitz et al., 2011; Kelleher, Chaffin, Hollenberg, & Fischer, 1994; Mustillo, Dorsey, Conover, & Burns, 2011).

Parent Depression and Substance Abuse

Children of parents with depression or substance abuse problems show a broad range of negative developmental outcomes including poor cognitive and motor skills (Petterson & Albers, 2001), higher likelihood of insecure attachment (Coyl, Roggman, & Newland, 2002; Hipwell, Goossens, Melhuish, & Kumar, 2000), and increased emotional and behavioral problems that include aggression (Hay, Pawlby, Waters, Perra, & Sharp, 2010; Mustillo et al., 2011). Children exposed to drugs prenatally, particularly to cocaine and methamphetamines, are more likely to have attention problems, language delays, cognitive limitations, and behavior problems that include aggression (Lester & Lagasse, 2010). Children of cocaine-addicted mothers are more likely to show insecure attachment (Strathearn & Mayes, 2010), which is related to early aggression (NICHD ECCRN, 2004). Toddlers and young children with alcoholic parents are more likely to be insecurely attached and also to show early aggressive behavior (Eiden, Edwards, & Leonard, 2002; Puttler, Zucker, Fitzgerald, & Bingham, 1998). These negative child outcomes are likely due to the higher probability of unsupportive parenting by parents facing challenges of poor mental health or addiction to drugs or alcohol (Eiden, Chavez, & Leonard, 1999; Eiden, Edwards, & Leonard, 2002; Hay et al., 2010). Unsupportive parenting is also more likely among parents who experience the stresses of poverty.

Poverty

Children living in poverty are more likely to have negative outcomes in their health and in multiple developmental areas (Aber, Bennett, Conley, & Li, 1997; Farah et al., 2006; Petterson & Albers, 2001; Rose-Jacobs et al., 2008; United Nations World Food Program, 2006). Specifically, household food insecurity puts young children at risk for poor developmental outcomes and behavior problems, including early aggression (Whitaker, Phillips, & Orzol, 2006). Internationally, even the slightest levels of household food insecurity have detrimental effects on children's early development (Chilton, Chyatte, & Breaux, 2007), not only among children in the world's poorest nations (Grantham-McGregor et al., 2007) but also among those in developed countries such as the USA and Brazil (Rose-Jacobs et al., 2008; Victora et al., 2003). Similarly to other sources of damaging stress, the effects of poverty on children are likely to be exacerbated due to poor parenting. Harsh, punitive, and insensitive parenting and developmentally unsupportive parenting are more likely when parents are under stress due to poverty (Engle & Black, 2008; Kiernan & Mensah, 2011; Korenman, Miller, & Sjaastad, 1995).

Parenting and Stress

A defining feature of damaging stress for infants and young children is that supportive parenting is lacking when children's stress responses are activated (Shonkoff, 2010). Parenting that is unresponsive, harsh, negative, and detached is potentially the most directly damaging source of stress for young children (Schore, 2001). Indeed, even mild forms of maternal maltreatment such as frequent punishment or emotional withdrawal in infancy have been associated with elevated stress hormones in toddlers (Bugental et al., 2003). High stress levels from these dysfunctional early relationships predict children's emotional and behavioral problems, including aggression, in school years (Essex, Klein, Cho, & Kalin, 2002). Such adverse early experiences in relationships with their parents place children on trajectories that involve poor self-regulation, negative emotion functioning, decreased social competence, and dysfunctional relationships (Taylor et al., 2004; Repetti, Taylor, & Seeman, 2002), which eventually lead to aggressive behavior (Lochman, Barry, Powell, & Young, 2010).

Responsive and supportive parenting, in contrast, can buffer children from the damaging effects of stress and resulting cortisol production (Ahnert, Gunnar, Lamb, & Barthel, 2004; Nachmias, Gunnar, Mangesldorf, Parritz, & Buss, 1996). Gunnar and Donzella (2002) suggest that regulation of the limbic hypothalamic-pituitary-adrenocortical (L-HPA) system is influenced by children's social experiences, particularly in their early relationships with their parents. Parents can help regulate infants' and young children's secretion of stress hormones through their relationships and presence with their children. Responsive parenting thus appears to help infants and toddlers adapt to stress and regulate the secretion of stress hormones, thereby reducing the effects of stress (Gunnar & Quevedo, 2007; Schore, 2001). Responsive parenting may also buffer children from stress by promoting secure attachment, which is associated with lower levels of childhood aggression (DeMulder et al., 2000; Finzy et al., 2001 Lyons-Ruth et al., 1993; NICHD ECCRN, 2004; Ooi et al., 2006; Weinfield et al., 1999), and serves as a protective factor against childhood aggression in young children with alcoholic fathers (Edwards, Eiden, & Leonard, 2006). Recent interventions have shown some promise in increasing supportive parenting, decreasing mothers' use of physical punishment, and/or reducing children's aggressive behavior (Duggan et al., 2004; Love et al., 2005). By intervening early, home visiting programs can help parents recognize their unique opportunity to positively influence children's early developmental outcomes through supportive interactions with their children during times of stress.

Research on Parenting to Support Child Development and Resilience

Specific kinds of parenting can support positive developmental outcomes and resilience in young children. The aim of developmental parenting home visiting is to increase parenting behaviors that research has shown can increase children's developmental competence and thereby increase their resilience to damaging stress (Bernier et al., 2010; Farah et al., 2008; Kim-Cohen et al., 2004; Masten, 2001). Although children's resilience in the face of severe adversity has sometimes been viewed as an unusual individual protective trait, research suggests that resilience is a normative adaptive system based on developmental competence that can be supported by positive parenting (Armstrong et al., 2005; Luthar, 2006; Masten, 2001; Wyman, Sandier, Wolchik, & Nelson, 2000). Recent considerations of resilience in infancy and early childhood have emphasized the basis of resilience not only in children's development but also in the parenting or the parent–child relationships that support it (Easterbrooks, Driscoll, & Bartlett, 2008; Howell, Graham-Bermann, Czyz, & Lilly, 2010).

Both children's own development and the parenting they experience can act as buffers for damaging stress and its long-term consequences. Children's developmental competence moderated the effect of damaging stress conditions (parent mental illness and chronic separations) on externalizing behavior problems that included aggression in a study of 4000 3-year-olds (Flouri, Tzavidis, & Kallis, 2010). Nurturant parenting and parent–child relationship quality in early childhood predicted better behavior and less aggression in early adolescence among over 200 boys from a severely impoverished urban neighborhood (Vanderbilt-Adriance & Shaw, 2008), and better parenting predicted better social-emotional development in young children from 56 families experiencing domestic violence (Howell et al., 2010). Developmentally supportive parenting thus appears to be a promising means by which parents can buffer children from damaging stress by promoting children's early development.

Research points to specific types of parenting that support early development, including warmth, responsiveness, encouragement, and cognitive stimulation (Dodici, Draper, & Peterson, 2003; Hart & Risley, 1995; NICHD ECCRN, 1999; Snow, Burns, & Griffin, 1998), and shows that supporting children's early development is especially critical for children most at risk for poor developmental outcomes (Bradley et al., 2001; Noble & McCandliss, 2005). Each of these domains of developmentally supportive parenting predicts more than one kind of developmental outcome (multi-finality), just as any particular developmental outcome can usually be predicted by parenting in more than one domain (multi-causality; Cicchetti & Rogosch, 1996; Masten, 2001). Also, a given parenting interaction may reflect multiple domains of parenting: A parent could smile warmly at a child playing with a toy, respond sensitively to the child's frustration with the toy, support the child's independent exploration of the toy, and talk to the child about the toy, all during the same few moments of interaction. Each of these parenting domains supports children's developmental competence under conditions of damaging stress. The first two domains—warmth and responsiveness—represent an affective dimension of parenting that differentiates between resilient and stress-affected children (Kilmer, Cowen, & Wyman, 2001), while the other two domains—encouragement and cognitive stimulation—represent a stimulation dimension of parenting important for preventing negative developmental outcomes among children at high risk for damaging stress (Brotman et al., 2009).

Warmth

Parental warmth involves the expression of affection, positive emotions, and positive regard toward the child (MacDonald, 1992; Rohner, 1986). During the early years, these positive expressions are an indicator of the quality of the mother–child relationship and are linked to positive outcomes for children (Grusec & Goodnow, 1994; Lay, Waters, & Parke, 1989). Parenting with warmth and affection is related to less aggressive behavior, more compliance, and better psychological adjustment (Caspi et al., 2004; Dodge, Pettit, & Bates, 1994; Dodici et al., 2003; MacDonald, 1992; Petrill & Deater-Deckard, 2004). Particularly for children at risk due to maternal drug abuse or severe poverty, high maternal warmth predicts better cognitive outcomes and fewer behavior problems including aggression (Farah et al., 2008; Kim-Cohen et al., 2004).

Responsiveness

Responsiveness involves reacting sensitively to a child's cues and expressions of needs or interests and interacting positively and contingently with the child. In the research literature, this and similar parenting behaviors predict children's secure attachment, cognitive development, social development, language development, emotion regulation, empathy, and socially appropriate behavior (Bernier et al., 2010; DeWolff & Van IJzendoorn, 1997; Hirsh-Pasik & Burchinal, 2006; Davidov & Grusec, 2006; Landry, Smith, Swank, Assel, & Vellet, 2001; Spencer & Meadow-Orlans, 1996; Tamis-LeMonda, Bornstein, & Baumwell, 2001; Volker, Keller, Lohaus, Cappenberg, & Chasiotis, 1999). Responsive parenting supports children's secure attachment, which then provides a foundation for children's positive development in multiple domains, including communication, exploration, and problem-solving (Booth, Rose-Krasnor, MacKinnon, & Rubin, 1994; DeWolff & Van IJzendoorn, 1997; Easterbrooks, Biesecker, & Lyons-Ruth, 2000; Kochanska, 1995; Suess, Grossman & Sroufe, 1992; van den Boom, 1994; Youngblade, Park, & Belsky, 1993). Even more specific to the developmental competence needed for resilience in the face of damaging stress, mothers' responsiveness, in high-risk communities in the USA and in other countries, is related to better executive function in infancy and to less aggression among children (Bernier et al., 2010; Brotman et al., 2009; Hart, Nelson, Robinson, Olsen, & McNeilly-Choque, 1998). These long-term positive outcomes extend into adolescence: Maternal responsiveness in infancy predicts substantially lower risk of adolescent conduct disorder, which includes aggressive behavior and other problems such as theft and property damage (Wakschlag & Hans, 1999).

Encouragement

Parental encouragement includes support not only of a child's growing independence but also of a child's efforts, exploration, creativity, and initiative. Parenting behaviors indicative of encouragement are associated with children who show greater willingness to try challenging tasks, less negativity, and better cognitive, language, and social development (Ispa et al., 2004; Hart & Risley, 1995; Landry, Smith, Miller-Loncar, & Swank, 1997; Kelly, Morisset, Barnard, Hammond, & Booth, 1996). Supportive and nonintrusive parenting interactions are particularly important for children's cognitive development in early childhood (Hubbs-Tait, Culp, Culp, & Miller, 2002). In addition, parent encouragement with infants at risk for damaging stress is an important predictor of executive function (Bernier et al., 2010), an important outcome for resilience in stressful early environments.

Cognitive Stimulation

Cognitive stimulation includes explanations, conversations, joint attention, and shared play. These and similar parenting behaviors are related to children's cognitive development, language development, and social development, as well as to their emergent literacy skills (Bingham, 2007; Farah et al., 2008; Hart & Risley, 1995; Hubbs-Tait et al., 2002; Kim-Cohen et al., 2004; Hockenberger, Goldstein, & Haas, 1999; Laasko, Poikkeus, Eklund, & Lyytinen, 1999; Tamis-LeMonda et al., 2001). Cognitive stimulation focuses on children's early learning of words and concepts and does indeed predict long-term academic success (Cook, Roggman, & Boyce, 2012). Lack of cognitive stimulation directly predicts more aggression in young children (Dodge et al., 1994). Among children at risk for damaging stress, cognitive stimulation is particularly important for better language development (Farah et al., 2008), which is associated with less aggressive behavior (Séguin, Parent, Tremblay, & Zelazo, 2009), and for behavioral control, including the inhibition of aggression (Brotman et al., 2009; Kim-Cohen et al., 2004). Cognitive stimulation is particularly important for children in highly stressful circumstances because they are likely to have fewer opportunities for the kinds of exploration and play that provide cognitive stimulation.

Parenting as a Focus of Home Visiting

The parenting behaviors that support children's early development—warmth, responsiveness, encouragement, and cognitive stimulation—support key child development outcomes that are the early foundations for resilience to stress, for later academic and life success, and for the prevention of childhood aggression that leads to later violence. And these are the parenting behaviors that are expected to increase as a result of a parent being present and engaged in the activities, interactions, discussions, and planning of developmental parenting home visits. Home visiting strategies to increase these key domains of parenting can help parents support their children's developmental competence in multiple areas of development. Indeed, a recent study of a home visiting program using a similar approach demonstrated not only increases in maternal sensitivity and cognitive stimulation but also reductions in children's cortisol stress reactivity and behavioral aggression in families involved with the judicial system because of an older sibling's aggressive behavior (O'Neal et al., 2010). These significant reductions in children's aggressive behavior were accounted for by the program's impact on improvements in parenting—increases in responsiveness and cognitive stimulation—that explained a significant amount of the intervention effect on children's aggression (Brotman et al., 2009).

Evidence for a *Developmental Parenting* Home Visiting Approach

Home visiting to families with infants and young children in stressful environments can help parents prevent childhood aggression and break the cycle of violence, but only if home visitors engage parents in the process of supporting their children's development. Home visitors often lack effective strategies to engage parents in developmentally supportive interactions with their children both during and between home visits. Developmental parenting home visiting practices can effectively engage parents by building relationships that focus on child development, responding to family strengths, facilitating developmental parenting behaviors, and collaborating nonintrusively. Based on experimental evidence and other research support, these home visiting practices comprise an evidence-based parenting intervention.

In two experimental design studies of separate samples, a home visiting intervention comprising these practices showed experimental impacts on positive parenting behavior. In an Early Head Start home visiting program using a developmental parenting approach, 161 qualified applicant families were randomly assigned to either the program or a comparison group. Children in the program group, compared with those in the comparison group, had significantly better cognitive development, more secure attachment, and less aggressive behavior, and their parents were significantly less likely to use harsh punishment (Roggman et al., 2009; Roggman & Cook, 2011). In another study, also using a developmental parenting home visiting approach, 75 mothers in a Migrant Head Start program were randomly assigned to receive either the usual program services or home visits to help them support their children's language development by engaging in meaningful interactions and conversations and then making books together about the interaction. These mothers, who were living in severe poverty and stressful community conditions, showed significantly more developmentally supportive parenting if they were in the intervention group rather than the comparison group (Boyce et al., 2010). In addition, a descriptive study of one of these home visiting practices, facilitating parent–child interaction, showed that greater facilitation of parenting, as observed by researchers, predicted significantly better family outcomes, as reported by program staff (Roggman et al., 2001).

These practices also have an evidence basis in other experimental studies. The practices that comprise the developmental parenting intervention are both common and important in the sense that one or more of them are frequently described as part of tested evidence-based home visiting programs that have been evaluated in randomized clinical trials, such as Early Head Start (Administration for Children, Youth, & Families (ACYF), 2002), Parents as Teachers (Wagner, Iida, & Spiker, 2001; Wagner & Spiker, 2001), Nurse–Family Partnership (Olds et al., 1998), or Healthy Families America (Duggan et al., 2007). These home visiting program models are supported by evidence from rigorous experimental designs in randomized clinical trials. Unfortunately, this rigorous testing of programs often reveals little of the variability in implementation of home visiting practices. Thus, these studies offer little information about what actually happens during home visits that leads to better outcomes for children and parents and even less about variations in home visiting practices that explain variations in parent and child outcomes from home visiting programs. Fortunately, a growing research literature points to several key home visiting practices that help parents provide more developmental support for their children.

Developmental Parenting Home Visit Practices

Several home visiting practices have evidence showing that they can promote developmentally supportive parenting and thus have the potential to prevent a cycle of violence that stems from poor early development and childhood aggression. The practices of the developmental parenting home visiting approach have research support from studies that have examined these practices in a variety of home visiting programs. Positive program outcomes for parents or children are more likely when home visitors do one or more of the following: engage parents in relationships focused on child development, respond to family strengths by engaging the whole family and incorporating learning into family activities, directly facilitate developmentally supportive parenting behaviors, and nonintrusively collaborate with parents (Dunst et al., 2006; Guralnick, 1989, 1998; Hebbeler & Gerlach-Downie, 2002; Mahoney, Boyce, Fewell, Spiker, & Wheeden, 1998; Mahoney & Perales, 2005; Raikes et al., 2006; Woods, Kashinath, & Goldstein, 2004). These home visiting practices are compatible with the mutual competence approach of Bernstein and colleagues (Bernstein, Campbell, & Akers, 2001) because the emphasis is on home visitors recognizing the competence of each parent and child, helping parents recognize their children's growing competence, and sharing the home visitor's competence by collaborating with families to help them support their children's development. Each of these practices reflects this emphasis.

Relationships Focused on Child Development

When home visitors build a partnership relationship with a family in which they enjoy doing things together that support the children's development, an implicit message of respect is sent to the parent. This message of respect assures parents that they can provide good developmental experiences for their infants or toddlers, even in difficult circumstances. Most home visiting practices promote positive relationships between the home visitor and parent, and several studies suggest that positive relationships promote trust and better parent–child relationships (Barnard, Morisset, Spieker, 1993; Bernstein, Hans, & Percansky, 1991; Emde, Korfmacher, & Kubicek, 2000). Maintaining a focus on child development in these relationships is important. When home visiting emphasizes child development, program outcomes are stronger (Guralnick, 1998; Raikes et al., 2006; Peterson et al., 2013). In developmental parenting home visiting, the home visitor–parent relationship focuses on supporting the child's early development and thereby preventing negative outcomes in stressful environments.

Partnership relationships between home visitors and parents are built using a mutual competence approach (Bernstein et al., 2001) of individualizing home visiting practices to each family's strengths, including their culture and values. Home visitors contribute their own strengths, expertise, and resources to the process, and instruction can be part of mutual competence, but home visitor–parent relationships remain central to effectively promoting developmental parenting. By using a mutual competence approach to build relationships with families, home visitors are able to use effective home visiting practices with respect for each family's unique strengths and resources. Several specific strategies to build relationships with families that focus on child development include remaining focused on parenting and a positive parent–child relationship (in contrast to modeling the "right" way to teach a child), building parent self-confidence by supporting the parent–child relationship (in contrast to parent training), and helping the parent see the impact of stressful events and family crises on their children, thereby strengthening the parent–child relationship in times of stress (in contrast to waiting until family problems are solved before addressing child development; Roggman, Boyce, & Innocenti, 2008).

Responsiveness to Family Strengths

Developmental parenting home visiting requires responsiveness to the parent's existing knowledge, values, culture, and unique challenges. Thus, it requires home visitors to have knowledge and skills related not only to infant/toddler development and methods to facilitate it but also to parenting and methods to facilitate adult learning. Responsiveness to family strengths and culture opens opportunities to increase children's developmental support by incorporating learning into regular family activities and involving fathers and other family members (Dunst et al., 2006; Lanzi, Terry, Guest, Cotton, & Ramey, 1999; Slaughter-Defoe, 1993; Smith, 1995; Woods et al., 2004).

Developmental parenting home visitors help parents employ the family's existing resources to help buffer their child from damaging stress by involving other family members to help support the child's development and by making use of regular family activities as learning opportunities. Cultural respect is an essential part of this approach because cultural values and traditions are viewed as family strengths and resources in this model. As with building partnership relationships with parents, responding to their strengths is also consistent with a mutual competence model (Bernstein et al., 1991, 2001) because it emphasizes individualizing practices to each family's knowledge, skills, culture, and values. Home visitors can respond to and build on family strengths by asking parents directly about family interests and knowledge, asking parents about past experiences with their own children and other children, asking what parents enjoy doing with their children, observing and commenting on parents' interests and ideas, and then using all of this information to plan home visit activities together with parents (Roggman et al., 2008).

Facilitation of Developmental Parenting

Planning activities to encourage positive parent–child interaction is a practice that is common across evidence-based home visiting programs. Research suggests that home visiting practices that focus directly on parenting and child development are more effective at promoting them both (Kagan & Neuman, 1997; Olds et al., 1997; Wagner & Clayton, 1999; Sweet & Appelbaum, 2004). Home visitor effectiveness with the highest-risk families thus relies on strategies that engage parents in developmentally supportive interactions with their children.

Facilitating parent–child interaction predicts more family improvement, and directly encouraging parents to teach, talk, and interact responsively and warmly with children can help parents improve child outcomes (Boyce et al., 2010; Chazen-Cohen et al., 2009; Hebbeler & Gerlach-Downie, 2002; Mahoney et al., 1998; Mahoney & Perales, 2005; Roggman et al., 2001, 2009). Effective home visitors elicit these kinds of parent–child interactions (Mahoney et al., 1998; Roggman et al., 2001) and directly encourage developmental parenting behaviors (Guralnick, 1989; Hebbeler & Gerlach-Downie, 2002; Mahoney & Perales, 2005). Specific practices that facilitate parent–child interaction in a developmental parenting home visiting approach include handing activity materials to the parent instead of the child; asking the parent about the child's skills, experiences, and interests; and observing and commenting on positive parent–child interactions, the child's response to the parent, and the parent's response to the child (Roggman et al., 2008).

Collaboration

Helping parents remain in their primary role to support their children's development is a key practice in the developmental parenting home visiting approach. Guiding parents to plan, implement, and review activities increases parent capacity to support development in the future and increases program capacity to have more lasting impacts (Dunst et al., 2006; Hebbeler & Gerlach-Downie, 2002). Rather than demonstrating "correct" interactions or interrupting positive interactions to tell parents exactly what to do, effective home visitors avoid these intrusive and ineffective practices and thereby avoid diminishing the parents' central importance in supporting their children's development. Collaboration with parents is also based on a mutual competence model (Bernstein et al., 2001), in which parent competence is recognized and fostered and home visitor competence is shared. To collaborate nonintrusively with parents, home visitors ask about typical family activities and regular routines, help parents choose family activities or routines to do together on home visits, help parents plan other activities for home visits, and plan together with parents how they will continue to support children's development between visits (Roggman et al., 2008).

Parent Engagement

Any intervention aimed at helping parents support their children's development depends on parent engagement. Home visiting programs have stronger outcomes when home visiting strategies keep parents present, active, interactive, and involved (Heinicke et al., 2001, 2006; Lieberman, Weston, & Pawl, 1991; Korfmacher et al., 1998; Raikes et al. 2006; Roggman et al., 2001). For high-risk families living in stressful environments, parent engagement may be even more important and more challenging: Parents under stress may find it difficult to be engaged in a program or even with their own child if struggling with poverty, mental illness, or substance abuse. In a case-analysis of participants in an Early Head Start program, parent engagement seemed to be a key factor in successful outcomes. Although case studies of both a "success" case and a "nonsuccess" case indicated parent mental-health problems, employment problems, chaotic home situations, and unreliable schedules that limited parent participation in home visits, parents in the "success" case were considerably more engaged in the program than the parents in the "nonsuccess" case (Roggman et al., 2001).

Parent engagement can be influenced not only by the approach and strategies used by the home visitors but also by parent, family, and child characteristics, such as fathers' or grandmothers' attitudes about the program or involvement with the child (Daro & Harding, 1999; Roggman, Cook, Boyce, & Hart, 2009). To effectively increase parenting that will promote children's early development and reduce the risk of aggression and subsequent violent behavior, home visiting practices need to be effective at engaging parents and other key family members in the home visit process.

Monitoring and Evaluating a *Developmental Parenting* Home Visit Program

Home visiting programs show considerable variability in quality in terms of how well and how consistently they are implemented and how families fare as a result (ACYF, 2002; Raikes et al., 2006; Roggman et al., 2001). A sustainable monitoring and evaluation system can increase the effectiveness of home visiting programs for at-risk families by monitoring home visiting practices and evaluating program outcomes both in children's early development and in parents' developmentally supportive behavior.

Monitoring Home Visiting Practices

As key practitioners delivering services in home visiting programs, home visitors often have adequate background in child development and activities that support early development, but little background in adult learning or practices that effectively support developmentally supportive parenting (Dunst et al., 2006; Hebbeler & Gerlach-Downie, 2002). In the US Early Head Start program, home visitors have, on average, as much education in early child development as the average Early Head Start classroom teacher in center-based programs (Vogel, 2011), but Early Head Start home visitors only rarely have training in working effectively with parents who have a mental illness or addiction, have been victims or perpetrators of family violence, or are extremely stressed (Tandon, Mercer, Saylor, & Duggan, 2008). And yet the children of these parents are the most at risk for damaging stress and will need the most support for their early development.

Home visitors may intend to help parents support their children's early development, but often plan activities they themselves do with the infant or child during a home visit. The implicit message is that the home visitor is the expert teacher and that the parent is unable to do activities to support the child's early development. A parent who infers this message may become even less likely to support the child's development between home visits, especially if struggling with adversity in a stressful environment. The infant or young child may respond positively to activities during a weekly home visit, but generally the few hours of services received each month is not enough time to make a lasting difference in the child's development.

Training and Supporting Home Visitors

Despite the strong research basis for the developmental parenting home visiting approach and the practices that comprise it, most home visitors need training to implement those practices effectively. A strong training and support system can increase home visitor effectiveness with the highest-risk families. Research by Bigelow and

Lutzker (2000) showed that when home visitors were given additional training, there were clear improvements in their work. To be effective at reducing the potential for violence in high-risk families, home visitors need initial training on effective research-based home visiting practices, ongoing coaching and problem-solving support to implement these practices with high-risk families, and opportunities to communicate with other home visitors in a community of practice. By initiating and implementing a system with these aspects of training and support for home visitors, home visiting programs are likely to become more effective.

Training for home visitors should integrate a strong content model, describing the key practices and intended outcomes of home visiting (Wechsler, Chap. 5, this volume). Training should focus on guided problem-solving using problems that are authentic, relevant, and personal (Gibbons, 2001; Merrill, 2002). Home visitors are usually motivated to do well and need to integrate new ideas with what they already know from their experiences with families and have their experiences, values, and cultures respected (Zemke & Zemke, 1981). Guided problem-solving can help home visitors generate practical solutions to the problems they face in their everyday work with families at high risk for damaging stress. Supportive reflective supervision and team support can help protect home visitors from feelings of exhaustion and frustration (Lloyd, King, & Chenoweth, 2002; Maslach, Schaufeli, & Leiter, 2001) and can help them be more supportive of parents who can, in turn, become more supportive with their children (Korfmacher, Chap. 6, this volume; Weatherston, 2007).

Measuring Home Visiting Practices

Supervisor or peer observations of home visits can help provide support for home visitors and identify training needs of home visitors. As part of an ongoing professional development, home visit observations can help supervisors identify positive examples of how home visitors are implementing effective practices. Feedback describing these examples can help home visitors expand their use of these practices in future home visits. A supervisor and home visitor can reflect on effective home visiting practices before and after a home visit to guide these observations.

A useful tool developed for measuring home visiting practices is an observational measure of home visiting, the *Home Visit Rating Scales* (HOVRS, Roggman et al., 2008; HOVRS-A, Roggman et al., 2010; HOVRS-A + v2, Roggman et al., 2014). All of the versions of the HOVRS list multiple quality indicators that can be observed during developmental parenting home visits. These indicators can be used to make ratings on seven scales representing four key home visiting practices (relationship with family, responsiveness to family strengths, facilitation of parent–child interaction, and nonintrusive collaboration) and three aspects of family engagement (parent–child interaction, parent engagement, child engagement). Scale indicators were originally developed from discussions with home visiting program staff about what happens on effective home visits and later corroborated with evidence from the research literature on home visiting practices in programs for families with infants and young children, as reviewed above. HOVRS scales were tested on 60 video observations of home visits made by two home-based Early Head Start programs in different areas of the USA. The scales demonstrate good reliability and validity. Two trained observers completed HOVRS ratings on 25 % of the videotaped home visits with 85 % agreement (*Kappa* >0.75), providing evidence of measurement reliability. Ratings of home visiting practices together predicted the quality of parenting on the *Home Observation Measure of the Environment* (Caldwell & Bradley, 1984) and also predicted children's language outcomes on the *Peabody Picture Vocabulary Test-III* (Dunn & Dunn, 1997) at the end of the program, providing evidence of measurement validity. Home visiting programs can use this measure, or another observational measure of home visiting practices, to monitor and evaluate effective home visiting practices and then use the measurement data to identify training and support the needs of home visitors.

Evaluating Child Outcomes

The ultimate aim of a developmental parenting home visiting program is the healthy early development of children living in environments that put them at risk for poor development. Thus, the ultimate outcome that should be measured is child development in multiple areas, including cognitive, language, and social-emotional development. When children's development is assessed regularly as part of home visiting program services, home visitors and parents can see if children are developing toward these outcomes. By using "family-friendly" child development measures, home visitors can help parents understand and appreciate their children's development in ways that will help parents provide more developmental support.

Family-friendly child development measures are those that are easy to understand, easy to use, practical in families' home environments, appropriate for a wide range of development, engaging for parents, and reliable and valid. By being involved in measuring child development, parents learn to better understand the child's behavior, to be more realistic about what the child can do, to become better observers of the child's play and activities, to keep the child safer, and to provide more positive parenting to support development. Several measures of children's early development are appropriate for use in home visiting programs. Some of the family-friendly child development measures used in the USA include the *Ages & Stages Questionnaires* (*ASQ-3*; Squires & Bricker, 2009), *The Ounce Scale* (Meisels, Marsden, Dombro, Weston, & Jewkes, 2003), *Parents Observations of Infants & Toddlers* (*POINT*; Mardell & Goldenberg, 2008), *Hawaii Early Learning Profile* (*HELP*; Park, 1999), and other assessments done in homes (e.g., *Individual Growth & Development Indicators (IGDIs)* Carta, Greenwood, Walker, & Buzhardt, 2010).

Evaluating Parenting Outcomes

The means by which developmental parenting home visiting improves child outcomes is by promoting developmentally supportive parenting. Thus, a practical measure of parenting is an essential tool for home visiting programs. Observations of parent–child interaction can help home visitors identify and give feedback on parenting behaviors that are known to support children's early development. An observational measure of parenting can both guide home visiting practice and evaluate program outcomes. The *Parenting Interactions with Children: Checklist of Observations Linked to Outcomes* (PICCOLO; Roggman, Cook, Innocenti, Jump Norman, & Christiansen, 2013a) is an observational measure that was designed for use by home visiting programs to observe positive parenting interactions with very young children, ages 1–3 years. PICCOLO measures four important domains of parenting interactions that promote children's cognitive, language, and social development: *Affection* (warmth, physical closeness, and positive expressions toward child), *Responsiveness* (responding to child's cues, emotions, words, interests, and behaviors), *Encouragement* (active support of play, exploration, curiosity, initiative, skills, and creativity), and *Teaching* (shared conversation and play, cognitive stimulation, explanations, and questions). PICCOLO parenting behaviors observed with children as young as 10 months predict good child development outcomes when those children are starting school, including better cognitive and language skills, better self-regulation, and lower rates of aggressive behavior (Innocenti, Roggman, & Cook, 2013; Roggman, Cook, Innocenti, Jump Norman, & Christiansen, 2013b).

Programs can use PICCOLO to assess parenting behaviors, to guide interventions with families, and to track program outcomes. Developed from over 4000 videotaped parenting interactions of over 2000 families, it is research-based, psychometrically strong, culturally relevant, and practical for home visiting programs. Independent observers, watching parent–child interactions separately, rate the items similarly, with an overall reliability coefficient of 0.80. Observations can be done from 5–10 min of observed parent–child interaction, and a variety of activities can be used. The measurement form includes detailed coding guidelines for each parenting behavior item. The items were developed from observations of low-income European-American, Latino, and African-American families in the USA, and the measure has been used in several other countries. All items are positive to help home visitors identify the parenting strengths they can encourage parents to do more. What parents do with children when they are being observed reflects what parents believe is important to do and are comfortable doing to support their children's early development. Therefore, observed parenting behaviors provide important opportunities for home visitors to help parents expand the developmental support available to their children.

Conclusion

A developmental parenting home visiting program can help parents support children's early development in ways that improve children's developmental outcomes and decrease children's risk of early aggression and later violence. Successful implementation of this approach requires a similarly "developmental" approach to monitoring and evaluating the program. A developmentally supportive process of monitoring and evaluating a home visiting program emphasizes home visitor and program strengths and changes as home visitors expand their skills and as programs become more consistently effective at making positive changes in parents and children. The process should be guided by observation and feedback and aligned with the program's logic model. Data from assessment of each component of the model is likely to reveal the factors that help or hinder the pathways between components—the links from program support to effective home visiting practices, from effective practices to developmental parenting outcomes, and from developmentally supportive parenting to positive child development outcomes. These factors may include the quantity of timing and duration of program activities and services, the sources of environmental stress in communities and families, and the level of support for change in the program and community. By using a parallel process for families and for home visitors, the process of monitoring and evaluating home visiting can be adapted with sensitivity and respect for community and culture.

References

Aber, J. L., Bennett, N. G., Conley, D. C., & Li, J. (1997). The effects of poverty on child health and development. *Annual Review of Public Health, 18,* 463–483.

Administration for Children, Youth, & Families (ACYF). (2002). *Making a difference in the lives of infants and toddlers and their families: The impacts of Early Head Start.* Washington, DC: Department of Health and Human Services.

Ahnert, L., Gunnar, M., Lamb, M., & Barthel, M. (2004). Transition to child care: Associations with infant-mother attachment, infant negative emotion and cortisol elevations. *Child Development, 75,* 639–650.

Anda, R., Felitti, V., Bremner, J. D., Walker, J., Whitfield, C., Perry, B., Dube, S. R., & Giles, W. H. (2006). The enduring effects of abuse and related adverse experiences in childhood. *European Archives of Psychiatry and Clinical Neuroscience, 256,* 174–186.

Armstrong, M., Birnie-Lefcovitch, S., & Ungar, M. T. (2005). Pathways between social support, family well-being, quality of parenting, and child resilience: What we know. *Journal of Child and Family Studies, 14*(2), 269–281.

Barnard, K. E., Morisset, C. E., & Spieker, S. (1993). Preventive interventions: Enhancing parent-infant relationships. In C. H. Zeanah (Ed.), *Handbook of infant mental health* (pp. 386–399). New York: Guilford.

Bernier, A., Carlson, S. M., & Whipple, N. (2010). From external regulation to self-regulation: Early parenting precursors of young children's executive functioning. *Child Development, 81,* 326–339.

Bernstein, V. J., Hans, S. L., & Percansky, C. (1991). Advocating for the young children in need through strengthening the parent–child relationships. *Journal of Clinical Child Psychology, 20,* 28–41.

Bernstein, V. J., Campbell, S., & Akers, A. (2001). Caring for the caregivers: Supporting the well-being of at-risk parents and children through supporting the well-being of the programs that serve them. In J. N. Hughes, A. M. La Greca, & J. C. Conole (Eds.), *Handbook of psychological services for children and adolescents* (pp. 107–132). New York: Oxford University Press.

Bigelow, K. M., & Lutzker, J. R. (2000). Training parents at risk or reported for child abuse and neglect to identify and treat their children's illnesses. *Journal of Family Violence, 15,* 311–330.

Bingham, G. (2007). Maternal literacy beliefs and the quality of mother–child book reading interactions: Associations with children's early literacy development. *Early Education and Development, 18,* 23–49.

Booth, C. L., Rose-Krasnor, L., McKinnon, J., & Rubin, K. H. (1994). Predicting social adjustment in middle childhood: The role of preschool attachment security and maternal style. *Social Development, 3*(3), 189–204.

Boyce, L. K., Innocenti, M. S., Roggman, L. A., Jump Norman, V. K., & Ortiz, E. (2010). Telling stories and making books: Evidence for an intervention to help parents in Migrant Head Start families support their children's language and literacy. *Early Education and Development, 21,* 343–371.

Boyce, L. K., Innocenti, M. S., Roggman, L. A., Price, C., Jump Norman, V. K., Cook, G. A., & Ortiz E. (2010). Family bookmaking: An approach to support parent–child language interactions in natural environments. *Review of Disabilities Studies: An International Journal, 6,* 42–53.

Bradley, R. H., Corwyn, R. F., Burchinal, M., McAdoo, H. P., & García Coll, C. (2001). The home environments of children in the United States Part II: Relations with behavioral development through age thirteen. *Child Development, 72*(6), 1868–1886.

Brotman, L., O'Neal, C. R., Keng-Yen, H., Gouley, K., Rosenfelt, A., & Shrout, P. E. (2009). An experimental test of parenting practices as a mediator of early childhood physical aggression. *Journal of Child Psychology & Psychiatry, 50*(3), 235–245.

Bryans, A., Cohen, R. C., & Raikes, H. H. (2011). *Hand in hand: Data, research, and quality.* Washington, DC: Presentation at the Birth to Three Institute.

Bugental, D. B., Martorell, G. A., & Barraza, V. (2003). The hormonal costs of subtle forms of infant maltreatment. *Hormones and Behavior, 43*(1), 237–244.

Caldwell, B. M., & Bradley, R. H. (1984). *Home observation for measurement of the environment (HOME).* Little Rock: University of Arkansas at Little Rock.

Cappell, C., & Heiner, R. B. (1990). The intergenerational transmission of family aggression. *Journal of Family Violence, 5*(2), 135–152.

Carta, J. J., Greenwood, C., Walker, D., & Buzhardt, J. (2010). *Using IGDIs: Monitoring progress and improving intervention for infants and young children.* Baltimore: Brookes.

Caspi, A., Moffitt, T. E., Morgan, J., Rutter, M., Taylor, A., Arseneault, L., et al. (2004). Maternal expressed emotion predicts children's antisocial behavior problems: Using monozygotic-twin differences to identify environmental effects on behavioral development. *Developmental Psychology, 40,* 149–161.

Chazan-Cohen, R., Raikes, H., Brooks-Gunn, J., Ayoub, C., Pan, B. A., Kisker, E. E., Roggman, L., & Fuligni, A. S. (2009). Contributions of the parenting environment during the first five years of life to child outcomes at kindergarten entry in a low-income sample. *Early Education and Development, 20*(6), 958–977.

Chemtob, C. M., Gudiño, O. G., & Laraque, D. (2013). Maternal posttraumatic stress disorder and depression in pediatric primary care: Association with child maltreatment and frequency of child exposure to traumatic events. *JAMA Pediatrics, 167*(11), 1011–1018.

Chilton, M., Chyatte, M., & Breaux, J. (2007). The negative effects of poverty and food insecurity on child development. *Indian Journal of Medical Research, 126,* 262–272.

Cicchetti, D., & Rogosch, F. A. (1996). Equifinality and multifinality in developmental psychopathology. *Development and Psychopathology, 8,* 597–600.

Cicchetti, D., Rogosch, F. A., Howe, M. L., & Toth, S. L. (2010). The effects of maltreatment on neuroendocrine regulation and memory performance. *Child Development, 81*(5), 1504–1519.

Cook, G. A., Roggman, L. A., & Boyce, L. K. (2012). Fathers' and mothers' cognitive stimulation in early play with toddlers: Predictors of 5th grade reading and math. *Family Science, 2*(2), 131–145.

Coyl, D. D., Roggman, L. A., & Newland, L. (2002). Stress, maternal depression, and negative mother–infant interactions in relation to infant attachment. *Infant Mental Health Journal, 23,* 145–163.

Daro, D. A., & Harding, K. A. (1999). Healthy families in America: Using research to enhance practice. *The Future of Children, 9*(1), 152–176.

Davidov, M., & Grusec, J. E. (2006). Untangling the links of parental responsiveness to distress and warmth to child outcomes. *Child Development, 77*(1), 44–58.

DeMulder, E. K., Denham, S., Schmidt, M., & Mitchell, J. (2000). Q-sort assessment of attachment security during the preschool years: Links from home to school. *Developmental Psychology, 36,* 274–282.

DeWolff, M. S., & Van IJzendoorn, M. H. (1997). Sensitivity and attachment: A meta-analysis of parental antecedents of infant attachment. *Child Development, 68*(4), 571–591.

Dodge, K. A., Pettit, G. S., & Bates, J. E. (1994). Socialization mediators of the relation between socioeconomic status and child conduct problems. *Child Development, 65,* 649–665.

Dodici, B. J., Draper, D. C., & Peterson, C. A. (2003). Early parent–child interactions and early literacy development. *Topics in Early Childhood Special Education, 23,* 124–136.

Dubowitz, H., Kim, J., Black, M. M., Weisbart, C., Semiatin, J., & Magder, L. S. (2011). Identifying children at high risk for a child maltreatment report. *Child Abuse & Neglect, 35*(2), 96–104.

Duggan, A., Fuddy, L., Burrell, L., Higman, S. M., McFarlane, E., Windham, A., & Sia, C. (2004). Randomized trial of a statewide home visiting program to prevent child abuse: Impact in reducing parental risk factors. *Child Abuse & Neglect, 28,* 623–643.

Duggan, A., Caldera, D., Rodriguez, K., Burrell, L., Rohde, C., & Crowne, S. S. (2007). Impact of a statewide home visiting program to prevent child abuse. *Child Abuse & Neglect, 31*(8), 801–827.

Dunn, L. M., & Dunn, L. M. (1997). *Examiner's manual for the PPVT-III: Peabody Picture Vocabulary Test* (3rd ed.). Circle Pines: American Guidance Service.

Dunst, C. J., Bruder, M. B., Trivette, C. M., & Hamby, D. W. (2006). Everyday activity settings, natural learning environments, and early intervention practices. *Journal of Policy and Practice in Intellectual Disabilities, 3,* 3–10.

Easterbrooks, M. A., Biesecker, G., & Lyons-Ruth, K. A. (2000). Infancy predictors of emotional availability in middle childhood: The role of attachment and maternal depression. *Attachment and Human Development, 2,* 170–187.

Easterbrooks, M., Driscoll, J., & Bartlett, J. (2008). Resilience in infancy: A relational approach. *Research in Human Development, 5*(3), 139–152.

Edwards, E. P., Eiden, R. D., & Leonard, K. E. (2006). Behavior problems in 18- to 36-month-old children of alcoholic fathers: Secure mother-infant attachment as a protective factor. *Development and Psychopathology, 18,* 395–407.

Eiden, R. D., Chavez, F., & Leonard, K. E. (1999). Parent–infant interactions in alcoholic and control families. *Development and Psychopathology, 11,* 745–762.

Eiden, R. D., Edwards, E. P., & Leonard, K. E. (2002). Mother–infant and father–infant attachment among alcoholic families. *Development and Psychopathology, 14,* 253–378.

Eigsti, I. M., & Cicchetti, D. (2004). The impact of child maltreatment on expressive syntax at 60 months. *Developmental Science, 7*(1), 88–102.

Emde, R. N., Korfmacher, J., & Kubicek, L. F. (2000). Toward a theory of early relationship-based intervention. In J. D. Osofsky & H. E. Fitzgerald (Eds.), *WAIMH handbook of infant mental health. Vol. Two. Early intervention, evaluation, and assessment* (pp. 3–32). New York: Wiley.

Engle, P. L., & Black, M. M. (2008). The effect of poverty on child development and educational outcomes. *Annals of the New York Academy of Sciences, 1136,* 243–256.

Essex, M. J., Klein, M. H., Cho, E., & Kalin, N. H. (2002). Maternal stress beginning in infancy may sensitize children to later stress exposure: Effects on cortisol and behavior. *Biological Psychiatry, 52,* 776–784.

Farah, M. J., Shera, D. M., Savage, J. H., Betancourt, L., Giannetta, J. M., Brodsky, N. L., & Hurt, H. (2006). Childhood poverty: Specific associations with neuro-cognitive development. *Brain Research, 1110*(1), 166–174.

Farah, M. J., Betancourt, L., Shera, D. M., Savage, J. H., Giannetta, J. M., Brodsky, N. L., Malmud, E. K., & Hurt, H. (2008). Environmental stimulation, parental nurturance and cognitive development in humans. *Developmental Science, 11*(5), 793–801.

Finzy, R., Anca, R., Har-Even, D., Shnit, D., & Weizman, A. (2001). Attachment styles and aggression in physically abused and neglected children. *Journal of Youth and Adolescence, 30,* 769–786.

Flouri, E., Tzavidis, N., & Kallis, C. (2010). Adverse life events, area socioeconomic disadvantage, and psychopathology and resilience in young children: The importance of risk factors' accumulation and protective factors' specificity. *European Child and Adolescent Psychiatry, 19*(6), 535–546.

Garner, A. S. (2013). Home visiting and the biology of toxic stress: Opportunities to address early childhood adversity. *Pediatrics, 132*(Suppl. 2), S65–S73.

Gibbons, A. S. (2001). Model-centered instruction. *Journal of Structural Learning and Intelligent Systems, 14,* 511–540.

Grantham-McGregor, S., Cheung, Y. B., Cueto, S., Glewwe, P., Richter, L., & Strupp, B. (2007). Developmental potential in the first 5 years for children in developing countries. *Lancet, 369,* 60–70.

Grusec, J. E., & Goodnow, J. J. (1994). Impact of parental discipline methods on child's internalization of values: A reconceptualization of current points of view. *Developmental Psychology, 30,* 4–19.

Gunnar, M. R., & Donzella, B. (2002). Social regulation of the cortisol levels in early human development. *Psychoneuroendocrinology, 27,* 199–220.

Gunnar, M., & Quevedo, K. (2007). The neurobiology of stress and development. *Annual Review Psychology, 58,* 145–173.

Guralnick, M. J. (1989). Recent developments in early intervention efficacy research: Implications for family involvement in P.L. 99–457. *Topics in Early Childhood Special Education, 9*(3), 1–17.

Guralnick, M. J. (1998). Effectiveness of early intervention for vulnerable children: A developmental perspective. *American Journal on Mental Retardation, 102,* 319–345.

Haller, J., Harold, G., Sandi, C., & Neumann, I. D. (2014). Effects of adverse early-life events on aggression and anti-social behaviours in animals and humans. *Journal of Neuroendocrinology, 26*(10), 724–738.

Hart, B., & Risley, T. R. (1995). *Meaningful differences in the everyday experience of young American children.* Baltimore: Brookes.

Hart, C. H., Nelson, D. A., Robinson, C. C., Olsen, S. F., & McNeilly-Choque, M. K. (1998). Overt and relational aggression in Russian nursery-school-age children: Parenting style and marital linkages. *Developmental Psychology, 34,* 687–697.

Hay, D. F., Pawlby, S., Waters, C. S., Perra, O., & Sharp, D. (2010). Mothers' antenatal depression and their children's antisocial outcomes. *Child Development, 81*(1), 149–165.

Hebbeler, K., & Gerlach-Downie, S. (2002). Inside the black box of home visiting: A qualitative analysis of why intended outcomes were not achieved. *Early Childhood Research Quarterly, 17,* 28–51.

Heinicke, C. M., Rineman, N. R., Ponce, V. A., & Guthrie, D. (2001). Relation-based intervention with at-risk mothers: Outcome in the second year of life. *Infant Mental Health Journal, 22*(4), 431–462.

Heinicke, C. M., Goorsky, M., Levine, M., Ponce, V., Ruth, G., Silverman, M., & Sotelo, C. (2006). Pre- and postnatal antecedents of a home visiting intervention and family developmental outcome. *Infant Mental Health Journal, 27,* 91–119.

Hipwell, A. E., Goossens, F. A., Melhuish, E. C., & Kumar, R. R. (2000). Severe maternal psychopathology and infant–mother attachment. *Development and Psychopathology, 12*(2), 157–175.
Hirsh-Pasek, K., & Burchinal, M. (2006). Mother and caregiver sensitivity over time: Predicting language and academic outcomes with variable- and person-centered approaches. *Merrill-Palmer Quarterly, 52,* 449–485.
Hockenberger, E. H., Goldstein, H., & Haas, L. S. (1999). Effects of commenting during joint book reading by mothers with low SES. *Topics in Early Childhood Special Education, 19*(1), 15–27.
Howell, K. H., Graham-Bermann, S. A., Czyz, E., & Lilly, M. (2010). Assessing resilience in preschool children exposed to intimate partner violence. *Violence and Victims, 25*(2), 150–164.
Hubbs-Tait, L., Culp, A. M., Culp, R. E., & Miller, C. E. (2002). Relation of maternal cognitive stimulation, emotional support, and intrusive behavior during head start to children's kindergarten cognitive abilities. *Child Development, 73,* 110–132.
Innocenti, M. S., Roggman, L. A., & Cook, G. A. (2013). Observing parenting interactions with children with a disability. *Infant Mental Health Journal, 34,* 307–318.
Ispa, J. M., Fine, M. A., Halgunseth, L. C., Harper, S., Robinson, J., Boyce, L., Brooks-Gunn, J., & Brady-Smith, C. (2004). Maternal intrusiveness, maternal warmth, and mother-toddler relationship outcomes: Variations across low-income ethnic and acculturation groups. *Child Development, 75*(6), 1613–1631.
Jaffee, S. R., Bowes, L., Ouellet-Morin, I., Fisher, H. L., Moffitt, T. E., Merrick, M. T., & Arseneault, L. (2013). Safe, stable, nurturing relationships break the intergenerational cycle of abuse: A prospective nationally representative cohort of children in the United Kingdom. *Journal of Adolescent Health, 53*(4), S4–S10.
Johnson, S. B., Riley, A. W., Granger, D. A., & Riis, J. (2013). The science of early life toxic stress for pediatric practice and advocacy. *Pediatrics, 131*(2), 319–327.
Kagan, S. L., & Neuman, M. J. (1997). Defining and implementing school readiness: Challenges for families, early care and education, and schools. In R. P. Weissberg, T. P. Gullotta, R. L. Hampton, B. A. Ryan, & G. R. Adams (Eds.), *Healthy children 2010: Establishing preventive services* (pp. 61–96). Thousand Oaks: Sage Publications.
Kelleher, K., Chaffin, M., Hollenberg, J., & Fischer, E. (1994). Alcohol and drug disorder among physically abusive and neglectful parents in a community-based sample. *American Journal of Public Health, 84,* 1586–1590.
Kelly, J. F., Morisset, C. E., Barnard, K. E., Hammond, M. A., & Booth, C. L. (1996). The influence of early mother–child interaction on preschool cognitive/linguistic outcomes in a high-social-risk group. *Infant Mental Health Journal, 17,* 310–321.
Kiernan, K. E., & Mensah, F. (2011). Poverty, family resources and children's early educational attainment: The mediating role of parenting. *British Educational Research Journal, 37,* 317–336.
Kilmer, R. P., Cowen, E. L., & Wyman, P. A. (2001). A micro-level analysis of developmental, parenting, and family milieu variables that differentiate stress-resilient and stress-affected children. *Journal of Community Psychology, 29*(4), 391–416.
Kim-Cohen, J., Moffitt, T. E., Caspi, A., & Taylor, A. (2004). Genetic and environmental processes in young children's resilience and vulnerability to socioeconomic deprivation. *Child Development, 75,* 651–668.
Kochanska, G. (1995). Children's temperament, mothers' discipline, and security of attachment: Multiple pathways to emerging internalization. *Child Development, 66*(3), 597–615.
Korenman, S., Miller, J. E., & Sjaastad, J. E. (1995). Long-term poverty and child development in the United States: Results from the NLSY. *Children and Youth Services Review, 17*(1–2), 127–155.
Korfmacher, J., Green, B., Staerkel, F., Peterson, C., Cook, G., Roggman, L., Faldowski, R. A., & Schiffman, R. (1998). Parent involvement in early childhood home visiting. *Child and Youth Care Forum, 37*(4), 171–196.
Laasko, M., Poikkeus, A. M., Eklund, K., & Lyytinen, P. (1999). Social interactional behaviors and symbolic play competence as predictors of language development and their associations with maternal attention-directing strategies. *Infant Behavior and Development, 22,* 541–556.

Landry, S. H., Smith, K. E., Miller-Loncar, C. L., & Swank, P. R. (1997). Predicting cognitive-linguistic and social growth curves from early maternal behaviors in children at varying degrees of biologic risk. *Developmental Psychology, 33,* 1040–1053.

Landry, S. H., Smith, K. E., Swank, P. R., Assel, M. A., & Vellet, S. (2001). Does early responsive parenting have a special importance for children's development or is consistency across early childhood necessary? *Developmental Psychology, 37,* 387–403.

Lanzi, R., Terry, K., Guest, K., Cotton, J., & Ramey, C. (1999). *Home visiting with families at risk for child abuse and neglect: Review of programs, findings, best practices, and lessons learned from the field.* Birmingham: Civitan International Research Center, University of Alabama at Birmingham.

Lay, K.-L., Waters, E., & Parke, K. A. (1989). Maternal responsiveness and child compliance: The role of mood as a mediator. *Child Development, 60*(6), 1405–1411.

Lester, B. M., & Lagasse, L. L. (2010). Children of addicted women. *Journal of Addictive Diseases, 29*(2), 259–276.

Lieberman, A. F., Weston, D., & Pawl, J. H. (1991). Preventive intervention and outcome with anxiously attached dyads. *Child Development, 62,* 199–209.

Lloyd, C., King, R., & Chenoweth, L. (2002). Social work, stress and burnout: A review. *Journal of Mental Health, 11,* 255–265.

Lochman, J. E., Barry, T., Powell, N., & Young, L. (2010). Anger and aggression. *Practitioner's Guide to Empirically Based Measures of Social Skills, ABCT Clinical Assessment Series, 3,* 155–166.

Love, J. M., Kisker, E. E., Ross, C., Raikes, H., Constantine, J., Boller, K., Brooks-Gunn, J., Chazan-Cohen, R., Tarullo, L. B., Brady-Smith, C., Fuligni. A. S., Schochet, P. Z., Paulsell, D., & Vogel, C. (2005). The effectiveness of Early Head Start for 3-year-old children and their parents: Lessons for policy and programs. *Developmental Psychology, 41,* 885–901.

Lupien, S. J., King, S., Meaney, M. J., & McEwen, B. S. (2000). Child's stress hormone levels correlate with mother's socioeconomic status and depressive state. *Society of Biological Psychiatry, 48,* 976–980.

Luthar, S. S. (2006). Resilience in development: A synthesis of research across five decades. In D. Cicchetti & D. J. Cohen (Eds.), *Developmental psychopathology (2nd ed.): Vol. 3 risk, disorder, and adaptation* (pp. 739–795). Hoboken: Wiley.

Lyons-Ruth, K., Alpern, L., & Repacholi, B. (1993). Disorganized infant attachment classification and maternal psychosocial problems as predictors of hostile-aggressive behavior in the preschool classroom. *Child Development, 64,* 572–585.

Lyons-Ruth, K., Easterbrooks, M. A., & Cibelli, C. D. (1997). Infant attachment strategies, infant mental lag, and maternal depressive symptoms: Predictors of internalizing and externalizing problems at age 7. *Developmental Psychology, 33,* 681–692.

MacDonald, K. (1992). Warmth as a developmental construct: An evolutionary analysis. *Child Development, 63,* 753–773.

Mahoney, G., & Perales, F. (2005). Relationship-focused early intervention with children with pervasive developmental disorders and other disabilities: A comparative study. *Journal of Developmental & Behavioral Pediatrics, 26*(2), 77–85.

Mahoney, G., Boyce, G., Fewell, R., Spiker, D., & Wheeden, C. A. (1998). The relationship of parent–child interaction to the effectiveness of early intervention services for at-risk children and children with disabilities. *Topics in Early Childhood Special Education, 18,* 5–17.

Mardell, C. D., & Goldenberg, D. S. (2008). *Parents' observations of infants and toddlers (POINT).* New York: Pearson Assessments.

Maslach, C., Schaufeli, W. B., & Leiter, M. P. (2001). Job burnout. In S. T. Fiske, D. L. Schacter, & C. Zahn-Waxler (Eds.), *Annual Review of Psychology*, 52, 397–422.

Masten, A. S. (2001). Ordinary magic: Resilience processes in development. *American Psychologist, 56,* 227–238.

Meisels, S. J., Marsden, D. B., Dombro, A. L., Weston, E. R., & Jewkes, A. M. (2003). *The Ounce Scale: An infant/toddler observational assessment.* New York: Pearson Assessments.

Merrill, M. D. (2002). First principles of instruction. *Educational Technology Research and Development, 50*(3), 43–59.
Middlebrooks, J. S., & Audage, N. C. (2008). *The effects of childhood stress on health across the lifespan*. Atlanta: Center for Disease Control and Prevention, National Center for Injury Prevention and Control.
Moss, E., Dubois-Comtois, K., Cyr, C., Tarabulsy, G. M., St-Laurent, D., & Bernier, A. (2011). Efficacy of a home visiting intervention aimed at improving maternal sensitivity, child attachment, and behavioral outcomes for maltreated children: A randomized control trial. *Development and Psychopathology, 23*(01), 195–210.
Mustillo, S. A., Dorsey, S., Conover, K., & Burns, B. J. (2011). Parental depression and child outcomes: The mediating effects of abuse and neglect. *Journal of Marriage and Family, 73*(1), 164–180.
Nachmias, M., Gunnar, M. R., Mangelsdorf, S., Parritz, R. H., & Buss, K. (1996). Behavioral inhibition and stress reactivity: The moderating role of attachment security. *Child Development, 67,* 508–522.
Nagin, D., & Tremblay, R. E. (2001). Parental and early childhood predictors of persistent physical aggression in boys from kindergarten to high school. *Archives of General Psychiatry, 58,* 389–394.
National Institute for Child Health and Development (NICHD) Early Child Care Research Network (ECCRN). (1999). Child care and mother–child interaction in the first three years of life. *Developmental Psychology, 35,* 1399–1413.
National Institute for Child Health and Development (NICHD) Early Child Care Research Network (ECCRN). (2004). Trajectories of physical aggression from toddlerhood to middle childhood. *Monographs of the Society for Research in Child Development*, *69*(4), vii–129.
Noble, K. G., & McCandliss, B. D. (2005). Reading development and impairment: Behavioral, social, and neurobiological factors. *Journal of Developmental & Behavioral Pediatrics, 26*(5), 370–378.
O'Neal, C. R., Brotman, L., Huang, K., Gouley, K., Kamboukos, D., Calzada, E. J., & Pine, D. S. (2010). Understanding relations among early family environment, cortisol response, and child aggression via a prevention experiment. *Child Development, 81*(1), 290–305.
Olds, D., Eckenrode, J., Henderson, C. R., Kitzman, H., Powers, J., Cole, R., Sidora, K., Morris, P., Pettitt, L. M., & Luckey, D. (1997). Long-term effects of home visitation on maternal life course and child abuse and neglect: 15-year follow-up of a randomized trial. *Journal of the American Medical Association, 278,* 637–643.
Olds, D. L., Henderson, C. R. Jr., Cole, R., Eckenrode, J., Kitzman, H., & Luckey, D., et al. (1998). Long-term effects of nurse home visitation on children's criminal and antisocial behavior: 15-year follow-up of a randomized trial. *Journal of the American Medical Association, 280,* 1238–1244.
Olson, S. L., Lopez-Duran, N., Lunkenheimer, E. S., Chang, H., & Sameroff, A. J. (2011). Individual differences in the development of early peer aggression: Integrating contributions of self-regulation, theory of mind, and parenting. *Development and Psychopathology, 23*(1), 253–266.
Ooi, Y. P., Ang, R. P., Fung, D. S. S., Wong, G., & Cai, Y. (2006). The impact of parent–child attachment on aggression, social stress, and self-esteem. *School Psychology International, 27,* 552–566.
Park, S. (1999). *Hawaii Early Learning Profile (HELP): Birth-3 years*. Palo Alto: VORT.
Peterson, C. A., Roggman, L. A., Green, B., Chazan-Cohen, R., Korfmacher, J., McKelvey, L., Zhang, D., & Atwater, J. (2013). Home visiting processes: Relations with family characteristics and outcomes. *Zero To Three, 33*(3), 39–44.
Petrill, S. A., & Deater-Deckard, K. (2004). Task orientation, parental warmth, and SES account for a significant proportion of the shared environmental variance in general cogntivie ability in early childhood: Evidence from a twin study. *Developmental Science, 7*(1), 25–32.
Petterson, S. M., & Albers, A. (2001). Effects of poverty and maternal depression on early child development. *Child Development, 72*(6), 1794–1813.

Puttler, L. I., Zucker, R. A., Fitzgerald, H. E., & Bingham, C. R. (1998). Behavioral outcomes among children of alcoholics during the early and middle childhood years: Familial subtype variations. *Alcoholism: Clinical and Experimental Research, 22,* 1962–1972.

Raikes, H., Green, B. L., Atwater, J., Kisker, E., Constantine, J., & Chazan-Cohen, R. (2006). Involvement in Early Head Start home visiting services: Demographic predictors and relations to child and parent outcomes. *Early Childhood Research Quarterly, 21,* 2–24.

Repetti, R. L., Taylor, S. E., & Seeman, T. E. (2002). Risky families: Family social environments and the mental and physical health of offspring. *Psychological Bulletin, 128,* 330–366.

Roggman, L. A., & Cook, G. A. (2011). Attachment, aggression, and family risk in a low-income sample. *Family Science, 1*(3–4), 191–204.

Roggman, L. A., Boyce, L. K., Cook, G. A., & Jump, V. K. (2001). Inside home visits: A collaborative look at process and quality. *Early Childhood Research Quarterly, 16,* 53–71.

Roggman, L. A., Boyce, L. K., & Innocenti, M. S. (2008). *Developmental parenting: A guide for early childhood practitioners*. Baltimore: Brookes.

Roggman, L. A., Cook, G. A., Jump Norman, V. K., Christiansen, K., Boyce, L. K., & Innocenti, M. S. (2008). Home Visit Rating Scales (HOVRS). In L. A. Roggman, L. K. Boyce, & M. S. Innocenti (Eds.), *Developmental parenting: A guide for early childhood practitioners* (pp. 209–217). Baltimore: Paul H. Brookes Publishing.

Roggman, L. A., Cook, G. A., Boyce, L. K., & Hart, A. D. (2009). *Father involvement as a moderator of intervention impacts on mothers' parenting behavior*. Paper presented at the Society for Research in Child Development, Denver, CO.

Roggman, L. A., Boyce, L. K., & Cook, G. A. (2009). Keeping kids on track: Impacts of a parenting-focused Early Head Start program on attachment security and cognitive development. *Early Education & Development, 20*(6), 920–941.

Roggman, L. A., Cook, G. A., Jump Norman, V. K., Christiansen, K., Boyce, L. K., Innocenti, M. S., Aikens, N., Boller, K., Paulsell, D., & Hallgren, K. (2010). *Home Visit Rating Scales version A (HOVRS-A)*. Princeton: Mathematica Policy Research.

Roggman, L. A., Cook, G. A., Innocenti, M. S., Jump Norman, V. K., & Christiansen, K. (2013a). *Parenting interactions with children: Checklist of observations linked to outcomes (PICCOLO)*. Baltimore: Brookes.

Roggman, L. A., Cook, G. A., Innocenti, M. S., Jump Norman, V., & Christiansen, K. (2013b). Parenting Interactions with Children: Checklist of Observations Linked to Outcomes (PICCOLO) in diverse ethnic groups. *Infant Mental Health Journal, 34,* 290–306.

Roggman, L. A., Cook, G. A., Innocenti, M. S., Jump Norman, V. K., Christiansen, K., Boyce, L. K., Aikens, N., Boller, K., Paulsell, D., & Hallgren, K. (2014). *Home Visit Rating Scales-adapted & extended: (HOVRS-A + v2)*. Unpublished measure.

Rohner, R. P. (1986). *The warmth dimension: Foundations of parental acceptance-rejection theory. New perspectives on family*. Thousand Oaks: Sage.

Rose-Jacobs, R., Black, M., Casey, P., Cook, J., Cutts, D., Chilton, M., et al. (2008). House-hold food insecurity: Associations with at-risk infant and toddler development. *Pediatrics, 121*(1), 65–72.

Schore, A. N. (2001). Effects of a secure attachment relationship on right brain development, affect regulation, and infant mental health. *Infant Mental Health Journal, 22,* 7–66.

Séguin, J. R., Parent, S., Tremblay, R. E., & Zelazo, P. (2009). Different neurocognitive functions regulating physical aggression and hyperactivity in early childhood. *Journal of Child Psychology and Psychiatry, 50*(6), 679–687.

Shonkoff, J. P. (2010). Building a new biodevelopmental framework to guide the future of early childhood policy. *Child Development, 81*(1), 357–367.

Shonkoff, J. P., Garner, A. S., Siegel, B. S., Dobbins, M. I., Earls, M. F., McGuinn, L., & Wood, D. L., et al. (2012). The lifelong effects of early childhood adversity and toxic stress. *Pediatrics, 129*(1), e232–e246.

Slaughter-Defoe, D. T. (1993). Home visiting with families in poverty: Introducing the concept of culture. *The Future of Children, 3,* 172–183.

Smith, L. (1995). *Healthy Families California: A review of standards and best practices in home visiting programs across California*. Sacramento, CA: California Consortium to Prevent Child Abuse.

Snow, C. E., Burns, M. S., & Griffin, P. (1998). *Preventing reading difficulties in young children*. Washington, DC: National Academy Press.

Spencer, P. E., & Meadow-Orlans, K. P. (1996). Play, language, and maternal responsiveness: A longitudinal study of deaf and hearing infants. *Child Development, 67,* 3176–3191.

Squires, J., & Bricker, D. (2009). *Ages & Stages Questionnaires, third edition: A parent-completed child-monitoring system*. Baltimore: Brookes.

Strathearn, L., & Mayes, L. C. (2010). Cocaine addiction in mothers: Potential effects on maternal care and infant development. *Annals of the New York Academy of Sciences, 1187*(1), 172–183.

Suess, G. J., Grossman, K. E., & Sroufe, L. A. (1992). Effects of infant attachment to mother and father on quality of adaptation in preschool: From dyadic to individual organization of self. *International Journal of Behavioral Development, 15*(1), 43–65.

Sweet, M. A., & Appelbaum, M. L. (2004). Is home visiting an effective strategy? A meta-analytic review of home visiting programs for families with young children. *Child Development, 75*(5), 1435–1456.

Tamis-LeMonda, C. S., Bornstein, M. H., & Baumwell, L. (2001). Maternal responsiveness and children's achievement of language milestones. *Child Development, 72,* 748–767.

Tandon, S. D., Mercer, C. D., Saylor, E. L., & Duggan, A. K. (2008). Paraprofessional home visitors' perspectives on addressing poor mental health, substance abuse, and domestic violence: A qualitative study. *Early Childhood Research Quarterly, 23,* 419–428.

Taylor, S. E., Lerner, J. S., Sage, R. M., Lehman, B. J., & Seeman, T. E. (2004). Early environment, emotions, responses to stress, and health. *Journal of Personality, 72,* 1365–1394.

Taylor, C. A., Guterman, N. B., Lee, S. J., & Rathouz, P. J. (2009). Intimate partner violence, maternal stress, nativity, and risk for maternal maltreatment of young children. *American Journal of Public Health, 99*(1), 175.

Thompson, R. A. (2014). Stress and child development. *Future of Children, 24,* 41–60.

Tremblay, R. E. (2000). The development of aggressive behaviour during childhood: What have we learned in the past century? *International Journal of Behavioural Develoipment, 24,* 129–141.

Tremblay, R. E., Nagin, D. S., Séguin, J. R., Zoccolillo, M., Zelazo, P. D., Boivin, M., Japel, C., et al. (2004). Physical aggression during early childhood: Trajectories and predictors. *Pediatrics, 114*(1), e43–e50.

United Nations World Food Program. (2006). *Hunger and learning*. Rome: United Nations.

van den Boom, D. C. (1994). The influence of temperament and mothering on attachment and exploration: An experimental manipulation of sensitive responsiveness among lower-class mothers with irritable infants. *Child Development, 65,* 1457–1477.

Vanderbilt-Adriance, E., & Shaw, D. S. (2008). Protective factors and the development of resilience in the context of neighborhood disadvantage. *Journal of Abnormal Child Psychology, 36*(6), 887–901.

Victora, C., Barros, F., Lima, R. C., Behague, D. P., Goncalves, H., Horta, B. L., et al. (2003). The Pelotas birth cohort study, Rio Grande do Sul, Brazil, 1982–2001. *Cad Saude Publica Rio de Janeiro*, 1241–1256.

Vogel, C. A., Boller, K., Xue, Y., Blair, R., Aikens, N., Burwick, A., Shrago, Y., Carlton, B. L., Kalb, L., Mendenko, L., Cannon, J., Harrington, S., & Stein, J. (2011). *Learning as we go: A first snapshot of Early Head Start programs, staff, families, and children. OPRE Report #2011-7.* Washington, DC: Office of Planning, Research, and Evaluation, Administration for Children and Families, U.S. Department of Health and Human Services.

Volker, S., Keller, H., Lohaus, A., Cappenberg, M., & Chasiotis, A. (1999). Maternal interactive behaviour in early infancy and later attachment. *International Journal of Behavioral Development, 23,* 921–936.

Wagner, M. M., & Clayton, S. L. (1999). The Parents as Teachers program: Results from two demonstrations. *The Future of Children, 9,* 91–189.

Wagner, M., & Spiker, D. (2001). *Multisite Parents as Teachers evaluation: Experience and outcomes for children and families*. Menlo Park: SRI, International.
Wagner, M., Iida, E., & Spiker, D. (2001). *The multisite evaluation of the Parents as Teachers home visiting program: Three-year findings from one community*. Menlo Park: SRI International.
Wakschlag, L. S., & Hans, S. L. (1999). Relation of maternal responsiveness during infancy to the development of behavior problems in high-risk youths. *Developmental Psychology, 35*(2), 569–579.
Weatherston, D. (2007). A home-based infant mental health intervention: The centrality of relationships in reflective supervision. *Zero to Three, 28,* 23–28.
Weinfield, N. S., Sroufe, L. A., Egeland, B., & Carlson, E. (1999). The nature of individual differences in infant-caregiver attachment. In J. Cassidy & P. Shaver (Eds.), *Handbook of attachment: Theory, research, and clinical application* (pp. 68–88). New York: Guilford Press.
Whitaker, R. C., Phillips, S. M., & Orzol, S. M. (2006). Food insecurity and the risks of depression and anxiety in mothers and behavior problems in their preschool-aged children. *Pediatrics, 118,* 859–868.
Woods, J., Kashinath, S., & Goldstein, H. (2004). Effects of embedding caregiver implemented teaching strategies in daily routines on children's communication outcomes. *Journal of Early Intervention, 26,* 175–193.
Wyman, P. A., Sandier, I., Wolchik, S., & Nelson, K. (2000). Resilience as cumulative competence promotion and stress protection: Theory and intervention. In D. Cicchetti, J. Rappaport, I. Sandier, & R. P. Weissberg (Eds.), *The promotion ofwellness in children and adolescents* (pp. 133–184). Washington, DC: Child Welfare League of America Press.
Youngblade, L. M., Park, K. A., & Belsky, J. (1993). Measurement of young children's close friendship: A comparison of two independent assessment systems and their associations with attachment security. *International Journal of Behavioral Development, 16*(4), 563–587.
Zemke, R., & Zemke, S. (July, 1981). 30 things we know for sure about adult learning. *Training*, 18(6), 45–46, 48–49, 52.

Lori Roggman (USA): Professor in the Department of Family, Consumer, and Human Development at Utah State University. She studies parenting and early intervention in relation to children's early social, cognitive, and language development. Dr. Roggman's career began as a Head Start home visitor and continued as a trainer and consultant for practitioners in infant/toddler and early childhood programs. She has conducted research on early parenting and on home visiting interventions to support parenting in Early Head Start and similar programs, and she coauthored *Developmental Parenting: A Guide for Early Childhood Practitioners*. She codeveloped the Parenting Interactions with Children: Checklist of Observations Linked to Outcomes (PICCOLO) scale using 4500 observations of parenting interactions to develop a valid, reliable, and easy-to-use measure for both researchers and practitioners that gauges affection, responsiveness, encouragement, and teaching. She also codeveloped the Home Visit Rating Scales of home visiting quality. She has served in several technical advisory groups developing methods and measures to study services for families of infants, toddlers, and young children.

Chapter 5
Developing the Home Visiting Workforce

Nick Wechsler

Home visiting is a strategy used in countries throughout the world to reach children in their earliest years of development. Through supporting and promoting meaningful parent–child experiences, home visiting maximizes the developmental opportunities that begin at birth. Every domain of human growth and development—neural, emotional, social, physical, and cognitive—is part of the professional home visitor's responsibility and scope of work.

This chapter explores a developmental approach to training and supporting the professional development of early childhood education home visitors. It highlights the parallels in the shared experience of children, parents, home visitors, and home visiting trainers. Recognizing these parallels grounds and informs the training process, guiding it for the best interests of young children and families. The chapter posits a perspective of professional training and support that identifies relationships as the driving force in learning and growing together and offers guidelines and resources for training home visitors.

Nina and Abbey

It is a still morning. The neighborhood has not awakened yet. Nina, an early childhood education home visitor, walks along the sidewalk looking for the right gate. Finding it locked, she[1] rises on her toes, stretches to look over the top, and calls,

[1] Note that although female pronouns were used in this example and throughout the chapter for simplicity and clarity, both women and men are home visitors. Likewise, both mothers and fathers can be served in home visiting programs.

N. Wechsler (✉)
Ounce of Prevention Fund, Chicago, IL, USA
e-mail: nickw@ounceofprevention.org

L. Roggman, N. Cardia (eds.), *Home Visitation Programs*,
DOI 10.1007/978-3-319-17984-1_5

"Abbey…Abbey…" She waits, and then tries again, "Abbey…" A dog on the other side of the gate barks, and a neighbor moves aside a curtain and peers out. Nina waits.

On the other side of the gate, Abbey waits, too, inside her small apartment alone with her young son, Marco. Imagine Abbey's emotions as she hears Nina calling. She knows that it is time for their scheduled home visit, and she remembers how she sometimes feels uneasy at the beginning of the visit. But she also remembers that she usually feels better by the end of the home visit. Not just better, but more comfortable—with Nina, with herself, and with Marco. Abbey wonders what this week's visit will be like. Will she feel Nina's approval or disapproval? Will she know what to say? Abbey is not sure if she is prepared to let the home visitor into her apartment, into her life.

Now, imagine Nina's thoughts as she waits on the other side of the gate. Imagine her feelings. Will Abbey have forgotten about their visit? Will Abbey ignore her, or open the gate and welcome her? Is Abbey safe? Is Marco safe? Will Abbey be eager or hesitant about the visit? Nina wonders if she might have said something during her previous visit to cause Abbey to retreat. She wonders if she will reconnect and spend meaningful time with Abbey and her toddler. Nina feels growing self-doubt. She wonders if she is prepared.

Waiting for Abbey to silence the dog and open the gate gives Nina time to become self-aware, to find an inner balance that helps her feel hopeful, helpful, and able. Her mind fills with recollections from past visits. She remembers occasions when she was left shaken by obstacles that came between her and Abbey. And she remembers her concern after witnessing obstacles between mother and child. Sometimes, she left worried about her ability to make a meaningful difference for this mother and child. She thinks about visits when she left concerned for Abbey's well-being and other times when she left afraid for Marco. After some visits, she felt emotional pain from her work with Abbey and Marco, and other times she wished that she could take both of them home to her own safe, warm, and caring life.

Nina thinks, too, about the many times she left visits with Abbey and Marco feeling great. She remembers sharing wonderful moments with Abbey learning together about Marco. Some visits left her feeling close to Abbey and aware of her own feelings of accomplishment from witnessing the warm, enjoyable, and responsive relationship that grew between Abbey and her son.

Nina smiles, remembering Abbey's look of pride last week as she calmly helped Marco come back from the brink of a temper tantrum. And Nina remembers her own pride when she left that visit—proud of their work together talking about how Abbey could help herself, and her son, during moments when one or both of them became overloaded or lost control. It was exciting to see the strategies they had developed together work. Nina thinks about her role in all of this—the happy times and the sad times, the successes and the frustrations, moments that felt like failure and successful moments they celebrated.

Abbey opens the gates and greets Nina for another home visit.

The Profession of Early Childhood Education Home Visiting

Home visitors and parents who meet each other in early childhood education home visiting programs anywhere in the world share moments like Nina and Abbey do. The door opens, meaningful connections are made, and relationships are nurtured. Parents grow more comfortable, knowledgeable, and able to do what all parents want to do—what is best for their child.

Doing what is best is no simple matter, for parents or home visitors. They begin their journey on opposite sides of the door, and join each other because they believe they can make a difference together. From their relationship with their home visitor, parents internalize a growing sense of confidence and self-esteem that becomes realized in their own relationship with their child. Gradually parents acquire knowledge, build greater self-awareness, and increase their capacity to foster the emotional, social, cognitive, and physical well-being of their young child. This is the goal of early childhood education home visiting.

In a special issue of *Infant Mental Health Journal* devoted to examining early preventive intervention and home visiting, Daniel Stern refers to a body of research that studied the elements of change and the impact of home visiting. He writes:

> …does any form of therapy/education (e.g., psychodynamic therapy, cognitive or behavioral therapies, or classes for mothers) have better or as good results as does home visiting with these populations? My impression of the literature is no! …The overwhelming non specific, positive factors lie in the relationship between the visitor and the family, especially the mother…. (Stern 2006, p. 1–2)

Although there is no university degree in home visiting, many home visitors have degrees in related fields, such as early childhood education, nursing, social work, psychology, counseling, or other human services. Many have studied parenting. Many are parents themselves and have learned from their own experiences. Some learned about home visiting from having been a recipient of early childhood education home visiting themselves in years past.

Training Home Visitors

Home visitor trainers are called upon to examine and propose strategies for building an effective professional work force to partner with parents in order to create positive early childhood outcomes. Professional development for home visitors can be viewed as mirroring all development in that it has a predictable pattern, builds on experience and mastery, and is not a linear or evenly paced experience. Like all development, it is individualized and often has periods of disorganization as new skills are being mastered (Brazelton & Sparrow, 2006). Professional development helps home visitors transform learning into executing. Learning experiences evolve from melding new concepts and ideas with personal and shared reflection on work experiences and exchanges. The various relationships that contribute to this style of active learning generate a dynamic process of internalizing and transforming learning into practice—a process that builds over time.

Professional development is more than a training program or a series of classes or workshops. Home visiting professional development is embedded in intersecting relationships that are experienced in supervision, in peer environments, at conferences and workshops, and in the self-reflection that home visitors practice to better understand what they experience with parents and young children (Cambrurn, 2010; Howe, Jacobs, Vukelich, & Recchia, 2012; Chu, 2012).

Relationships are the driving force in effective professional education for home visitors, just as they are in child development and home visiting. Infants rely on consistent and repeated experiences with their caregivers, and those experiences reinforce the caregivers' availability, responsiveness, and sensitivity in support of the infants' ability to navigate the world. The same can be said for what the home visitor trainee looks for from the trainer.

We are all in a process of development. Just as how Nina is with Abbey, becomes a working model for how Abbey can be with Marco, the way that Nina's trainers were—and are—with her became a model for how she can be with Abbey and the other families she visits. The relationships that began in Nina's training eventually settled with Marco.

A Developmental Trajectory for Training

When parents enroll their children in early childhood home visiting programs, they enroll themselves as well. No matter the parents' age, raising children is a hard job. It is often confusing, sometimes frightening, and always challenging. Parenthood is filled with ambiguity and learning by trial and error. The hours are unforgiving. No matter how experienced or prepared a parent may be, the constant swing between deep emotional energy and joy, and deep emotional exhaustion and uncertainty can undo anyone. Home visitors experience that complexity, ambiguity, and emotional swing in their work with children and families.

In the first months of their career, home visitors confront many of the same challenges that new parents and very young children experience when coming face to face with their new life. How a mother feels about herself, and the way in which she understands and participates in relationships with her own parents, peers, and now her home visitor, shapes the opportunities and risks her child will experience. An early childhood education home visitor encourages a mother to recognize that she is capable, competent, and loveable—first in the eyes of others who care about her, and then in the eyes of her child. The home visitor helps her understand her importance and value to her child, and helps her recognize the genuine feeling of being in love with and loved by her child. These may be the only positive messages some mothers hear.

The range and intensity of the experiences home visitors encounter in their new professional capacity can easily undo novice professionals. They need a safe place to be heard and accepted amid the onslaught of new experiences as they begin working with families. Their professional development must begin with providing this safe place.

New home visitors—like infants and new parents—can be easily overwhelmed by new stimuli. Each visit may bring home visitors to a new neighborhood where they are outsiders. Each family presents a new system of family dynamics. Each parent brings a different history of how she was parented or established relationships with others. Often a parent's own history of relationships has been difficult (Korfmacher, Adam, Ogawa, & Egeland, 1997; Korfmacher et al., 2008).

Each child a home visitor encounters stirs her compassion. And each family constellation that surrounds a child makes her hope that risk will not become the child's destiny. While the home visitor absorbs this cacophony, she is most often alone at home with the family, and the isolation compounds the danger of emotional overload.

The ability to self-regulate and accept co-regulation is an accurate metaphor for a new home visitor's survival mechanisms. Training and support for the developing professional must help her navigate new and unknown experiences without becoming undone by them. The home visitor, too, benefits from consistent and repeated experiences with her professional development partners that help her gain skills and navigate her new professional role and world (Birman, Desimone, Porter, & Gartet, 2000; Lanigan, 2010).

A comprehensive approach to professional development requires a broad context with special emphasis on self-learning accomplished through ongoing reflective supervision and learning interactions with peers. Tables 5.1 and 5.2 are resources for designing and implementing home visitor training.

Table 5.1 Home visitor training

Home visitor training—key points to consider
Formal training of home visitors modulates learners' exposure to content and regulates their learning experiences
Training design should flow from learning to executing and rely on home visitors becoming active in cocreating their professional development
The wide scope of topics—and the interplay between content and practice—challenges and rewards trainers and home visitors alike
Training requires a substantial commitment of time and staff resources
Training should be characterized by a repeated cycle of exposure to new ideas, opportunities for practicing new strategies, and consistent reflection on new practices
Home visitor training benefits from even pacing over time
Seasoned home visitors often support, coach, and mentor newer visitors, which sharpens their own knowledge and skills as they pass them on to their colleagues

Table 5.2 Designing home visitor training

A good training design reinforces the elegant interplay of the home visitors' role: what they know, how they are, and what they do with families
Construct the training design so that it flows from learning to executing and relies on home visitors cocreating their professional development
Develop a training plan that provides what new home visitors need, when they need it
Be intentional in providing visitors with a clear orientation to their roles and practice to reduce their uncertainty and help them become grounded in their work
Choose content that meets emerging needs in the early stage of the home visitors' development
Add more complex content and training structure as the home visitor matures
Begin with child development—an ideal entry point to training
Add professional use of self and understanding the parents' developmental status and its impact on parenting concurrently with child development
Convey program, practice, and curricula information in a concrete, detailed fashion that provides home visitors with a place and way to enter their work
Give home visitors an opportunity to see, experience, and practice interactions with families through the use of video and role playing
Encourage home visitors to bring their own work experiences into the training as they become able to move beyond vignettes and role playing alone
Structure training so that a majority of seasoned home visitors' training is focused on sharing their work and exploring different responses to situations they encounter

Training to Build a Secure Base

Home visitor training must provide the visitor with experiences that lead her to trust and feel secure in her learning environments. This trust in others evolves into trusting the emergence of her professional self and becoming secure in her abilities to forge meaningful relationships with families and add value to the parents' nurturing of their children.

At this stage of her training, the home visitor needs to feel safe sharing her experiences. She should be encouraged to express frustrations and fears and to reflect on personal and professional bravery, strengths, and success. She needs a place to be heard and accepted for what she is going through and how it is affecting her. Training and support for the new home visitor can be appreciated as a "holding environment," a place where the home visitor can be emotionally held as the trainer partners with her to process, understand, and cope with all of the new experiences she is encountering (Freshwater & Robertson, 2002; Winnicot, 1975).

Much like parenting, the initial goal of the training relationship is to cocreate a secure base. New roles, new experiences, new learning, and new practices require the learner to be ready to move from the known, to the unknown, and back again. She must be willing to face her own vulnerabilities and to risk change. Because home visiting can put her emotional, professional, and even physical safety at risk, she must trust that her trainer has her best interests in mind. She must experience from the start that she will be protected in the process.

Thinking about what secure base behaviors look like between parents and children is an effective way to frame what they should look like in the training experience (Cassidy, 1999; Simmons, Gooty, Nelson, & Little, 2009). Each trainer brings a unique history and capacities to the training relationship. She is able to read, understand, and respond to a broad range of signals from the trainee such as distress, openness, self-discovery, and success. The trainer expresses over and over: "You communicate well. I understand, and I am there for you. I will help you work it out." No matter what the form of training or supervision is, the trainer must demonstrate by her words and actions that she values what the trainee brings to the training—a specific experience and point of view that broadens mutual understanding and learning.

Once that secure base has been established, the trainer and trainee are able to step outside the training process to examine what and how each has contributed to building it. Then, they can apply that same approach to what the home visitor will do with parents to bring the parents to the same kind of safe place where the parents feel invited, heard, emotionally held, and accepted. The home visitor's own training experiences are transformed into her practice with families, and the experiences that parents have with home visitors become similar to those that the home visitors have had with their trainers (Bernstein, Hans, & Percansky, 1991; Bronfenbrenner, 1979).

Families and home visitors are ready to learn and grow together after repeated experiences that are safe, secure, and mutually respectful and trusting. Each brings something of value to the learning relationship—their knowledge, experience, values, and so much more that adds depth and meaning to the work they do together. The same is true for the home visitor and the home visitor trainer. It is the trainer's responsibility to seize and expand on what the home visitor brings. This is the essence of sharing power: Each is more effective with the other.

New home visitors may find it challenging to identify and expand on what parents bring to their work together—their beliefs, experiences, and parenting practices. Supervision and training are ideal places for home visitors to explore this. Just as trainers and home visiting trainees grow to value sharing power and responsibility in the learning process, home visitors and parents benefit from the same balance in their supportive relationship.

Core Training Content: Nine Learning Strands

Because there are so many critical areas of knowledge to address, it is essential to construct home visitor training in a way that protects the home visitor from becoming overwhelmed by the training experience. A strategic training design offers home visitors with what they need first and most to be able to provide meaningful experiences for the parents and children they encounter. Areas of study expand over time as the training proceeds, and the pedagogical design also matures as the professional matures. The parallel with co-regulation is an effective guiding principle in organizing and presenting home visitor training.

The following nine core topic areas comprise key learning strands for the early childhood education home visitor:

- Child development
- Skillful use of self
- Stages of the helping relationship
- Adolescent and parent development
- Parenting in the context of family history, systems, and dynamics
- Communicating with parents
- Parental problem-solving
- Accessing and coordinating community resources
- Professional and personal self-care

Although this list may seem daunting, it is the foundation of what early childhood home visitors must know. Other chapters in this book address the work of home visitors, in particular, settings and circumstances that affect children's development and require specific training content and delivery to build professional practice. This specialized curriculum and training adds to the foundation described in this chapter.

Child Development

Training in child development can help home visitors become less judgmental in their observations and more accepting of the families they meet. It helps home visitors become attuned to valuing parents' expertise about their child and can help them become curious to learn more about children, families, and themselves and their home visiting practice. It can teach home visitors about parenting behaviors that foster secure attachment and early learning and make them more capable to help parents build secure relationships with their children.

Children rely on caring adults to be there for them in the ways that matter most. They depend on parents and caregivers to nurture their well-being. But a parent's emotional well-being influences her openness to engaging as an active partner in the home visiting experience. How the parent feels about herself in the presence of the home visitor contributes to opening or closing their partnership on behalf of the child. Knowing that the fear of negative judgment and issues of control permeate new working relationships, a home visitor does well to introduce a safe space for parent and home visitor to share their mutual interest and commitment to the child's development. Supporting and promoting a child's healthy development becomes the common ground that unites parent and home visitor. This makes child development an ideal entry point for home visitor training. The home visitor can intentionally address unspoken concerns by honoring the parent's perspective and sharing her own knowledge (Jack et al. 2005; Korfmacher et al. 2007; Wechsler 2004).

Starting training with child development works for the home visitor, too. While much of home visitor training will be highly personal and complex, child development is an emotionally safe topic for the trainee. It also builds on the trainee's existing knowledge and experiences, which allows the trainer to demonstrate a foundational principle from the start—an appreciation for what the trainee brings to the training experience. The manner in which the trainer draws out the trainee's expertise and nurtures her feeling of confidence and competence sets the tone for her ongoing training and work with families.

Child development training requires the home visitor's nonjudgmental observation of child behavior and reflective exploration of these observations in order to sharpen understanding. This understanding adds value to the home visitor's usefulness and success with parents. As training evolves to become more personal and more challenging, remembering that added value can keep the home visitor open to those later training challenges.

Developmental Screening Many home visiting programs include developmental screening, which the home visitor is trained to administer in partnership with parents. Screening accomplishes two purposes. First, it joins the parents and home visitor in observing the child's development. Second, the screening and related discussions are an opportunity to build a secure base in the home visitor's relationship with the parent.

Screening is a sensitive time for most parents, and how the home visitor facilitates the screening affects how open the parent will be with the home visitor—then and later. Professional development prepares the home visitor to protect and support parents' emotions during screening and to use the screening discussions as an opportunity to talk about the child's continuing development, which evolves into understanding the parent–child relationship.

Resilience During Change When the home visitor understands the parent's perspective and adds information to what the parent is already feeling, the parent's self-esteem and belief in herself grows, as does the secure base between the parent and home visitor (Allen, 2007; Whittaker & Cowley, 2012). This resilience is critical for protecting and encouraging parents through the disequilibrium of growth and the disorganization that comes with a child's rapidly changing development.

Children and parents are continuously challenged by the emotional upheaval of development as they move back and forth between mastery and uncertainty. These typical periods of disorganization can cause tension between parent and child, as neither is yet comfortable with what is ahead. Home visitors are uniquely positioned to help parents anticipate what to expect in their child's development, when to expect it, how it may affect them, and what they can do to support their child's growth. By teaching parents that regression usually precedes bursts of new development and competence, home visitors help parents make sense of what they are going through. Home visitors grow to use their relational understanding of child development to help calm, inform, guide, and support parents in their parenting (Brazelton & Sparrow, 2006).

Home visitors must learn to understand the developmental ebb and flow and to build relationships with parents that foster understanding of how the child and parent feel in the presence of each other.

Skillful Use of Self

Training makes the home visitor more self-aware and supports her professional use of self—how she builds working alliances with each family she encounters. Imagine the challenge of a home visitor preparing to make it work with many varied families!

Every time a home visitor knocks on a door and waits, she faces the same tests that Nina faced with Abbey. Will she be invited to enter? Will the parent grow comfortable enough in the course of the visit to share and explore her knowledge of her child and her experience of parenting? Will she partner with the home visitor to explore sensitive areas and be willing to experiment with new behaviors? Will she be motivated to practice parenting strategies that may cause her to feel uncertain or vulnerable?

Two wise clinicians who have heavily influenced the training and practice of early childhood specialists framed a foundation for working with parents. Jeree Pawl maintains, "How you are is as important as what you do" (Pawl & St. John, 1998). Sally Provence gives a bit more directive guidance: "Don't just do something. Stand there and pay attention. Your child is trying to tell you something" (Slade, 2008, p. 225). The cartoonist Nancy Drew illustrates this theory in a single -panel cartoon. She writes, "Every woman and child in the neighborhood came to mama for advice. The funny thing was that her best advice was really none at all. She simply listened."

Listening may well be the pinnacle of professional use of self. But how do trainers impart this skill? They do it best by listening themselves as trainers. But listening is not simple. What informs one's listening and the manner in which one listens give meaning to what one hears.

Trainers begin in the beginning, as do home visitors with parents, by seeking to learn about the experiences, knowledge, attitudes, feelings, and strengths that new home visitors bring to their work. They explore by learning about the home visitors' strengths, inquiring how they came to be, and considering how those strengths and that history affect the home visitors' work with families. The key for home visitors and trainers, as for home visitors and parents, is expanding communication and understanding. Open-ended questions encourage the other to describe, wonder, and discover. Each engages the other in an ever-deepening self-awareness through repeated reciprocal exchanges. This is a methodology that home visitors can be encouraged to practice with families, and then to share their experiences in a reflective environment supported by trainers, supervisors, and peers.

Asking open-ended questions is a receptive posture, a way of listening that draws on one's voice, touch, eyes, mind, and body. Words do not convey everything, especially in the beginning of a relationship when both partners are figuring out the other. Being open to observe, to sense, and to receive the full communication—far beyond words—is much more enlightening (Cardone, Gilkerson, & Wechsler, 2008).

Home visitors learn through practice and experience to employ specific techniques using a receptive posture with parents. How home visitors mirror and frame what they hear can bring deeper meaning for the parents and emphasize the importance of what the parents are expressing. When parents or home visitors are uncertain, clarifying and asking to learn more help parents express what they wish to communicate. These are all teachable techniques that bring meaning to what home visitors hear. Home visitors learn to use this receptive posture with parents by inviting, encouraging, elaborating, discussing, and guiding the discussion. Listening in this manner is not a passive interaction. The home visitor must practice being highly attuned, taking in all of the spoken and nonverbal communication, making connections between expressions and meaning, and guiding the discussion to accomplish the goals and focus of the work. Even as the home visitor learns and practices the receptive posture, parents must be able to experience her as fully present and entirely focused on them (Cardone, Gilkerson, & Wechsler, 2008).

Training helps home visitors sharpen their receptive posture, bring greater clarity to their observations, and better interpret the multiple messages they receive. Training also allows home visitors to practice conversing with families beyond the surface—to understand more without making parents feel self-conscious or retreat. Instead, parents feel drawn into the opportunity for self-expression and shared discovery. It takes courage for a home visitor to invite others to speak the unspeakable—negative or frightening thoughts a parent views as unacceptable and fears that, if voiced, might cause a negative reaction from the home visitor, such as "my baby hates me" or "sometimes I can't stand my child." Entering gently into a conversation that helps a parent put her feelings into words requires the kind of readiness that grows from training. Training becomes a safe place for the home visitor to practice hearing a parent's unedited feelings while maintaining her own emotional equilibrium. Home visitors learn to receive and hold what parents share, maintaining a safe space for parents to share both the delights and demons that occupy their mind.

Because home visitors work alone, training is a safe place to experience being held in someone's mind. Even when they are away from the training situation, home visitors gain self-confidence by drawing on their awareness that someone knows what they are experiencing, someone believes they can do this work, and someone is holding the hard moments with them. Training eventually becomes a place where home visitors, too, can develop self-awareness to practice holding someone else—a parent and child—in their mind (Pawl, 1995).

Stages of the Helping Relationship

Home visitors benefit from a framework to guide their ongoing work with parents, and their working relationship with parents becomes the primary tool of their trade. Exposure to Bernstein's (2002–2003) five stages of the helping relationship in home visiting early in their training reinforces that framework. While a receptive posture provides the new home visitor with a way of being, the stages of a helping relationship guide the home visitor in a process of doing.

As home visitors transform their training into practice, those stages structure a working process that helps them join with families and reflect on the shared power between parents and home visitors. Experimenting with each stage of the helping relationship in the context of their work provides repeated opportunities to discover what makes help helpful.

Stages 1 and 2: Orientation and Acceptance Home visitors and parents have common thoughts at the onset of their relationship. What will it be like to work together? Will they want to continue? What a parent reads or hears about a home visiting program pales in comparison to how she feels about herself in the presence of the home visitor.

Sharing power requires letting go of deficit-based views of parents and families. Home visitors whose education, training, program experience, personal values, or professional insecurity incline them to deficit perspectives may find this difficult. There is a false sense of safety in the unbalanced relational approach. Home visitors bring to their relationships with families a history of how they experience comfort in their role and how they express knowledge and program authority. These inform their manner of organizing and controlling the working relationship and may act to deny them the opportunity to engage and build on the parents' investment in their children. Training, supervision, and peer support help home visitors understand that they and parents contribute equally to the success of their work together.

Orientation is reciprocal. Home visitors explicitly and clearly explain program goals, describe what parents and children will experience as part of the program design, explain the home visitor's role, and share expectations for parent and child participation. Program policies, including confidentiality, reporting suspected abuse and neglect, and parental behaviors and conditions that might exclude them from program participation, must also be shared in orientation. The home visitor also uses orientation as a time to intentionally draw the parent into orienting the home visitor to her child, her extended family, her support network, and her hopes, dreams, and desires for herself and her child.

Orientation is also a time for the home visitor to reflect on her experience of being in the presence of the parent and the extent to which the parent is comfortable in the new relationship. Thinking about what it is like for that parent to work with her begins their work together. As the home visitor is trained in the orientation process, she develops professional patience and pacing. The home visitor comes to appreciate that orientation continues and, often, repeats itself over several visits. Training teaches the home visitor how to use this stage to begin building openness and trust, and to listen more than tell.

Acceptance—the second stage—typically coincides with the exchanges that begin in orientation and continue as the home visitor gets to know the parent over time. Training supports this acceptance by helping the home visitor genuinely accept the stories, values, beliefs, and practices she hears about from a particular family. Training helps the home visitor recognize that accepting is different from agreeing with what she hears.

Home visitors who have felt accepted in their own disclosure of self in the course of training more easily accept values and practices different from their own, even behaviors and parenting practices that they are uncomfortable with or know are not optimal. Acceptance allows parents and home visitors to work toward change together.

In some instances, consciously or unconsciously, parents may test home visitors by trying to shock or challenge them, by shutting down, or simply by missing appointments. Training teaches home visitors to depersonalize these events and appreciate the parents' need to test the new relationship or protect themselves. Training also offers strategies on how best to respond to these tests and turn them into opportunities for visitors to demonstrate, by their actions, that they care about the parents and respect them for who and how they are.

Stage 3: Shared Understanding Home visitors' intentional use of self contributes to parents experiencing home visitors as curious and invested in learning from them at the same time that home visitors are supporting them and helping them understand child development. Home visitors employ specific skills to expand parents' understanding. They guide the discussion with their own observations and prompts based on their knowledge of child development and parent–child interactions. Home visitor training for this stage of the helping relationship elevates those discussions to professional exchanges aimed at strengthening the development of the child.

Training is a place for home visitors to experience guided self-discovery and to share and examine their own practice. Just as parents benefit from self-discoveries, so do professional home visitors. The trainer guides home visitors' self-reflection, understanding, and experimentation with this stage of the helping relationship.

Stage 4: Agreement The home visitor and parent must agree on the focus of their work together, and the agreement stage defines the goals and a plan of action for that work. The action plan addresses roles, strategies for reaching goals, measures to determine if goals have been met, and a timeframe for accomplishment.

Training helps home visitors learn and practice a delicate balance—guiding, supporting, and sharing ideas, information, and resources with parents in a way that both inform and respect parents' own goals. Cocreating plans with home visitors leads to parents feel successful and experience themselves as competent and effective on behalf of their child—a life lesson that can propel planning and decision -making success in the future. Training once again becomes a place for home visitors to appreciate the benefit of shared power with parents.

Stage 5: Review and Recommitment This stage creates a space for parents to pause and evaluate how home visiting is working from their perspective. It is an opportunity for them to celebrate success and to redirect their agreement with the home visitor if necessary. The review may lead to a recommitment to continue, to establish new goals, or even to terminate the working relationship. Parents need to know that they are in charge of their own choices and decisions. Parents hold responsibility for the work when they know that their home visitor welcomes periodic self- and co-evaluation. Training prepares the home visitor for facilitating the review and for accepting and responding positively to what parents say.

The professional helping relationship in home visiting is developmental. It builds on experience and becomes deeper, more complex, and more mature over time. Similarly, learning, practicing, and becoming more masterful with these five stages of the helping relationship develops in the home visitor over time (Bernstein, 2002–2003; Bernstein, Percansky, & Wechsler, 1996).

Adolescent and Parental Development

Children depend on their parents to understand, nurture, and protect them and to motivate them to explore and grow. What parents bring to their child's experiences matters and directly affects the child's development.

Home visitors who work with teenage parents quickly realize that there are two developmental processes underway—the parent's and the child's. Both are in the midst of a growth spurt marked by rapid change: neural, emotional, physical, cognitive, and social. Both need a tremendous amount of patience, understanding, and support. Because home visitors also are experiencing a period of rapid change and growth as they develop their professional abilities, they, too, have similar needs for support.

Home visitor training can do much to counter negative assumptions about adolescent parents. Teenagers have great strengths and many attributes that make them just what their child needs. The structure of an adolescent's brain is in transition. While some executive functions are not fully developed in adolescence, there appears to be a greater ability to learn new things during this period. Teenagers are open and able to learn about parenting. They may be energetic, active, fun loving, and creative—all useful qualities for a parent. They also are often passionate in their devotion to the ones they love, which is the thing children need most from their parents (Dahl, 2004).

Home visitors who work with teenagers need accurate information about all aspects of adolescent development, and trainees need to learn to identify the full range of developmental traits they witness in the teenagers they visit. Working with teenagers is often challenging, and home visitors may be confused by the contradictions that teenagers express when connecting with adults, especially adults on whom they depend. Teenagers can easily push home visitors' buttons, but knowledge, perspective, and the ability to depersonalize the affront can reduce the reactive pain (Blakemore and Choudhury 2006).

Training provides home visitors with a broad view of typical adolescent growth and development that helps them understand and appreciate the behaviors they observe and come to terms with their interactions with teenage parents. The better the home visitor understands the young parent, the more opportunity she has to connect and become useful in their working relationship.

All parents—no matter their age—learn as they go. All parents are affected by personal and social relationships and bring varied emotional histories and styles to their parenting role. Home visitors may find themselves reacting negatively to parents of any age as they look for ways to match and connect. When home visitors are able to take a professional perspective and step aside from their own reactions, they can develop greater empathy and a clearer understanding of what defines, guides, and motivates parents.

Parenting in the Context of Family History, Systems, and Dynamics

Home visitors, by the very nature of their work, find themselves in the midst of other people's lives. Children grow and become a reflection of their parents and other family members. Relationships and experiences shape them. Children carry the dreams of those who care for and about them. They personify the results of that caring, bearing witness to the past while entering into a world of new experiences, relationships, and possibilities that combine with their uniqueness.

Raising children is a profound experience—the passing of family values, beliefs, customs, and practices from generation to generation. Every parent has been parented. A parent's sense of self has been marked by her past, and it influences the next generation and how she will function as a parent. Developmental Psychologist Mary Main found that how a mother experienced her relationship with her own parents affects her relationship with her child. A mother has a high probability—greater than 70 %—of experiencing the same degree of secure attachment with her child that she experienced with her own mother (Main & Goldwyn, 1985; Siegel & Hartzell, 2003).

Main's research also showed that when parents encounter positive and empowering relationships, they are able to experience what she calls "earned attachment." This suggests that benefits parents may have missed in their relationship with their own parents can now be experienced with their home visitor. Parents then can draw on these positive experiences with the home visitor to create more secure relationships with their child (Siegel & Hartzell, 2003).

Fathers and Maternal Elders Two family members in particular are critical to the home visitor's success—the baby's father and the maternal elder, most often the mother's mother. The child will be affected both by the relationship that the father and grandmother have with the mother and by the relationship that each of them has with the home visitor. These relationships also will affect the home visitor's ability to contribute to the child's healthy growth and development.

In most instances, a father has a right to be part of his child's life. Both child and father benefit when they are involved with each other. When the father does not live at home, the home visitor needs strategies to discover from the mother how she wants the father to be involved. Training provides the home visitor with opportunities to learn about fathers' rights and unique contributions and how to understand and navigate the mother's relationship with the father as either a bridge or a barrier to the child's development and to her own life.

The maternal head of the family is often a gatekeeper who can help or hinder the home visitor, especially when the mother is a teen. Grandmothers understandably may have concerns about having an outsider, the home visitor, be so active in what is traditionally the grandmother's role—preparing and supporting her daughter for motherhood.

Home visitors benefit from examining their feelings toward these influential family members. In order for their work to build on a family's history, dynamics, and shared interests, home visitors must consider what it means to fathers and grandmothers to have a home visitor enter into the family constellation and how the home visitor is experienced by these influential others.

Training Opportunities Training supports this reflection and understanding by providing opportunities for home visitors to consider where they fit into the families they meet, how others experience them, how to come to terms with their place in the family dynamics, and how to use these relationships in the best interest of the child. Training also supports home visitors as they practice fitting into and supporting the family system. This is an example of how training becomes personal when the home visitors' emotions surface as they understand themselves in the context of their work.

The difficulties and complexities of families' lives can blur home visitors' strength-based vision. When this happens, home visitors find it helpful to share those experiences with colleagues who can support their efforts and empathize with their feelings and struggles. Trainers, supervisors, and peers are the ideal people for home visitors to turn to in times like this. Understanding a strength-based approach as a strategy for entering into deeper self-discovery, rather than an end unto itself, prepares home visitors to explore concerns they may be keeping at a safe distance.

Communicating with Parents

Communication involves receptive and expressive interactions, including nonverbal and verbal exchanges. The parent and the home visitor are each receiving and sending messages. The home visitor communicates most effectively when she is both self-aware and fully attuned to the parent. Home visitor training incites curiosity, provides content to consider, and protects the process of self-discovery.

Training also should provide ample opportunity for home visitors to consider the temperamental styles of young children and adults. Parents and home visitors bring their basic style into the relationship, just as happens in parent–child relationships. Home visitors know what it is like to meet with a parent who is slow to warm, quiet, unforthcoming, or reluctant to try new ideas. Such interactions can leave the home visitor feeling as if she is working harder than the parent or not making an impact. Home visitors also know what it is like to work with a parent whose thoughts, speech, and actions are always on the move and who are hard to keep focused on one idea at a time. A home visitor may leave a visit like this questioning whether she is making an impact and feeling confused and exhausted.

When a home visitor finds a parent's style uncomfortable, it is the home visitor's professional role to adapt to the parent's style. The security a home visitor feels in training and during supervision allows her to examine her part in difficulties she experiences with a parent. At the same time, training and supervision bolster her self-confidence by helping her recognize the positive contributions she is making. Training helps home visitors better appreciate interpersonal challenges and develop strategies to transform them into opportunities.

Home visitors also benefit from knowledge about how individuals learn. There are well-developed theories of adult learning styles (Pitts, 2009) that are valuable tools in the home visitor's repertoire, but training must go beyond simply identifying styles. It must help the home visitor recognize her comfort zone and preferred teaching style while also encouraging her to practice less familiar and comfortable styles. Imagine the challenge both parties would face if a home visitor relies on the printed word with parents who do not learn well by reading. Consider their mutual frustration if a home visitor encourages parents to learn by doing, but the parents learn best in another way. To be successful with families, the home visitor must be willing and able to match how she is with the parents' learning styles.

Training, reflective supervision, and ongoing peer support become more critical as the home visitor realizes that her success connecting with parents depends largely on her ability to adapt. They give her the courage to stretch how she communicates, learn more about herself, and experiment with the unknown. This means that as a home visitor develops she must become comfortable being many different ways in order to connect with many different parents. As she becomes more experienced, the home visitor develops professional dexterity in a broad range of communication, temperament, and teaching styles.

Parental Problem-Solving

Negotiating and solving problems are a big part of a parent's job. A parent must make decisions that are good for both parent and child. These decisions begin in pregnancy and continue throughout life. Some are minor, and some are important. Learning how to manage all of the planning and decisions of parenting is hard, and home visitors can help to do so.

Parents respond to their child's needs in a passionate manner. How parents regulate their emotions is critical for their success in facing and resolving conflict and in making decisions. Home visitors help parents see the impact of their interactions and develop a long view of planning for success. They provide parents with understanding, support, a different perspective, and guidance on how to make the most of difficult situations.

Working with parents on conflict resolution requires the same attention and sensitivity called for in building the working relationship. The trust that the home visitor and parent developed while connecting and learning about each other and the child contributes to the ongoing comfort and openness between home visitor and parent. Parents grow to trust that home visitors can help with other difficulties in parenting and in relationships with others. The work then focuses on helping parents master the relationships that create inner strength and lead to better social support.

Home visitor training includes opportunities for home visitors to develop an understanding of how parents face conflict, negotiate differences, and make decisions and plans. It introduces effective strategies and activities for partnering with parents to address concerns and solve problems. Home visitors also learn to use tools and methods, such as problem-solving methodologies, that can be adapted to their work with families (Schmidt, van der Molen, te Winkl, & Wijnen, 2009). Most of these methodologies depend on the kind of sequenced interactions that home visitors are already having with parents and come with specific training to build additional skills.

It is essential that parents feel a growing sense of success while they are learning and enhancing their problem-solving skills. This motivates parents to believe in themselves and to continue to grow and change. Training teaches the home visitor to protect and guide the parent in this process to increase the likelihood of success.

Accessing and Coordinating Community Resources

Families often need assistance that is outside a program's scope or that home visitors are not trained or prepared to provide. As home visitors mature in their role, they become more comfortable with the limitations and boundaries of their practice, but it is common for new home visitors to wish they could respond to all of a family's needs. The safe and reflective environment of training is an ideal place for home visitors to come to terms with their limitations and learn how to stay within their roles. Failure to honor those limitations can lead to professional burnout.

No one can do this work alone. Home visitors must be able to find resources in other community settings and in colleagues outside of their own work environment. Training helps visitors examine their motives, recognize that knowing their limits is a personal strength, and learn to identify others who are more skilled at addressing specific situations beyond the home visiting role. In much the same manner that home visitors build independence, resourcefulness, and self-sufficiency within parents, professional development builds independence, resourcefulness, and self-sufficiency within home visitors.

A critical part of this professional self-sufficiency is learning how to build and nurture networks and collaborations to support their work with families. But knowing where to refer parents for other services is only useful when the home visitor also knows how to actually connect families to them—to be the bridge that supports parents in reaching out and accepting other services. Training must prepare home visitors to do both. Home visitors with these skills help parents feel competent and successful in building broader bases of support. The initial secure base that parents have developed with their home visitor is a foundation for reaching out to additional supportive relationships and services. Parents and their children will depend on success in this area throughout their lives. The intimacy of the home visiting relationship is an ideal place to begin.

Professional and Personal Self-Care

Home visitors carry the lives of others around with them. Home visiting reaches into the home visitor's emotions, touching them in inspiring and traumatizing ways. Thinking about and caring for others takes a toll. The personal cost of caring is the single greatest risk of the profession, and training and supervision must prepare the home visitor to navigate that risk from the beginning of her training to the end of her career. Home visitors need special attention devoted to their physical, emotional, and professional well-being.

Early in their careers, home visitors also need to explore their own comfort with coming into neighborhoods and visiting homes that are not their own. Danger is real for them. In addition to opportunities that support self-awareness and self-expression, home visitors need safety skills training in topics, such as traveling safely, assessing danger in home settings, deescalating conflict and other dangerous situations, and using basic self-defense strategies. Most importantly, home visitors must know that their trainers and supervisors put their physical well-being first so that they are more able to care for others.

Emotional safety is also a key factor. Home visitors take their work to heart, and it is often painful. Their training and supervision should be a safe place to own and share the pain. The first step in training is support for the home visitor in accepting and voicing her vulnerabilities, fears, and disappointments. If the home visitor is to share all of herself, the training environment must foster safety. Feeling understood and protected in training, supervision, and among peers helps her face and express her concerns. This is a delicate process, underpinned by respect for each trainee's pace for self-disclosure. Hearing, holding, and confronting insecurities become the norm when the process begins during training and continues as a regular aspect of learning and growing in the professional role throughout supervision and staff development.

Navigating others' pain is an occupational hazard of home visiting. The intimacy of their experiences with families can contribute to vicarious or secondary trauma (Figley, 1995) for home visitors. If not addressed, these feelings compromise the home visitor's ability to partner with parents. To address her own or the parents' pain, she may find herself trying to resolve issues that are beyond her ability or scope. Or, she may shut down and protect herself from feeling what the parents feel because it is too painful. Professional development prepares home visitors for these common experiences and begins the process of protecting them from emotional injury.

Caring for the professional self requires that the training experience grows alongside the home visitor's experiences. To the extent that training is responsive—in both the content and process—and changes as needs change, the home visitor knows that she will be understood and supported throughout her professional journey.

The Power of Training

This chapter explored consistent themes for training and supporting the home visitor, who in turn supports the parent–child relationship. Home visitor trainees benefit from an environment in which they are secure and willing to explore their strengths and their insecurities, biases, and blind spots. Home visitors seek concrete information that helps them understand experiences that are new and complex. They seek partnerships with trainers, supervisors, and peers that are supportive and empowering. They thrive on training relationships that give them the courage to venture into new practices and new ways of being with families. And they learn from ongoing reflection on new feelings, new knowledge, new skills, and new experiences.

Think back to the story of Nina's visit to Abbey and Marco at the beginning of this chapter. Nina's work comes with equal parts confusion and certainty, opportunity and challenge, despair and hope. Home visitors work alone, but they rely on partners to help them believe in their own power and potential. Their work makes lives better. It can even save lives. Their faith in what they know and how they are with parents and children brings them to the door believing in themselves and the success to come. When they knock on the door, they have the power of that knock. When the door is opened and the parent welcomes them, they step into the home bringing with them all that they have experienced in the course of training. They have the power of training as their co-visitor. They are not alone.

Acknowledgments The author thanks the hundreds of home visitors and many trainers he has learned from over the years. Special appreciation to Mary J. McGonigel, Sarah Mudd, Nancy Sinclair, and Kelly Woodlock.

References

Allen, S. F. (2007). Parents' perceptions of intervention practices in home visiting programs. *Infants & Young Children, 20*(3), 266–281.

Bernstein, V. (2002–2003). Strengthening families through strengthening relationships: Supporting the parent-child relationship through home visiting. *Newsletter of Infant Mental Health Promotion Project* (IMP), *35*, 1–5.

Bernstein, V. J., Hans, S. L., & Percansky, C. (1991). Advocating for the young child in need through strengthening the parent-child relationship. *Journal of Clinical Child Psychology, 20*, 28–41.

Bernstein, V., Percansky, C., & Wechsler, N. (1996). *Strengthening families through strengthening relationships: The ounce of prevention fund developmental training and support program*. Mahwah: Lawrence Erlbaum.

Birman, B. F., Desimone, L., Porter, A. C., & Gartet, M. S. (2000). Designing professional development that works. *Educational Leadership, 57*(8), 28–33.

Blakemore, S. J., & Choudhury, S. (2006). Development of the adolescent brain: Implications for executive function and social cognition. *Journal of Child Psychology and Psychiatry, 47*(3), 296–312.

Brazelton, T. B., & Sparrow, J. D. (2006). *Touchpoints birth to three: Your child's emotional and behavioral development* (2nd ed.). Boston: Da Capo Press.

Bronfenbrenner, U. (1979). Toward an experimental ecology of human development. *American Psychologist, 32*, 513–531.

Cambrurn, E. M. (2010). Embedded teacher learning opportunities as a site for reflective practice: An exploratory study. *American Journal of Education, 116*, 463–489.

Cardone, I., Gilkerson, L., & Wechsler, N. (2008). *Teenagers and their babies: A perinatal home visitor's guide*. Washington, DC: ZERO TO THREE.

Cassidy, J. (1999). The nature of the child's ties. In J. Cassidy & P. Shaver (Eds.), *Handbook of attachment: Theory, research, and clinical applications* (pp. 3–20). New York: Guilford Press.

Chu, M. (2012). Observe, reflect, and apply: Ways to successfully mentor early childhood educators. *Dimensions of Early Childhood, 40*(3), 20–28.

Dahl, R. E. (2004). *Adolescent brain development: A period of vulnerabilities and opportunities*. New York: New York Academy of Science.

Figley, C. R. (1995). Compassion fatigue: Toward a new understanding of the costs of caring. In B. H. Stamm (Ed.), *Secondary traumatic stress* (pp. 3–28). Brooklandville: Sidran Press.

Freshwater, D., & Roberston, C. (2002). *Emotions and needs*. Buckingham: Buckingham Press.

Howe, N., Jacobs, E., Vukelich, G., & Recchia, H. (2012). In-service professional development and constructivist curriculum: Effects on quality of child care, teacher beliefs, and interactions. *Alberta Journal of Educational Research, 57*(4), 353–378.

Jack, S. M., DiCento, A., & Lohfeld, L. (2005). A theory of maternal engagement with public health nurses and family visitors. *Journal of Advanced Nursing, 49*(2), 182–190.

Korfmacher, J., Adam, E., Ogawa, J., & Egeland, B. (1997). Adult attachment: Implications for the therapeutic process in a home visitation intervention. *Applied Developmental Science, 1*(1), 43–52.

Korfmacher, J., Green, B., Spellman, M., & Thornburg, K. R. (2007). The helping relationship and program participation in early childhood home visiting. *Infant Mental health Journal, 28*(5), 459–480.

Korfmacher, J., Green, B., Staerkel, F., Peterson, C., Cook, G., Roggman, L., Faldowski, R.A., & Schiffman, R. (2008). Parent involvement in early childhood home visiting. *Child & Youth Care Forum, 37*, 171–196.

Lanigan, J. D. (2010). Family child care providers' perspectives regarding effective professional development and their role in the child care system: A qualitative study. *Early Childhood Education Journal, 38*, 399–409.

Main, M., & Goldwyn, R. (1985). *Adult attachment classification system*. Unpublished manuscript. Berkeley: University of California.

Pawl, J. (1995). *The therapeutic relationship as human connectedness: Being held in another's mind* (Vol. 15, issue 94, pp. 2–5). Washington, DC: ZERO TO THREE.

Pawl, J., & St. John, M. (1998). *How you are is as important as what you do*. Washington, DC: ZERO TO THREE.

Pitts, J. (2009). Identifying and using a teacher-friendly learning-styles instrument. *The Clearing House, 82*(5), 225–231.

Schmidt, H. G., van der Molen, H. T., te Winkel, W. W. R., & Wijnen, W. H. F. W. (2009). Constructivist, problem-based learning does work: A meta-analysis of curricular comparisons involving a single medical school. *Educational Psychologist, 44*(4), 227–249.

Siegel, D. J., & Hartzell, M. (2003). *Parenting from the inside out*. New York: Tarcher/Putnam.

Simmons, B. L., Gooty, J., Nelson, D. L., & Little, L. L. (2009). Secure attachment: Implications for hope, trust, burnout, and performance. *Journal of Organizational Behavior, 30*, 233–247.

Slade, A. (2008). Working with parents in child psychotherapy: Engaging the reflective function. In F. Busch (Ed.), *Mentalization: Theoretical considerations, research findings, and clinical implications* (pp. 207–234). New York: Analytic Press.

Stern, D. (2006). Introduction to the special issue on early preventitive intervention and home visiting. *Infant Mental Health Journal, 27*(1), 1–4.

Wechsler, N. (2004). Turning a "me" thing into a "we" thing: Early Head Start and teen parents. In J. Lombardi & M. M. Bogle (Eds.), *Beacon of hope: The promise of Early Head Start for America's youngest children* (pp. 108–126). Washington, DC: ZERO TO THREE.

Whittaker, K. W., & Cowley, S. (2012). A survey of parental self-efficacy experiences: Maximizing potential through health visiting and universal parenting support. *Journal of Clinical Nursing, 21*, 3276–3286.

Winnicott, D. W. (1975). The concept of a healthy individual. In C. Winnicott, R. Shepherd, & M. Davis (Eds.), *D. W. Winnicott: Home is where we start from: Essays by a psychoanalyst* (pp. 21–39). New York: Penguin.

Nick Wechsler (USA): Infant specialist and the director for program development for the Ounce of Prevention Fund in Illinois, USA. For the Ounce he has developed, trained, and supported numerous program strategies and services to promote secure parent–child relationships in both home and center-based programs. These activities include video intervention, doula services, the community-based family-administered neonatal activities (C-B FANA, a perinatal guide for home visitors), infant mental health services and consultation, reflective supervision, and Dr. T. Berry Brazelton's *Touchpoints*.

Chapter 6
Supporting the Paraprofessional Home Visitor

Jon Korfmacher

As home visiting programs for families of young children expand in the USA and around the world, increased attention is being placed on what might be considered the most important element of the home visiting program: the home visitor. This is not to say that other aspects of the program are optional. There are many elements that must go right for a home visiting program to be of high quality and make a meaningful difference for the families who participate in it. The curriculum or program content must be relevant and the information accurate. The program must have appropriate administration and management. Care must be taken so that expectations for the amount of home visiting are reasonable and sufficient. And families must be carefully recruited, so that services are targeted appropriately to those who need them the most.

But the home visitor is at the center of all of this. They are the "face" of a home visitation program to the families who participate. Home visitors deliver the program content and information, make sure they are visiting the families enough (but not overwhelming them), provide referrals and resources to other services, and collect the data that programs need to ascertain whether or not they are showing fidelity to the program model. Most importantly, the home visitor is the one who is there for the family, who shows up and says that she wants to help, and lets the family know it is deserving of help and support.[1] Home visiting programs cannot exist without the home visitor.

[1] In most cases I refer to the home visitor as female for convenience, but this does not have to be the case. There are male home visitors, but in my experience they are rare. I also sometimes refer to the parent as the mother, since most often the parent participating in a home visiting programs is the mother. Again, this does not have to be so. Fathers do participate in home visiting, and programs should make efforts to recruit fathers in greater numbers, a topic that deserves greater attention than can be provided here (see, for example, Raikes & Bellotti, 2006).

J. Korfmacher (✉)
Erikson Institute, Chicago, IL, USA
e-mail: jkorfmacher@erikson.edu

L. Roggman, N. Cardia (eds.), *Home Visitation Programs*,
DOI 10.1007/978-3-319-17984-1_6

For this reason, we should know as much about the home visitor as possible, so that we can find ways to support this provider as she goes about the difficult task of supporting and possibly even transforming the life of a family with a young child. A central question that emerges from this is: Who should be a home visitor? What background is necessary for home visitors to do this work, and how does this background influence the work they do?

The Paraprofessional as Home Visitor

In the USA, there has been considerable debate about the professional identity of the home visitor (see Hans & Korfmacher, 2002, for review). As noted by Halpern (1999), home visiting emerged, in part, from the grassroots family-support movement, which promoted using relatively untrained or "lay" workers from the community to visit families as a form of both community empowerment and a way to engender trust in the family with the social services being provided (see below). As paraprofessional home visiting became a more common element of early childhood services, it brushed up against other service systems that used professionals as visitors, such as nurses and social workers. A question became how well could paraprofessionals "do" the job that others, who had received advanced schooling and training, were (at least in rough approximation) also doing?

This is a gross simplification of the issue (although US human service policies have been based on grosser simplifications), partly because I have not yet defined what I mean by professional and paraprofessional. To start with, what makes a professional? There are four main features of helpers that let us consider them to be professional:

1. They have a higher educational background, such as a degree from a college or university.
2. With that degree usually comes some specific training in their field, although it is rare for someone to be taught in their formal schooling about how to be a home visitor, at least in the USA.
3. The professionals have a history of experience in their field that is closely monitored and supervised.
4. The professionals, because of all of the above, typically have some kind of license, certification, or formal recognition of their qualifications.

The paraprofessional, in contrast, lacks some or all of these qualifications. Paraprofessionals are essentially defined by what they are not, although there are qualities that paraprofessionals often have that professionals themselves are not expected to have, such as a similar background to the clientele. The line between professional and paraprofessional is not always clear, and it is important to acknowledge this. A program using community-based doulas is an illustration of this.

Doulas are women who help other women with the birth of their child, not as medical professionals, but as helpers who are concerned about the mother's physical comfort and emotional experience of the birth (Klaus, Kennell, & Klaus, 2002). Their primary job is helping during labor and delivery, but they also often work with mothers before birth to help them plan what they want their birth to be. They may also work with mothers after birth to help with the transition of being a new parent (see also Abramson, Breedlove, & Isaacs, 2007).

The doulas in this program came mostly from the same community of the poor young moms with whom they worked. Most did not have college degrees or previous experience doing this sort of work. So they were very much paraprofessionals. But, on the other hand, they received very intensive, specialized, hands-on training in being a doula—the equivalent of a month of full-time training. Over the course of the research trial they were involved in, they also sought out additional trainings as much as possible, some of which led to certification in breastfeeding counseling and family life education. They were also employed by a university hospital and were even given white coats to wear like other medical staff.

So, are they professionals, or not? The doulas would see themselves as professionals, certainly, but they also saw their role as the need to advocate for young women whom they felt could easily be swallowed up by the medical system during the labor and delivery process, which could put them in conflict with the higher-level professionals (e.g., doctors, nurses, and hospital social workers) with whom they worked. In the USA, few educational or certification programs prepare you specifically to be a home visitor in early childhood programs, so this ambiguity will likely continue.

Paraprofessionals are used as home visitors in the USA for both practical and theoretical reasons. It is important to understand the different motivations behind these reasons, as they have implications for how paraprofessionals may be used in other areas of the globe, including in developing nations. First, paraprofessionals typically work at lower wages than visitors with degrees or professional certifications, so a program can have more visitors for less money. In the USA, you might be able to hire four paraprofessionals for the cost of one nurse, so it can be a significant difference, and this difference may be even greater in developing nations. Second, paraprofessionals may be hired to support the development of a workforce in a distressed area, providing empowerment and employment to (usually) women within their own community. In countries with shortages of professionals in the workforce, it may be that paraprofessionals are the best resource to deliver services. Finally, because paraprofessionals share common experiences and culture with the families they serve, they might understand the families better, and the families are more likely to trust and relate to them. Under this reasoning, there is a decreased social distance between the paraprofessional and family that makes it easier to form relationships.

There are also *challenges* to using paraprofessionals that must be considered. Although these challenges are not universally true, they have been noted in reports on programs that have used paraprofessionals as home visitors (e.g., Musick & Stott, 2000; Hiatt, Sampson, & Baird, 1997). One of these challenges is an increased risk for a lack of professionalism. That is, home visitors with less formal education and experience may not yet understand the culture of professionals, so certain tasks that lead to a smoothly running program may be harder for them. They may not be good at organization and time management. They may struggle more with record keeping and making sure all forms on each family are filled out correctly. They may show an inappropriate or too casual appearance, which may lead to a lack of respect from other professionals with whom they interact (a reason the doulas wanted white lab coats when in the hospital) or even from families themselves.

Some home visitors hired from lower income communities, if exposed to the same educational problems as those of the families they see, may struggle with their own literacy issues and have trouble reading all the program material that is now expected of them. Musick and Stott (2000) also note that if these communities have high exposure to violence and trauma, then paraprofessionals from these communities may have unresolved issues around their own exposure. If left unexamined by the paraprofessional (quite possible in typical supervision sessions), these issues can create "domains of silence" (p. 446), in which the home visitor becomes afraid to or incapable of providing help and support to families who need assistance in this area.

A second challenge to consider is that *professionals* are so called because they have a certain level of knowledge and expertise that they have received from all of their education, training, and supervised experience. There are areas where they might simply have more knowledge and understanding, such as mental health concerns, specific health symptoms, or case management, which allows them to go deeper in their help to families. Paraprofessionals are less likely to have had formal training about these topics, so they may only know what has been given to them as a part of their in-service training within the program.

Figure 6.1 shows a simple example, from one of the few studies that has directly compared paraprofessionals to professionals, using the same program model. Nurse Family Partnership is a popular home visitation program model for first-time, low-income parents that traditionally uses public health nurses as home visitors (Olds,

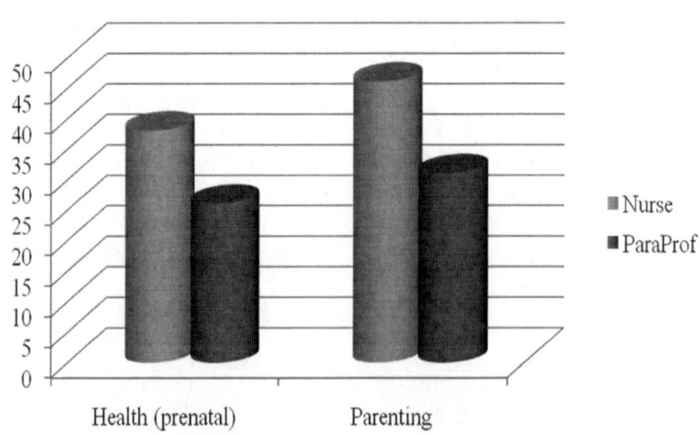

Fig. 6.1 Percentage of time home visitors, on an average, spent on prenatal health concerns and on issues of parenting (postnatal)

2002; see also nursefamilypartnership.org). About 15 years ago, however, the model was tested in a randomized trial comparing implementation and outcome when the program was delivered by nurses versus paraprofessionals, most of whom were women from the same community as the mothers and did not have a college degree (Korfmacher, O'Brien, Hiatt, & Olds, 1999).

One of the many results that came out of this trial was that nurses, as compared with paraprofessionals, spent considerably more time dealing with health issues of the mother, particularly during the prenatal period, and spent much more time focused on parenting. The reason for this is likely that nurses had the training and background that led them to spend more time on physical health and on basic caregiving concerns that the mothers had.

Third, it is possible that being a professional brings more respect whether one actually has more expertise or not. For example, although pediatricians in the USA receive extensive training in child health and physiology, they receive relatively less training about child development beyond a focus on developmental milestones.[2] Surveys show, however, that parents trust their child's doctor more than anybody else when they have questions about their child's development (e.g., Melmed, 1998), most likely because of the high status our society offers the medical profession. Most societies have hierarchies that value some helpers over others. Some in the USA have argued that home visiting will be taken more seriously by policymakers if the home visitors have professional background, training, and degrees. Recent trends suggest that infancy and early childhood services in the USA, including home visitation, are focusing on career lattices or ladders to promote the development of an educated and competent workforce (e.g., Gebhard, Jones, & Ochshorn, 2011).

Finally, a challenge in using paraprofessionals is the way they form relationships with the families. This may seem ironic, given that a prime motivation for hiring paraprofessionals is because they possibly understand the families better and are more likely to be trusted by the families. But there are challenges to this decreased social distance, as will be shown later in this chapter.

The issue is *not* whether paraprofessional home visitors are more challenged at forming relationships with families than professionals. My experience of talking to home visitors of many different backgrounds has convinced me that almost all home visitors want to engage with families and work hard to do so. Most parents report strong satisfaction with their home visitor when you ask them, to the point that many self-report forms show very little range in responses (Korfmacher, Green, Spellmann, & Thornburg, 2007). But, I do believe that home visitors from different backgrounds approach relationships with families differently, and we need to pay attention to those differences.

[2] Developmental pediatrics is a subspecialty that does provide more extensive training in child development, but makes up a relatively small percentage of the pediatric workforce in the USA.

The Importance of the Helping Relationship

There are two parts of the home visitor that are important: what they do and who they are. In most programs, home visitors "do" by teaching parents about their child's development, providing activities and games (or teaching parents these activities and games) to help the child's development, and helping parents problem-solve aspects of their life—their family, their school and work, and their own future. But equally important is not just *what* they do, but *how* they do it (Pawl & St. John, 1998).

In other words, the way in which the home visitor spends time with the family, interacts with the family, and relates to the family has as much, if not more, meaning as what content is actually transferred to the family. For example, there was a study of a home visiting program for high-risk mothers in the USA where the mothers were asked to rank in order 32 different program elements in terms of importance to them (Pharis & Levin, 1991). The strongest ranked answer was "a person to talk to who really cared." More than any assistance in daily living, problem-solving around crisis issues, or developmental guidance, the mothers most appreciated the feeling that came from knowing that there was someone available who "really cared" about them. This is one piece of evidence pointing towards the importance of the helping relationship in early childhood interventions. But the next question that may occur to you is this: What does it mean to "really care?"

These two simple words carry enormous weight, and my experience suggests it means different things to different home visitors. For the remainder of this chapter, I will provide examples of the differences in how helping relationships are thought about through interviews I did with home visitors and their clients in three different early childhood programs. The first program is a home visiting program for adolescent mothers run through high schools in a large urban school district (see Korfmacher & Marchi, 2002). The home visitors were paraprofessional. They did not have formal training in providing help, but they came from the same community as the mothers. The goals of the program were to help young mothers stay in school, delay future pregnancies, and promote their children's development. The second program was also for young mothers, but used doulas who were trained birth helpers (see Humphries & Korfmacher, 2012). As noted earlier, the doulas were hospital employees with formal training in how to assist mothers during labor and delivery; they also had similar backgrounds as the young mothers they helped. Third, I interviewed therapists at a mental health center that focused on working with families with young children.[3] The therapists were mostly social workers and did not have backgrounds similar to most of the families they served at this agency. The families they saw were referred because of concerns about the child's or the mother's mental health. The therapists not only did home visits but also met the families at their office.

[3] Unlike the other two studies, I was not able to interview the families of the mental health therapists. The results from these interviews with the therapists have not been published, but were the focus of a doctoral dissertation by Bonnie Schwartz (2005).

Across these three programs, one can see an increasing level of professionalization, from the family advocates (as they were called) in the high school program to the doulas, to the social workers. As this professionalization increased, however, there was also an increase in the social distance between the family and the service provider, with the social workers having the least similar background to the families they helped. Although the helpers in each of these programs were interviewed as a part of separate study, a similar interview protocol was used in each to allow some comparison across the providers. All interviews focused on how the helping relationship was defined by the providers and the families they visited, how a good relationship was conceived, and how differences between the provider and the helper was seen to influence the quality of the relationship.

To begin with, I will provide an example from each of the three types of providers.[4] Here is a quote from a paraprofessional where she comments about how she knows the relationship is going well with her client:

> …[I]t's very comfortable. I feel relaxed when I'm around her. I'm not nervous. I feel like I'm home…It's like I'm going to some of my relatives' house. That's how the relationship is with her…she calls me when I don't visit…I like it because she makes me smile. I like her a lot.

Notice she is focusing on feeling comfortable and happy ("I like it because she makes me smile") when she thinks about a good relationship with a mother—she compares the experience to being with a member of her own family. Compare this to the following quote from a doula about her client:

> I believe she's starting to trust me more because her mother will come up the stairs [and say]: "Natalie have a discharge" …And Natalie would just look at her weird, and say, "Why did you tell her that?" So now *Natalie* calls me and says, "You know, I'm having a discharge. What do you think it is?" So now, it's like I believe the trust is going.

In this example, the doula is focusing on signs that the young mother is seeking her out and trusts her to be helpful as a sign of the positive relationship. Finally, the following is a quote from a mental health therapist, a psychologist with a considerable formal training in therapy, particularly with families of young children, discussing a client she was currently seeing:

> [S]he couldn't believe that I really cared…she would start laughing and rolling her eyes. And I think that she always feels so humiliated, and she does a good job of pushing people away and humiliating them. But in the last few sessions that has really changed dramatically and she has not been doing so much laughing or eye-rolling at all. The past session was the first time in a long time that she did not mention not coming back.

Compared to the other two helpers, the therapist is focusing on very small or subtle signs, including body language, that the client feels safe and is not defensive. Across all three of these quotes, there is a sense of the client wanting help from the helper, whether it is calling the family advocate on the phone, presenting a physical symptom to the doula, or simply not responding in a defensive way to the therapist.

---

[4] Many of the quotes used in this chapter have been the focus of previous articles (Korfmacher, 2001; 2007; Korfmacher & Marchi, 2002; Humphries and Korfmacher, 2012).

All three of these helpers are paying attention to the emotional tone of their interactions with their client surrounding this help-seeking behavior, but the area of their focus is quite different.

The Personal–Professional Relationship

The three quotes used above are illustrative. But when I and my colleagues systematically reviewed and coded the transcribed interviews of the helpers and the participating mothers, several themes emerged. One of the strongest differences across the interviews between professionals and paraprofessionals was the willingness of the paraprofessionals and the doulas to put themselves personally into the relationship so that their helping relationships had a more familiar and intimate flavor than the mental health therapists. They were more willing to share details of their private life, such as talking about their own past or their own children (sometimes even bringing their children with them on home visits). They often wanted to be seen as a member of the family, such as an elder sister or a second mother. They talked about the importance of feeling comfortable when spending time with their client mothers. They also were willing to say that they love the mother and feel touched when a mother loves them back, a theme I explore more below. One doula noted that this personal connection was a strategic decision she made, as a way to increase the likelihood that the young mothers would see her as a source of support:

> You have to give a little to get from them…You have to share to let them realize that you are not an alien, you are not by yourself, there is someone that understands.

The doula here is saying that the mother will not talk about herself if the doula does not talk about herself first, a clear articulation of the importance of a reduced social distance in forming a strong alliance with the mother. The doulas in this study overall tried very hard to be seen as different from other professionals (such as doctors and nurses), whom they believed often did not respect these teenage mothers and did not understand the lives and circumstances of the young mothers. By letting the young mothers know that she herself, for example, had been a teen mother, the doula is fostering a sense of closeness, and modeling for the young mothers that it is possible to be successful in life despite similar personal challenges. The mental health therapists, on the other hand, had strong rationales for *not* sharing aspects of their personal lives with their clients, as shown in the following quote:

> The reason why we may not be talking about my own personal information is that it may take up too much space and then the focus would be on me, and I really want the focus of treatment to be on her.

In other words, the more the therapist talks about herself, the more she takes attention away from the client, who should be the focus of the session. In another example, a therapist realized that her client wants to view her as a friend as a way of avoiding talking about important issues.

> In her becoming comfortable with me…she still is resistant against wanting to go any deeper, so she's kind of keeping me at a friendship arm's length or distance.

The therapist saw this sharing as a problem with the relationship, not as a sign of closeness. Although therapists would talk about whether or not they liked a client when directly asked, they did not see it as central to their work. Their training had taught them to be suspicious of relationships that get too friendly.

As noted above, love was frequently mentioned in the interviews with the doulas and the family advocates, but not the mental health therapists. Admission of love towards a client is not normally heard from the mouths of doctors, or nurses, or social workers, or psychologists. This level of closeness or strong feelings is not encouraged by their professional training. But, the doulas and the family advocates had no such qualms. The following two quotes highlight this. One doula discusses the feelings she had after a particularly difficult labor and delivery by a young mother with whom she felt a particularly strong alliance.

> It [birth] almost made me go against my big rule to never cry…and after everything was over she hugged me so tight and she says, "I love you." And I said, "Oh I love you."

The young mother, in recounting the labor and delivery, had this to say about her doula:

> She's just like a friend. We've been through like everything. Labor was really hard, but she was there for me though. I actually asked if she would be my baby's godmother. That's because I feel that close to her now.

The baby's godmother is typically a very important role for the families who participated in this program. It places the doula not merely as a helper but as an honored member of the family and assumes that the doula would be in this child's life (and by extension, the mother's life) indefinitely.

The concerns of early childhood are intimate concerns. Home visitors are spending time with a parent at their home, surrounded by the client's personal life. They are often witnessing the birth of a child and then supporting the parent as she struggles with feeding or breastfeeding, sleeping, changing the newborn, and later promoting the young child's security and exploration. So perhaps, we should not be surprised by a feeling of love that emerges between a mother and someone who works with her so closely.

Given the training and the focus on emotional boundaries in the helping professions, however, it is not surprising that we are also uncomfortable about the concept of love in the helping relationship. Across the interviews of the mental health therapists, love was mentioned only one time, and only as a superlative, with a therapist noting that she "loves to be around" a particular mother and her young children. The word "love" has a different meaning in this case. It is used to express enjoyment with the family (also an infrequent theme for therapists), but not intimacy.

When the paraprofessional family advocates and the doulas and their client mothers use "love" when discussing their relationship, it conveys a level of emotional closeness in the interviews. But how should we define this love? Social psychologists have been studying a concept called *compassionate love* which is defined

Table 6.1 Comparing dimensions of positive relationships and compassionate love

Positive relationship	Compassionate love
Caring	Caring
Trust	Trust
Available	Desire to spend time together
Understanding	Understanding
Feeling helped or feeling helpful	Helping

as a love that is not romantic, spiritual, or familial, but love where one is concerned about another person's well-being (Fehr & Sprecher, 2008). As Table 6.1 shows, the constructs of compassionate love (as described by Fehr & Sprecher) align very closely with the major positive relationship themes emerging from the interviews in my studies.

When the participants talk about love in the helping relationship, I believe that it is this kind of love that emerges. This is one of the motivators or drivers of the relationship. It is something that paraprofessionals are more willing to acknowledge than professionals, and it is something that families respond to.

Challenges of the Personal Relationship

On the other hand, there are challenges associated with this personal relationship. As pop singers from past to present have often noted, love is not always kind. When you are let down or disappointed by someone you love, it can be very difficult, and it can be difficult to be objective. Along with the positive aspects of strong emotional connections between home visitors and their families, negative elements emerged from the interviews as well. Both the mothers and the home visitors could feel disappointed and be taken for granted by each other.

Here is one example from a young mother, talking about her family advocate, who had reduced the frequency of visitation so that the family advocate could focus time on clients she was more concerned about:

> She'll go visit [other clients] before she go visit me, because she thinks I'll understand because I know how sometimes they get busy. And I feel like, no, I won't understand.

When elements of a personal relationship enter a working alliance, it can be difficult for the helpers to not see reactions and choices of the client as a referendum on themselves and what they mean to the client. For example, when asked what made the most difference for a young mother she worked with, one of the doulas noted that the mother became very emotional when presented with an infant carrier. Although this was part of the program model and a very specific way that the doula helped the mother, the doula was unsettled by this strong emotional reaction, a reaction she did not see before in the ongoing contact together:

> [W]hen you think that you've made an impact on them, that might not be the impact... When I saw her I said "Man, I thought I was really getting down with her," but I've never seen no expression like that coming out of her...It wasn't my doing. It was the carrier. She really needed it at the time. But I think that's what makes a difference.

Although the doula is working at being equanimous about this realization, there is a sense that she is jealous of the mother's reaction ("It wasn't my doing. It was the carrier.") to the point that she cannot take credit for this intervention.

In more extreme cases, some of the paraprofessionals became so disappointed in the life choices that the young mothers made that they reacted more like angry friends than as helpers. In the following example, the family advocate was upset that she arrived for a home visit to find the teen mother sleeping and the child needing care.

> I had come over and the baby's pamper would be soaking wet...And I say, "Get up off your ass and put him in a pamper!" And that's how you have to talk to her.

In another example, a family advocate refuses to visit a client until she changes her mind about school.

> I just tell her, "I'm just gonna block you out!"...Until she really gets herself back into school, I think me and her gonna be like that.

Both of these cases were mothers who dropped out of school, and it felt like a betrayal to the home visitors. The mothers let them down, and the visitors had a hard time coming back from that. Although the first family advocate quoted is still engaged with the mother, the second family advocate notes that she would refuse to see the mother—she would "block her out," which defeats the whole purpose of the intervention. The very real anger that this family advocate is expressing seems to be interfering with her ability to help the young mother.

Support for the Paraprofessionals

There are ways to support the paraprofessional as they struggle with these challenges. These forms of assistance are not just for paraprofessionals but also for all home visitors as they form alliances with families. Home visiting is a difficult job no matter the level of the visitor's experience and training. One important support to home visitors is having a caseload of reasonable size. If you think about the work of visitors as relationship building, then a caseload of 20 or more is a lot of relationships for a helper to keep in his or her head.

Many program models in the USA limit the number of families with whom a home visitor may work. As in one example, Early Head Start, the federally funded early childhood program, requires maximum caseloads of 12 families for weekly home visits (Early Head Start National Resource Center, 2009). But other program models specify the maximum number of *visits per month* that a home visitor is expected to make across their entire caseload, without attention to the number of families. This is done to allow more families on caseloads who might have reduced visitation schedules (e.g., monthly instead of weekly visits). The tension in many programs is allocation of resources. If there is a high demand for home visiting, setting limits on caseloads can create waitlists, with some families receiving no services at all.

Another way to support the home visitor is to have clear expectations of their role and what they are supposed to do with families. This seems like a simple suggestion, but the role of the home visitor is often not clear. Home visitation is a service field that emerged from many different human service professions, including infant mental health, public health, nursing, early intervention, social work, early education, and community advocacy. Each of these professions advocates attention to different aspects of family life and well-being. Unless home visitors have a good understanding of their role and the limits to their roles, they may feel compelled to do everything for the families. Often home visitors are the primary face of human services for families, precisely because they are willing to make the effort to meet the parents in their homes, which increases the pressure to be a little bit of everything to the families. But, paraprofessionals should not be expected to know what nurses know, or do what social workers do, even if there are ways they can support the family and assist in the child's development.

It can be argued that having increased structure and precise session-by-session manuals is one way to promote these clear expectations. This may be helpful for some, especially new visitors with less experience. Manuals, however, tend to focus on what home visitors should do. As has been pointed out throughout this chapter, this is only one half of the equation. *How* home visitors are with families is equally important and less subject to manualization. Many home visiting program models in the USA also adopt a family-centered approach and emphasize the need to attend to the individual needs and strengths of families. Ultimately, home visitors must be able to go beyond rigid program protocols as they individualize services to families.

In short, home visiting is a mixture of science and art. As much as we wish we could be prescriptive about what home visitors should do with families based on carefully controlled empirical studies, it is an art to figure out a family and know how to help them. There will always be some mystery in determining what works. Because of this mystery, ongoing experiential training is important. Programs in the USA are moving beyond a focus on intensive introductory trainings and planning more for the professional development of home visitors over time.

And finally, supervision is essential to the process of supporting home visitors. There are different models of supervision, including administrative, educational, and reflective supervision (Heffron & March, 2010). There has also been increased attention towards incorporating direct observation of practice and feedback (e.g., video recording of home visits for later review) as part of supervision (Roggman, Boyce, & Innocenti, 2008). Reflective supervision is currently seen as a key component of supporting home visitors in their work with families and in their own professional development. One principle of infant mental health that is worth noting in home visiting programs that promote a relationship-based orientation is the parallel process. A good supervisor helps the home visitors make sense of their feelings,

Fig. 6.2 Parallel process in support

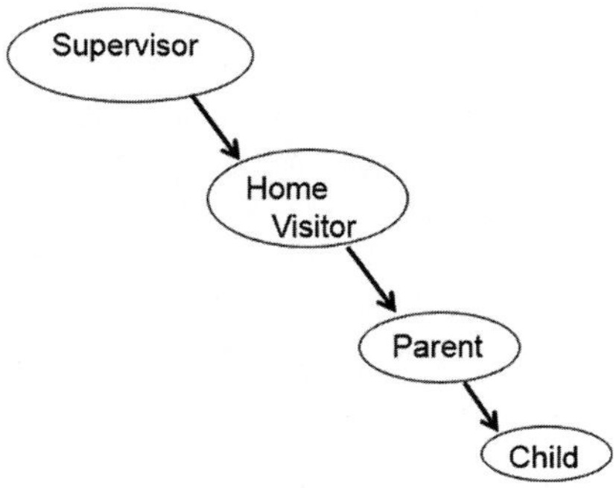

just as the home visitors may help the parents with their feelings, as the parents help their children make sense of the world.

Jeree Pawl, an infant mental health theorist in the USA, takes the Golden Rule—an ethical notion of reciprocity attributed to different prophets in religious texts—and extends it to incorporate this parallel process (Pawl, 1994). Instead of "Do to others as you would have others do to you," the message promotes looking forward and outward: Do to others as you would have others do to others. As the supervisor is to the home visitor, the home visitor can be to the parent, and the parent can be to the child (see Fig. 6.2).

Deborah Daro, a leading home visiting expert in the USA, has summarized the ways that parents help their children into four categories: (1) teaching them, (2) helping them to problem-solve, (3) regulating their feelings, and (4) scaffolding or supporting them as they explore and take risks (Daro, 2011).

These same processes are involved when home visitors provide help to a parent. Home visitors teach parents about child development. They help parents to problem-solve issues in caring for their children and their own life. They can help regulate the feelings of parents when they are overwhelmed with the stresses of caregiving. And they provide scaffolding to the parent as she takes risks in her relationship with her child (such as providing activities that mother can do with her child to promote bonding) or in seeking out further help and support (such as accompanying parents when they interact with other providers). Furthermore, these are the same processes involved when a supervisor provides support to the home visitor. A supervisor teaches, problem-solves, regulates, and scaffolds the home visitor as they do the difficult job of supporting the parent.

Conclusion

In this chapter, I have attempted to provide a brief overview of how paraprofessionals are used in home visiting programs and the issues that arise in their professional development and training. The ways that many paraprofessional home visitors relate to families, particularly with an orientation that is flexible in incorporating more personal qualities into their help-giving, has both strengths and challenges. It is important to recognize both. As home visiting becomes more "professionalized" in the USA, with increasing numbers of home visitors having college education and specific training to prepare them for working with families, it will be interesting to see if such a personal orientation to their work remains. If home visiting becomes a viable service model for supporting families of young children in other parts of the world, especially in developing countries, more research will be needed to examine the extent how the cultural and national context influences the way that home visitors spend time with their families, and how we support them in their work.

Acknowledgments The studies noted in this chapter were funded by grants from the Spencer Foundation, the US Maternal and Child Health Bureau, and the Irving B. Harris Foundation.

Thank you to Isabela Marchi, Marisha Humphries, and Bonnie Schwartz for their assistance in collecting, transcribing, coding, and analyzing the data across the three studies.

References

Abramson, R., Breedlove, G. K., & Isaacs, B. (2007). *The community-based doula: Supporting families before, during, and after childbirth*. Washington, DC: ZERO TO THREE.

Daro, D. (2011). *Sustaining home visiting programs: Critical considerations and challenges*. Invited presentation to the International Seminar on Home Visitation. São Paulo, Brazil (May, 2011).

Early Head Start National Resource Center. (2009). *Early Head Start tip sheet, No. 31: EHS home visitor caseload*. http://www.ehsnrc.org/Publications/English%20Tip%20Sheets/TIP_SHEET_31.PDF. Accessed 2 Nov 2011.

Fehr, B., & Sprecher, S. (2008). Compassionate love: Conceptual, measurement, and relational issues. In B. Fehr, S. Sprecher, & L. G. Underwood (Eds.), *The science of compassionate love: Theory, research, and applications* (pp. 27–52). San Francisco: Wiley-Blackwell.

Gebhard, B., Jones, L., & Ochshorn, S. (2011). 10 policy recommendations to build a strong infant-toddler workforce. *Zero To Three, 32*(1), 44–45.

Halpern, R. (1999). *Fragile families, fragile solutions: A history of supportive services for families in poverty*. New York: Columbia University Press.

Hans, S., & Korfmacher, J. (2002). The professional development of paraprofessionals. *Zero To Three, 23*(2), 4–8.

Heffron, M. C., & March, T. (2010). *Reflective supervision and leadership in infant and early childhood programs*. Washington, DC: ZERO TO THREE.

Hiatt, S. W., Sampson, D., & Baird, D. (1997). Paraprofessional home visitation: Conceptual and pragmatic considerations. *Journal of Community Psychology, 25,* 77–93.

Humphries, M. L., & Korfmacher, J. (2012). The good, the bad, and the ambivalent: Quality of alliance in a support program for young mothers. *Infant Mental Health Journal, 33*(1), 22–33.

Klaus M. H., Kennell J. H., & Klaus P. H. (2002). *The doula book: How a trained labor companion can help you have a shorter, easier, and healthier birth*. New York: Da Capo Press.

Korfmacher, J. (2001). *Harder than you think: Understanding what works, for whom, and why in early childhood interventions*. Occasional Paper published by the Herr Research Center, Erikson Institute. http://www.erikson.edu/PageContent/en-us/Documents/HRC/op_korfmacher.pdf. Accessed 2 Nov 2011.

Korfmacher, J. (2007). The heart of relationship-based care. *IMPrint: Newsletter of the Infant Mental Health Promotion Project*, 48 (Spring). http://www.sickkids.ca/pdfs/IMP/21459–48IMPReprint-Korfmacher.pdf. Accessed 2 Nov 2011

Korfmacher J., & Marchi, I. (2002). The helping relationship in a teen parenting program. *Zero To Three, 23*(2), 21–26.
Korfmacher, J., O'Brien, R., Hiatt, S., & Olds, D. (1999). Differences in program implementation between nurses and paraprofessionals in prenatal and infancy home visitation: A randomized trial. *American Journal of Public Health, 89,* 1847–1851.
Korfmacher, J., Green, B., Spellmann, M., & Thornburg, K. R. (2007). The helping relationship and program participation in early childhood home visiting. *Infant Mental Health Journal, 28,* 459–480.
Melmed, M. (1998). Talking with parents about emotional development. *Pediatrics, 102*(Supplement E1), 1317–1326.
Musick, J., & Stott, F. (2000). Paraprofessionals revisited and reconsidered. In J. P. Shonkoff & S. J. Meisels (Eds.), *Handbook of early childhood intervention* (2nd ed., pp. 439–453). Cambridge: Cambridge University Press.
Olds, D. L. (2002). Prenatal and infancy home visiting by nurses: From randomized trials to community replication. *Prevention Science, 3,* 153–172.
Pawl, J. (1994). On supervision. *Zero to Three, 15*(3), 21–29.
Pawl, J. H., & St. John, M. (1998). *How you are is as important as what you do…In making a positive difference for infants, toddlers, and their families*. Washington, DC: ZERO TO THREE.
Pharis, M. E., & Levin, V. S. (1991). "A person to talk to who really cared": High-risk mothers' evaluations of services in an intensive intervention research program. *Child Welfare Journal, 70,* 307–320.
Raikes, H. H., & Bellotti, J. (2006). Two studies of father involvement in early head start programs: A national survey and a demonstration program evaluation. *Parenting: Science & Practice, 6*(2), 229–242.
Roggman, L. A., Boyce, L. K., & Innocenti, M. S. (2008). *Developmental parenting: A guide for early childhood practitioners*. Baltimore: Paul H Brookes.
Schwartz, B. (2005). *Therapists' experiences of the working alliance in early childhood and infant mental health intervention: A qualitative analysis*. Dissertation Submitted to the Faculty of The Chicago School of Professional Psychology.

Jon Korfmacher PhD. (USA): Associate Professor at the Erikson Institute. His research focuses on differential responses of children and families to early childhood intervention programs. He is interested in understanding why families participate in these programs, what the experience is like for them, and what types of services work best for different families under different circumstances. He also studies the training and professional development of early childhood service providers. He is also a faculty associate with Herr Research Center for Children and Social Policy and a graduate fellow of ZERO TO THREE.

Chapter 7
Engagement and Retention in Home Visiting Child Abuse Prevention Programs

William M. McGuigan and Breanna Gassner

Introduction of Study of Program Engagement

Home visiting is a common strategy used throughout the USA and many other countries to assist high-risk families in the prevention of child maltreatment and abuse. Nonetheless, a summary of the home visiting literature (Gomby, Culross, & Behrman, 1999; Sweet & Applebaum, 2004) showed that most home visiting programs reported only moderate success in changing parental risk behaviors. Program success and effectiveness may be undermined by a lack of active parental participation since the success of home visiting programs is reliant upon parental involvement. While no studies have been conducted to demonstrate the exact number of home visits or exact amount of time in the program that is necessary to create change, there is evidence that increased participation results in greater benefits (Daro, McCurdy, Falconnier, & Stojanovic, 2003; Olds et al., 1999; Wagner & Clayton, 1999). Therefore, studies that seek to explain why families engage and remain active in home visiting programs are extremely important.

This chapter is a review of the findings from two previous studies of engagement and retention in a home visiting program (McGuigan, Katzev, & Pratt, 2003a; McGuigan, Katzev, & Pratt, 2003b). Both studies used data from the Oregon Healthy Start (OHS) program, a voluntary home visiting family support program designed to prevent poor child outcomes, including child maltreatment. The OHS program was modeled after Healthy Families America (HFA), a national child abuse prevention initiative of Prevent Child Abuse America (1999). From 1994 to 2003, the OHS program used the 15-item Hawaii Risk Indicators (HRI) checklist (Hawaii Family Stress Center 1994) to screen approximately 80% of all first-birth mothers in 15 participating Oregon counties. Mothers were screened at or near the time of their first child's birth. Screening items included known

W. M. McGuigan (✉) · B. Gassner
Pennsylvania State University—Shenango, Sharon, USA
e-mail: wmm11@psu.edu

L. Roggman, N. Cardia (eds.), *Home Visitation Programs*,
DOI 10.1007/978-3-319-17984-1_7

risks for child maltreatment, such as a mother who has not completed high school, is unmarried, and who received late or no prenatal care. All families who were screened received one "welcome baby" home visit, a list of community resources, a packet of child development information, and various free baby supplies (diapers and baby blanket). Approximately one half of all mothers screened showed two or more risks on the HRI checklist. Two or more risks qualified these mothers for further assessment using the Kempe Family Stress Inventory (KFSI). The KFSI is an in-depth interview that assessed ten psychosocial factors related to child maltreatment including history of childhood abuse and history of substance abuse (Korfmacher, 2000; McGuigan & Pratt, 2001).

The purpose of the first study was to examine factors that contribute to active engagement in home visitation services. National surveys report that parents generally approve of the idea of home visiting family support programs (Taffee-Young, Davis, & Schoen, 1996). Visiting families at home allows those families to receive support services in the convenience of their own home, eliminating potential barriers such as the need for childcare and transportation costs. Still, many eligible parents do not participate in these voluntary services (Daro & Gelles 1992). Reaching and enrolling target families in services is a common problem for programs designed to support children and families, especially for those serving high-risk populations (Larner, Halpern, & Harkavy, 1992). A number of studies report that up to 25 % of eligible parents decline to enroll in home visiting family support programs (Gomby, Culross, & Behrman, 1999; National Committee to Prevent Child Abuse (NCPCA), 1996).

Even when parents enroll in home visitation programs, it is no guarantee they will engage in services (Daro & Harding, 1999). Many home visiting programs consider parents enrolled if they agree to participate when services are initially offered. Agreeing to participate in a program is different from actively engaging in services. For example, evaluation of Hawaii's Healthy Start program found that beyond the 15 % of "initial refusals," there was an additional 15 % of "secondary refusals" (NCPCA 1996). These were parents who initially enrolled in services, but who dropped from the program after receiving very few, if any, home visits during 3 months of intensive outreach efforts. Other studies confirm that a substantial portion of parents drop out of home visiting programs within the first few weeks after enrollment (Marcenko & Spence, 1994; Myers-Walls, Elicker, & Bandyk, 1997).

Studies have not differentiated degrees of participation by separating non-engaging families from engaging families. Instead, one study of program participation combined families who enrolled but were dropped or withdrew after receiving few, if any, home visits (non-engaging families) with other families who received ongoing home visits but dropped out at some point prior to program completion (Clark & Winje, 1998). This might be because most studies focus on factors that contribute to overall attrition or any premature departure from services (McCurdy & Daro, 2001) rather than specifically examining program engagement.

By focusing almost exclusively on why parents leave programs, researchers ignore an equally fundamental question: Why do some eligible parents who enroll in home visitation programs never fully engage in services? More specifically, what factors in the community and in the family influence the decision to engage in services? As stated by McCurdy and Daro (2001), early research "suffered from a restrictive conceptual framework…in terms of the areas explored" (p. 113). The vast majority of researchers limited their scope to one or two potential determinants of program participation (primarily participant and provider characteristics), rather than acknowledging that participants and providers live in communities. Focusing strictly on participant and provider characteristics ignores the potential influence that community factors might have on families' engagement in home visiting programs (McCurdy & Daro, 2001).

We add to the discussion of engagement in home visiting programs that past research is restricted in the methods of analysis. Researchers understand that individual factors (e.g., income, age, and ethnicity) and community factors (e.g., community health characteristics) can influence where parents live. However, individual and community factors also are likely to influence which services a parent seeks out and uses. The "nested" structure of these levels of influence (individuals within communities) requires recognition of the interdependence of these causal agents and movement from a reliance on conventional linear or main effect models.

Researchers have long suspected that community factors influence mothers' commitment to engage in home visitation services (Damashek, Doughty, Ware, & Silovsky, 2011). Yet to date, there remains a paucity of research that has addressed specifically which community factors affect mothers' engagement in home visitation services. Comparisons across community areas on established health outcomes may be one way to broaden our understanding of the effectiveness and practices of programs within the communities. Examining community health factors exemplifies an "outcome orientation" that communities can affect families positively or negatively, and this effect can be measured in higher or lower rates of positive outcomes for the population living in the area (Coulton, Korbin, & Chow, 1995).

On an individual level, if teenage mothers had conflictive and non-supportive families, they were less likely to fully engage in a home visiting parenting program (Josten, Mullett, Savik, Campbell, & Vincent, 1995). Studies report higher rates of engagement in family support programs among mothers whose infants displayed health risks at birth (Josten, Mullett, Savik, Campbell, & Vincent, 1995; Olds & Kitzman, 1993). Lower rates of engagement in home visitation services are reported for mothers who experienced family conflict or family problems (Josten, Mullett, Savik, Campbell, & Vincent, 1995). High-risk pregnant women who abused substances (Damashek, Doughty, Ware, & Silovsky, 2011; Navaie-Waliser et al., 2000) and mothers who knew they would soon be moving to another house or neighborhood also were found to be less likely to engage in home visiting services (NCPCA, 1996).

One early study of participation in parent education programs found that after initial enrollment mothers who were raising their children without a supportive network of family and friends perceived greater benefits and fewer costs of program involvement than did mothers with extensive support networks (Powell, 1984). In contrast, a later study focusing on the health outcomes of participants in a home visiting program found that family and friendship networks had the opposite effect on program engagement. Luker and Chalmers (1990) reported that after an initial decision to enroll in home visitation, mothers with a limited network of maternal support were more likely to withdraw from the program early.

Beyond individual risk factors, we suspect that the overall health of the community would influence the decision of mothers with newborns to engage in home visitation services. Although there are many possible paths of influence, one plausible explanation is that in areas of high community health, mothers may see supports for healthy family conditions as common. We concur with McCurdy and Daro's (2001) speculation that in communities where the dominant ethos views healthy families as an asset, mothers may be more likely to engage in services. In contrast, mothers raising their newborns in areas with poor community health may be more wary and less likely to expect positive results from a social service program. These mothers may see the family deficits present in their community (i.e., high infant death rate and high number of low-birth-weight infants) as normal conditions families should expect to endure alone. An adequately large sample allowed us to statistically control for several factors related empirically to participation in home visiting programs while testing the following two hypotheses:

- H_1: After initial enrollment, mothers raising their newborn infant in areas with poorer community health are less likely to actively engage in home visiting family support services.
- H_2: After initial enrollment, mothers experiencing greater maternal isolation are less likely to actively engage in home visiting family support services.

In this study, the data came from OHS. One of the mandates from the Oregon legislature was that OHS seek to improve health outcomes for the families they served, such as ensuring access to preventative health care and improving immunization rates for children. Public health departments were active collaborators in the OHS programs. In many counties, the OHS program was physically housed within the public health building. Whereas other community factors such as social cohesion and social disorganization can impact families, community health factors were particularly important to the OHS home visiting program.

Methods of Study of Program Engagement

To improve the health and welfare of Oregon families, OHS offered regular home visits to high-risk families during the first 5 years of raising their firstborn child. Home visits were scheduled based on the family's needs, beginning with weekly visits and graduating to monthly visits. Home visitors offered parenting education, support, and referrals to any needed services such as mental health services, alcohol and drug treatment programs, childcare, food, housing, and transportation. All OHS home visitors received at least 96 hours of initial training and over half (53 %) had college degrees, some with degrees in nursing.

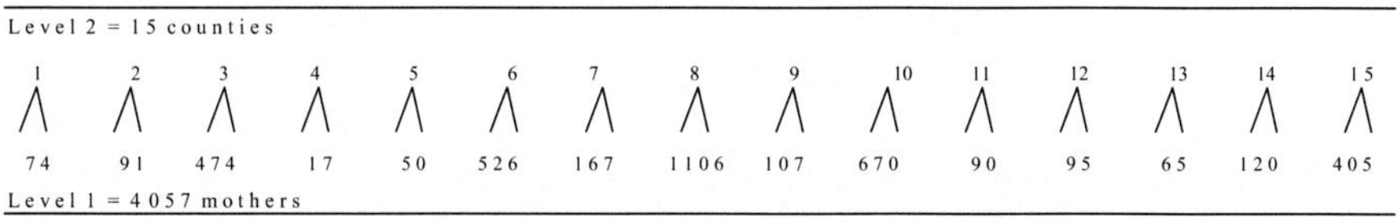

Fig. 7.1 Engagement study: two-level model predicting engagement in home visits for 4057 mothers residing in 15 counties

From January 1, 1995 to December 31, 1998, a total of 4341 families were assessed as high risk and offered regular home visitation services. Of these, 284 (7%) refused any further service. The remaining 4057 (93%) mothers gave their written consent to participate in home visitation and were considered enrolled in the OHS program. These mothers lived in 15 Oregon counties and made up the study sample (n=4057). There were no significant differences in risk or assessment scores between those who refused and those who initially accepted OHS services (Fig. 7.1).

Mothers in the study sample resided in semirural or small metropolitan areas and were predominantly single (78%). Over half had low incomes (58% with gross monthly family incomes <US$1000) and less than a high school education (54%). The sample was predominantly White (77%) with 23% minorities (18% Hispanic, 5% African-American, Native American, Asian, or other). On average, mothers were 20.6 years old (*SD*=5.0) when their child was born, and most did not work outside the home (82%). Over half of the mothers (58%) lived with their husband or boyfriend; one third (33%) lived with parents, relatives, or friends; and the remaining 9% lived only with their newborn child.

The OHS program followed HFA guidelines when dealing with families who had accepted the program but were reluctant to fully engage in services or difficult to contact. For the first 3 months after enrollment, OHS workers used "creative outreach" techniques to connect with families. These included repeated mailings, telephone calls to the home, work, and message numbers, and drop-by visits to the home. After 3 months of intensive outreach efforts, families were discharged from the program if (a) home visitors were not able to schedule a visit, (b) families were consistently absent after scheduling home visits, or (c) the families said they no longer wanted to participate.

Based on these established HFA guidelines and the fact that OHS was designed to provide 5 years of supportive services, involvement in the program beyond 3 months was accepted as a legitimate definition of program engagement. Engagement was coded as received services more than 90 days (0) and received services for 90 days or less (1). Thus, the dependent variable was non-engagement in home visitation services. Of the 4057 families who initially accepted services, 745 (18.4%) remained enrolled in the program from 1 to 90 days, for an average of 34 days (*SD*=31). The number of home visits completed by these 745 families ranged from 0 to 4, with an average of 0.48 home visits (*SD*=0.72). With that being said, we considered these 745 families as never actively engaging in the OHS home visiting programs.

A five-item maternal isolation index was constructed with each item being 0=no (not an indication of isolation) and 1=yes (an indication of isolation). Self-report items included the following: single, no spouse or partner; mother lives alone with newborn; mother has no phone; mother lists no emergency contact person. The fifth item on the maternal isolation index was assessed during the KFSI interview. This was "mother is isolated with few lifelines, low self-esteem, or depression." This combination of few lifelines, low self-esteem, or depression has always been part of the KFSI (Orkow, 1985). It is a global measure that reflects the mother's standing on two psychosocial components of maternal isolation: being socially isolated from others through a lack of lifelines and being personally isolated from immediate others due to low self-esteem and depression. Trained family assessment workers (FAWs) rated this item as not an issue for this mother, somewhat of an issue, or a significant issue. For this study, ratings were dichotomized as not at all an issue for this mother (0), and at least somewhat of an issue for this mother (1) to match the response categories of the other index items. The five items were summed to produce a total range of 0–5. Overall, mothers did not report high levels of maternal isolation; however, there was variation between engaging and non-engaging mothers at the lower levels of the index (see Table 7.1).

To control for the association between mother's age and engagement, the mother's age in years was included. Mother's ethnicity was included as Hispanic (0) and other ethnicity (1). Infant health status was assessed using information from birth records that indicated whether the child was premature (gestation <37 weeks), of low birth weight (≤ 2500 g), or had any other medical risks at birth. Of the 4057 newborns in the study families, 320 (7.9%) displayed at least one of these three health concerns at birth. Infant health status was included in the analysis as at least one health concern present at birth (0) and no health concerns present at birth (1). As previously mentioned, retention may be affected by marital or family problems, maternal history of substance abuse, or living in unstable housing. These three items were included as additional control variables and coded as not an issue for this family (0) and an issue for this family (1).

Families in the same community were not differentiated on the measure of community health, so standard logistic regression would have introduced the possibility of bias by violating the assumption of independence. Families were not random-

Table 7.1 Engagement study: Means (standard deviations) or percentages of all variables by engagement status

Variables	Engaged (n=3312)		Never engaged (n=745)	
Poor community health index	0.63	(0.88)	0.86	(0.75)
Maternal isolation index	1.53	(0.82)	1.78	(0.93)
Mother's age (years)	20.63	(4.97)	20.46	(4.93)
Mother is non-Hispanic	81%		88%	
No infant health risks at birth	92%		94%	
Marital or family problems	47%		54%	
History of substance abuse	32%		31%	
Unstable housing	25%		29%	

ly assigned to family support programs nor were families or programs randomly assigned to communities. This lack of independence required a statistical method that could estimate non-independent community and individual level effects. Our outcome variable had a Bernoulli distribution (engaged: yes/no), so we used the hierarchical general linear model (HGLM) for the nonlinear analysis of binary outcomes (Raudenbush, Bryk, Cheong, & Congdon, 2000). The HGLM Bernoulli model was used to estimate the unique effect of poor community health and the unique effect of maternal isolation on mothers' engagement in the OHS program while holding constant the effects of the six control variables. This model allowed for the examination of all possible moderator effects within and across individual and community levels. Tolerance tests indicated no problems with multicollinearity.

Results of Study of Program Engagement

Results of the multilevel analysis for engagement provided support for our first hypothesis: Mothers living in counties with poorer community health were significantly less likely to engage in home visitation services. The multilevel analysis also provided support for our second hypothesis: Isolated mothers were less likely to engage. For every one-unit increase in the five-item maternal isolation index, the odds of engaging in home visitation services decreased by 39 %.

Further, the multilevel model revealed that non-Hispanic mothers (95 % White) were 82 % less likely to engage in home visitation services than Hispanic mothers. When controlling for the significant effects of community health, maternal isolation, and mother's ethnicity, program engagement was not significantly related to any of the other variables: mother's age, history of substance abuse, unstable housing, family problems, or infant health.

While the sizes of the odd ratios were modest (Table 7.2), it is understood that without collinearity the additive log-odds of significant predictors are multiplicative. The addition of each risk factor "multiplies" the likelihood of non-engagement.

Table 7.2 Engagement study: Community- and family-level factors contributing to non-engagement ($n=4057$)

Variables	Coefficient	*t*-ratio	Odds-ratio
Poor community health index	0.31	2.86	1.36*
Maternal isolation index	0.33	6.63	1.39**
Mother's age (years)	0.01	0.04	1.01
Mother is non-Hispanic	0.60	4.71	1.82**
No infant health risks at birth	0.24	1.40	1.27
Marital or family problems	0.07	0.85	1.07
History of substance abuse	0.10	1.11	1.10
Unstable housing	0.10	1.01	1.10

*$p \leq 0.01$
**$p \leq 0.001$

Consequently, a White mother who had any one of the five indices of maternal isolation and lived in a county that scored one standard deviation above the average on the index of poor community health was nearly 3½ times (3.44) less likely to engage in services than mothers with none of these characteristics.

1.82	×	1.39	×	1.36	=	3.44
White mother		Living in isolation		Poor community health		

Introduction for Study of Program Retention

As previously stated, getting high-risk families to engage in home visiting programs can be a difficult task. An equally important hurdle to overcome is retaining families in home visiting programs once they have engaged. Reviews of home visiting programs (Guterman, 2000) found that 8–51 % of families leave home visiting programs within 12 months of service. The specific factors that contribute to these low rates of program retention remain unclear, but it is suspected that multiple levels of influence effect retention rates (McCurdy & Daro, 2001).

The underlying empirical rationale for the current study is that program retention is linked to program efficacy. The current study focused on the associations between retention in a voluntary home visiting child abuse prevention program and (1) the attributes of the communities in which the program was offered, (2) attributes of the home visitors, and (3) attributes of the enrolled mothers. Previous studies have been unable to estimate these multiple effects within the same statistical model due to the violation of independence. Mothers who receive visits from the same home visitor are not statistically independent of each other nor are visitors working within the same community. This lack of independence required a statistical method that could simultaneously estimate "non-independent" community, visitor, and maternal level effects while considering all possible interactions. It is only in the past decade that such robust statistical methods have become available. Hierarchical General Linear Modeling (HGLM; Raudenbush, Bryk, Cheong, & Congdon, 2000) is one such statistical technique appropriate for this type of multilevel analysis. This study used HGLM to obtain an accurate assessment of the unique roles that community, visitor, and maternal level attributes play in retaining families in a voluntary home visiting child abuse prevention program.

Community level attributes, such as community violence, contribute to the overall quality of family and community life and may have a strong impact on program retention. Community violence has a negative effect on children's healthy growth and development (Vig, 1996) and has been associated with increased family violence (Osofsky, 1995) and increased child maltreatment (Lynch & Cicchetti, 1998). An extensive body of research also shows that high levels of community violence contribute to a "toxic environment" detrimental to both families and the community as a whole (Osofsky, 1995). Garbarino and Kostelny (1992) found that in the most socially toxic communities, residents reported less family involvement, fewer positive interactions with neighbors, and a lower quality of life. In contrast, residents in less toxic communities were more hopeful, reported more available services, and were more likely to participate in both formal and informal family support services.

In their cardinal study assessing the effects of community on child maltreatment, Garbarino and Sherman (1980) compared the help-seeking behavior of mothers living in high-risk, lower-quality-of-life communities to mothers living in low-risk, higher-quality-of-life communities. They reported that mothers living in high-risk communities were less likely to rely upon experienced helpers for support, and, when they did so, they were more likely to demonstrate an "incomplete" use of support services. These studies suggest that families raising children in violent communities may be difficult to retain in a voluntary home visiting child abuse prevention program.

There are limited accounts of how retention rates are influenced by the home visitor's age (Damashek, Doughty, Ware, & Silovsky, 2011), education, and training (Korfmacher, O'Brien, Hiatt, & Olds, 1999; Olds & Kitzman, 1993; Wasik, 1993). One study (Korfmacher, O'Brien, Hiatt, & Olds, 1999) found higher rates of program retention for nurse home visitors than for non college-degreed paraprofessional home visitors. However, it remains unclear how home visitors with other educational degrees, such as master of social work, master of public health, or bachelor's degrees in social sciences, might influence retention rates.

Lacking any standardized credentials or licensing, home visitors are often hired based on personal attributes thought to contribute to an effective helping relationship (Wallach & Lister, 1995). In a national survey of home visitation programs, staff identified maturity, warmth, empathy, and a non judgmental orientation as essential home visitor attributes (Wasik, 1993). However, it remains unclear which, if any, of these attributes affect program retention. An important home visitor attribute notably absent from previous studies is the amount of supervision the home visitor receives (Duggan et al., 2000). Supervision is especially important for home visitors serving at-risk families that experience chaotic lifestyles, multiple stresses, and difficulty in maintaining active service (Wallach & Lister, 1995).

The few studies that examined interactions between home visitor and maternal attributes identified some promising influences on retention. These included matching home visitors and participating mothers on ethnicity (Barth, Ash, & Hacking, 1986), establishing mutual perspective taking (Luker & Chalmers, 1990), and developing an empathetic helping relationship (Wallach & Lister, 1995). However, these findings have yet to be sufficiently replicated across studies.

Previous studies of intervention programs identified several notable maternal attributes that influenced program retention, but with little agreement about the direction of influence. While some studies reported that younger mothers tended to engage and remain in parenting programs (Olds & Kitzman, 1993), other studies reported younger mothers were more likely to drop out (Josten, Mullett, Savik, Campbell, & Vincent, 1995). Still another study reported that teens who had not finished high school were most likely to remain in home visiting services (Duggan et al., 2000). Married mothers were more likely to remain in a parent training intervention (Dumka, Garza, Roosa, & Stoerzinger, 1997), while single mothers were more likely to engage in a statewide home visitation program (Myers-Walls, Elicker, & Bandyk, 1997). Ethnicity had no significant effect on retention in some home visiting parenting programs, while other studies with adequate samples of minority participants found significantly higher retention rates for Hispanic and African-American parents (Daro, McCurdy, Falconnier, & Stojanovic, 2003; Dumka, Garza, Roosa, & Stoerzinger, 1997; Navaie-Waliser et al., 2000). Several studies have found mothers of low-birth-weight preterm infants were more likely to remain in home visiting programs than mothers whose full-term infants had no special health-care needs (Duggan et al., 2000; Josten, Mullett, Savik, Campbell, & Vincent, 1995; Olds and Kitzman, 1993).

Methods for Study of Program Retention

Using an ecological framework (Bronfenbrenner, 1979), this study investigated the effects of community, visitor, and maternal attributes on retention in a voluntary home visiting program.

Mothers were nested within home visitors, and both were nested within communities (Fig. 7.2). A review of the literature indicated that attributes from each of these three levels could influence program retention. Accordingly, analyses were conducted to examine the effect of community violence on program retention, key home visitor attributes that influence program retention, key maternal attributes that influence program retention, and all possible interactions within and across these three levels.

Exploratory techniques were warranted because this study was part of an ongoing program evaluation. The immediate intent was to inform program-funding agents, administrators, and providers of the distinct attributes at each of these levels that may impact retention in voluntary home visiting child abuse prevention programs. As outlined in the introduction, the underlying empirical rationale for this study is that program retention is linked to program efficacy. By knowing what factors influence program retention, program staff could develop strategies to increase retention rates and, thereby, increase program effectiveness.

Healthy Start FAWs conducted the KFSI interviews after receiving extensive training in the KFSI interview protocols. Scores on the KFSI can range from 0 to 100 with scores above 25 considered at risk for poor child outcomes. Approximately 75% of all families assessed with the KFSI scored above 25 and were offered weekly home visits and extensive family support services by trained family support workers (FSWs). Each year over 92% of the families who were assessed as high risk on the KFSI accepted regular home visits and were considered enrolled in the Healthy Start Program.

FSWs, most with bachelor's degrees, received 96 hours of training before providing home visits to higher-risk families with firstborns, as they begin parenting. Nurses and multidisciplinary teams of professionals supervised FSWs. Further-

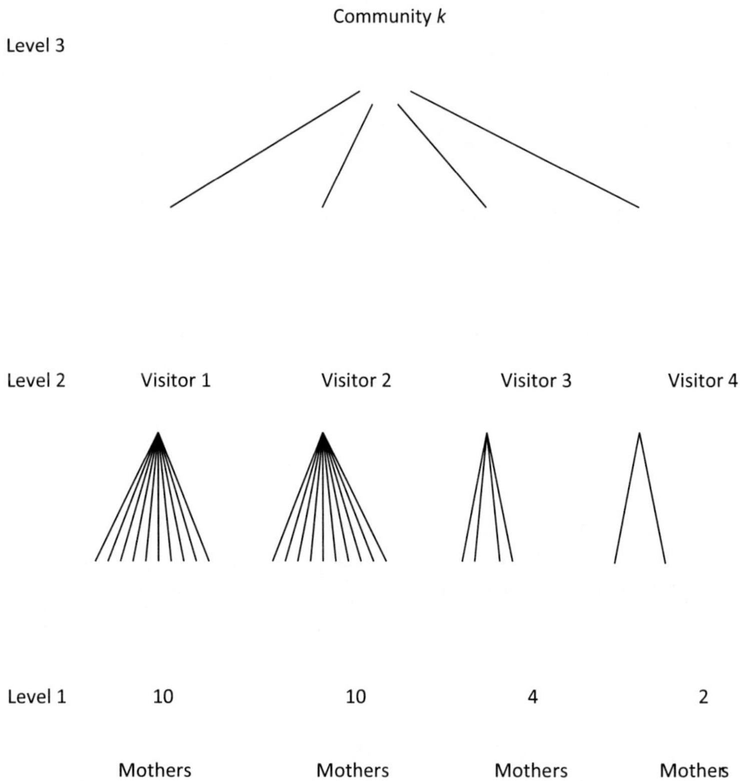

Fig. 7.2 Retention study: diagram of the multilevel structure of one community's home visiting program

more, this study was part of that ongoing evaluation and represents families who received home visits between February 1, 2000 and February 1, 2001.

Research has shown that the first year families begin parenting to be especially stressful (Belsky & Rovine, 1990). National statistics show the highest percentage of child abuse fatalities occur during the child's first year (US Department of Health and Human Services, 2000). Accordingly, OHS begins services either during the prenatal period or immediately after the first child's birth, starting with weekly home visits. Home visitors work with parents to set service-plan goals and refer parents to needed services (i.e., health care, counseling). During the first year, children in OHS families are linked to a primary health-care provider, begin the immunization sequence, are screened for developmental delays, and are referred to early intervention or other necessary services (Katzev, Pratt, & McGuigan, 2001). As families make progress toward service goals, they graduate to a lower intensity of service and less frequent visits throughout the first 5 years of child-rearing.

Because families drop out at varying times, the challenge for program evaluators is to define a level of retention that is meaningful to the specific program under review. This study used the crucial first-year time point as a meaningful measure of retention in the OHS home visiting program. This 1-year time point closely parallels the mean number of months (M= 13.7) all OHS families received services during the 1999–2000 fiscal year (Katzev, Pratt, & McGuigan, 2001). Retention was dichotomized as families who received services at least 1 year (1) and families who stopped receiving services, for any reason, prior to 1 year (0).

The community attributes included in this study were four indices of community violence: the number of homicides, assaults, and forcible rapes known to police and the number of domestic violence arrests. The most reliable data available on the number of homicides, assaults, and forcible rapes known to police in each county were obtained from the Bureau of the Census (1999). Data on the number of domestic violence arrests in each county were obtained from the Oregon Department of Human Resources (1999). Data were based on 1995 rates per 1000 adults in each county's population.

On February 1, 2000, a staff questionnaire was mailed to all OHS site administrators, who made the questionnaire available to home visitors. The questionnaire included a cover page explaining that participation was voluntary. The questionnaire did not ask for home visitors' names, but did require home visitor ID numbers to match visitors with the families they served. Of the 73 home visitors employed across the 12 OHS sites, 71 (97%) completed the questionnaire. The staff questionnaire contained demographic questions including age, race, gender (all home visitors were female), and educational attainment. Job-specific questions were also included, such as prior experience conducting home visits and hours of individual supervision received per month. In addition, the questionnaire included two scales from the Interpersonal Reactivity Index (IRI; Davis, 1983).

The IRI is a self-report measure of empathy consisting of four seven-item scales. The staff questionnaire included the seven-item Perspective Taking scale that assessed the tendency to adopt the point of view of others and the seven-item Empathic Concern scale that assessed feelings and concern for others. Questions on the Perspective Taking scale included "I believe there are two sides to every question and try to look at them both." A typical question from the Empathic Concern scale was "I am often quite touched by things I see happen." Responses were on a five-point scale indicating level of agreement. Both scales had good internal reliabilities (Cronbach's alphas of 0.70 and 0.77) and established convergent and discriminant validity (Davis, 1983).

The Perspective Taking and Empathic Concern scales were included in exploratory analyses with five other home visitors attributes thought to affect program retention. Visitor's age was measured in years. Visitor's ethnicity was included as Hispanic (1) and other ethnicity (0). Education was recorded as bachelor's degree or higher (1) and less than a bachelor's degree (0). Experience conducting home visits prior to employment with OHS was measured as prior home visiting experience (1) and no prior home visiting experience (0). While the same service program employed the home visitors working in each community, workers in a given program could experience very different hours of supervision. The final home visitor attribute in the analyses was the hours of individual supervision received per month (Table 7.3).

Table 7.3 Retention study: Means and standard deviations or percentages of all attributes

	m	*SD*	%
Community level (n=12)			
Community violence index	7.85	2.22	
Home visitor level (n=71)			
Visitor is Hispanic			18.3
Bachelor's degree or higher			53.5
Prior experience conduction home visits			41.0
Visitor's age in years	39.25	9.54	
Monthly hours of supervision	1.75	0.70	
Perspective Taking scale	3.10	0.38	
Empathic Concern scale	3.00	0.51	
Maternal level (n=1093)			
Mother is Hispanic			19.5
Mother has HS diploma or GED			43.0
Mother is currently married			20.0
Child born premature (<37 weeks) and low birth weight			8.5
Child not premature but low birth weight			4.0
Child had no health risks at birth			87.5
Mothers age in years	20.35	4.43	

m mean, *SD* standard deviation, *HS, GED*

Next, bivariate analyses were used to identify home visitor attributes to include in the multivariate analysis. Mothers were significantly more likely to remain in the program for at least 1 year if their home visitor was Hispanic, had less than a bachelor's degree, and received more hours of monthly supervision. These three home visitor attributes were included as level-2 predictors in the initial HGLM multivariate analysis. Bivariate analyses showed that remaining in the OHS home visiting program at least 1 year was not significantly related to the home visitor's age, prior home visiting experience, or scores on the Perspective Taking or Empathic Concern scales. These home visitor attributes were excluded from the multivariate analysis.

Results indicated a significant community level effect on program retention. With every one-unit increase in the index of community violence, mothers were 14% less likely to remain in home visiting services at least 1 year. The odds of remaining in the OHS program for at least 1 year increased by 89% with every 1-hour increase in the amount of monthly supervision the home visitor received. In this multivariate analysis, remaining in home visiting services for at least 1 year was not significantly related to the home visitor's ethnicity or whether the visitor had a college degree (Table 7.4).

On the maternal level, the HGLM analysis revealed that Hispanic mothers were 48% more likely than non-Hispanic mothers to remain in the OHS program for at least 1 year. With every year of age, mothers were 4% more likely to remain in the OHS program ($OR=1.04$, $p=0.01$). After considering the significant effects of community violence, home visitor supervision, and mother's age and ethnicity, results of the multilevel analysis showed that mother's marital status and infant health

Table 7.4 Retention study: Final hierarchical general linear model (HGLM) analysis of attributes effecting retention in a home-visiting program

	Coefficient	*t*-ratio	Odds-ratio	*p*-value
Community level ($n=12$)				
Community violence index	−0.14	−2.70	0.87	0.02
Home visitor level ($n=71$)				
Monthly hours of supervision	0.64	5.79	1.89	<0.001
Maternal level ($n=1093$)				
Mother is Hispanic	0.39	2.50	1.48	<0.01
Mothers age in years	0.04	2.76	1.04	<0.01

risks were not significantly related to remaining in home visiting services for 1 year or more. This model was used to examine all possible interactions within and across the three levels. There were no significant interactions.

Conclusion

Using different samples, these two studies sought to deepen our understanding of how multiple factors influence engagement and retention in home visiting child abuse prevention programs. These findings suggest that program engagement and retention are just as much a function of the community and provider as they are a function of the individuals receiving services. Community health and community violence should be considered when providing services. One method to address these issues is to promote family involvement in community health and safety organizations. Mothers who live in isolation may require additional efforts to secure their engagement in program services. Enlisting the support of other family members could enhance engagement. Providing home visitors with regular and ongoing supervision is crucial in increasing family retention. Supervisors should periodically shadow home visitors and provide visitors opportunities to discuss difficult cases. Regular supervision and ongoing staff training would promote a sense of value and reduce the likelihood of staff burnout.

Limitations

The findings are based on non-Hispanic (77 %) and Hispanic (19.5 %) families who received home visits in semirural and small metropolitan areas. Although this sample parallels the characteristics of many young Oregon families, future studies may wish to examine these relationships in a more ethnically diverse or urban sample. Moreover, although counties were a meaningful focus for these studies, future studies may wish to narrow their focus to attributes at the zip code, school district, or census block level. This would provide a more rigorous investigation of how community violence influences retention rates and allow multiple community factors, such as social integration and social cohesion (McCurdy & Daro, 2001), to be included in the analyses. Despite these limitations, these studies illustrate the utility of considering community, home visitor, and maternal attributes when developing strategies for engaging and retaining families in home visiting child abuse prevention programs.

References

Barth, R., Ash, J., & Hacking, S. (1986). Identifying, screening and engaging high-risk clients in private non-profit child abuse prevention programs. *Child Abuse & Neglect, 10,* 99–106.

Belsky, J., & Rovine, M. (1990). Patterns of marital change across the transition to parenthood. *Journal of Marriage and the Family, 52,* 5–19.

Bronfenbrenner, U. (1979). *The ecology of human development: Experiments by nature and design.* Cambridge: Harvard University Press.

Bureau of the Census. (1999). *USA counties 1998 on CD-ROM* (machine-readable data files) prepared by the Bureau of the Census. Washington: The Bureau (Producer and distributor). http://govinfo.library.orst.edu/ stateis.html. Accessed 1 May 2001.

Clark, J., & Winje, C. (1998). *Participant engagement and retention in health related programs: Literature review.* Unpublished manuscript, National Committee to Prevent Child Abuse, Chicago, IL.

Coulton, C., Korbin, J., Su, M., & Chow, J. (1995). Community level factors and child maltreatment rates. *Child Development, 66,* 1262–1276.

Damashek, A., Doughty, D., Ware, L., & Silovsky, J. (2011). Predictors of client engagement and attrition in home-based child maltreatment prevention services. *Child Maltreatment, 16,* 9–20.

Daro, D., & Gelles, R. J. (1992). Public attitudes and behaviors with respect to child abuse prevention. *Journal of Interpersonal Violence, 7,* 517–531.

Daro, D., & Harding, K. (1999). Healthy families America: Using research to enhance practice. *Future of Children, 9,* 152–176.

Daro, D., McCurdy, K., Falconnier, L., & Stojanovic, D. (2003). Sustaining new parents in home visitation services: Key participant and program factors. *Child Abuse & Neglect, 27,* 1101–1125.

Davis, M. H. (1983). Measuring individual differences in empathy: Evidence for a multidimensional approach. *Journal of Personality and Social Psychology, 44,* 113–126.

Duggan, A., Windham, A., McFarlane, E., Fuddy, L., Rohde, C., Buchbinder, S., & Sia, C. (2000). Hawaii's healthy start program of home visiting for at-risk families: Evaluation of family identification, family engagement, and service delivery. *Pediatrics, 105*(1), 250–260.

Dumka, L., Garza, C., Roosa, M., & Stoerzinger, H. (1997). Recruitment and retention of high-risk families into a preventive parent training intervention. *The Journal of Primary Prevention, 18*(1), 25–39.

Garbarino, J., & Kostelny, K. (1992). Child maltreatment as a community problem. *Child Abuse & Neglect, 16,* 455–464.

Garbarino, J., & Sherman, D. (1980). High-risk neighborhoods and high-risk families: The human ecology of child maltreatment. *Child Development, 51,* 188–198.

Gomby, D., Culross, P., & Behrman, R. (1999). Home visiting: Recent program evaluations—Analysis and recommendations. *The Future of Children, 9,* 4–26.

Guterman, N. B. (2000). Enrollment strategies in early home visitation to prevent physical child abuse and neglect and the "universal versus targeted" debate: A meta-analysis of population-based and screening-based programs. *Child Abuse & Neglect, 23,* 863–890.

Hawaii Family Stress Center. (1994). *Early identification training materials: Healthy families America*. Honolulu: Hawaii Family Stress Center.

Josten, L., Mullett, S., Savik, K., Campbell, R., & Vincent, P. (1995). Client characteristics associated with not keeping appointments for public health nursing home visits. *Public Health Nursing, 12*(5), 305–311.

Katzev, A. R., Pratt, C. C., & McGuigan, W. (2001). *Oregon healthy start 1999–2000 status report*. Corvallis: Oregon State University.

Korfmacher, J. (2000). The Kempe Family Stress Inventory: A review. *Child Abuse & Neglect, 24*(1), 129–140.

Korfmacher, J., O'Brien, R., Hiatt, S., & Olds, D. (1999). Differences in program implementation between nurses and paraprofessionals providing home visits during pregnancy and infancy: A randomized trial. *American Journal of Public Health, 89*(12), 1847–1851.

Larner, M., Halpern, R., & Harkavy, O. (1992). The fair start story: An overview. In M. Larner, R. Halpern, & O. Harkavy (Eds.), *Fair start for children: Lessons learned from seven demonstration projects* (pp. 3–22). New Haven: Yale University Press.

Luker, K. A., & Chalmers, K. I. (1990). Gaining access to clients: The case of health visiting. *Journal of Advanced Nursing, 15,* 74–82.

Lynch, M., & Cicchetti, D. (1998). An ecological-transactional analysis of children and contexts: The longitudinal interplay among child maltreatment, community violence, and children's symptomatology. *Development and Psychopathology, 10,* 235–257.

Marcenko, M., & Spence, M. (1994). Home visitation services for at-risk pregnant and postpartum women: A randomized trial. *American Journal of Orthopsychiatry, 64,* 468–478.

McCurdy, K., & Daro, D. (2001). Parent involvement in family support programs: An integrated theory. *Family Relations, 50,* 113–121.

McGuigan, W. M., & Pratt, C. C. (2001). The predictive impact of domestic violence on three types of child maltreatment. *Child Abuse & Neglect, 25,* 869–883.

McGuigan, W. M., Katzev, A. R., & Pratt, C. C. (2003a). Multi-level determinants of retention in a home-visiting child abuse prevention program. *Child Abuse & Neglect, 27,* 363–380.

McGuigan, W. M., Katzev, A. R., & Pratt, C. C. (2003b). Multi-level determinants of mothers' engagement in home visitation services. *Family Relations, 52,* 271–278.

Myers-Walls, J. A., Elicker, J., & Bandyk, J. (1997). *Which families stay and which ones leave an early home visiting program?* Paper presented at the 105th annual convention of the American Psychological Association, Chicago.

National Committee to Prevent Child Abuse. (1996). *Intensive home visitation: A randomized trial, follow-up and risk assessment study of Hawaii's healthy start program*. Chicago: National Committee to Prevent Child Abuse (now known as Prevent Child Abuse America).

Navaie-Waliser, M., Martin, S. L., Campbell, M. K., Tessaro, I., Kotelchuck, M., & Cross, A. W. (2000). Factors predicting completion of a home visitation program by high-risk pregnant women: The North Carolina maternal outreach worker program. *American Journal of Public Health, 90,* 121–124.

Olds, D., & Kitzman, H. (1993). Review of research on home visiting for pregnant women and parents of young children. *The Future of Children, 3*(3), 53–92.

Olds, D., Henderson, C., Kitzman, H., Eckenrode, J., Cold, R., & Tatelbaum, R. (1999). Prenatal and infancy home visitation by nurses: Recent findings. *The Future of Children, 1,* 44–65.

Oregon Department of Human Services. (1999). *Oregon's 1998 county profiles. Office of alcohol and drug abuse programs*. Salem: Oregon Department of Human Services.

Osofsky, J. D. (1995). The effects of exposure to violence on young children. *American Psychologist, 50*(9), 782–788.

Powell, D. (1984). Social network and demographic predictors of length of participation in a parent education program. *Journal of Community Psychology, 12,* 13–20.

Prevent Child Abuse America. (1999). *Healthy families America: A snapshot view*. Chicago: Prevent Child Abuse America.

Raudenbush, S., Bryk, A., Cheong, Y. F., & Congdon, R. (2000). *HLM5 hierarchical linear and nonlinear modeling*. Lincolnwood: Scientific Software International, Inc.

Sweet, M. A., & Applebaum, M. I. (2004). Is home visiting an effective strategy? A meta-analytic review of home visiting programs for families with young children. *Child Development, 75,* 1435–1456.

Taafee-Young, K., Davis, K., & Schoen, C. (1996). *The Commonwealth fund survey of parents with young children.* New York: The Commonwealth Fund.

US Department of Health and Human Services. (2000). *Child maltreatment 1998: Reports from the states to the National Child Abuse and Neglect Data System. Administration on children, youth, and families.* Washington, DC: US Government Printing Office.

Vig, S. (1996). Young children's exposure to community violence. *Journal of Early Intervention, 20,* 319–328.

Wagner, M., & Clayton, S. (1999). The parents as teachers program: Results from two demonstrations. *The Future of Children, 9,* 91–115.

Wallach, V. A., & Lister, L. (1995). Stages in the delivery of home-based services to parents at risk of child abuse: A healthy start experience. *Scholarly Inquiry for Nursing Practice: An International Journal, 9*(2), 159–173.

Wasik, B. H. (1993). Staffing issues for home visiting programs. *The Future of Children, 3*(3), 140–157.

William M. McGuigan (USA): Associate professor of human development and family studies at the Pennsylvania State University—Shenango Campus. He is a certified family life educator and a member of the American Professional Society on the Abuse of Children, the American Sociological Association, and the National Council on Family Relations. He has served on the review board of *Child Abuse & Neglect, The International Journal.* His research focuses on child abuse, family violence, and the effectiveness of home visitation programs.

Breanna Gassner (USA): Graduate student with a master's degree in American studies and a degree in human development and family studies. She has worked as a research assistant and data analyst on projects related to bias and racial prejudice and has presented her research at national conferences. Currently, she works as an administrative assistant and tutor in the Learning Center at the Pennsylvania State University—Shenango Campus.

Chapter 8
Addressing Psychosocial Risk Factors Among Families Enrolled in Home Visitation: Issues and Opportunities

S. Darius Tandon

Home visitation (HV) for expectant and new mothers is one of the largest avenues through which perinatal women come to the attention of service providers. HV is prevalent in North America as well as in Asia, Africa, Europe, and South America and uses both professional and paraprofessional models. HV programs are focused on improving maternal and child health outcomes such as reducing infant mortality, child abuse, neglect, and improving infant and young child development and access to pediatric and primary care. HV program services may be provided by paraprofessional and/or professional staff. Paraprofessional home visitors are often individuals from the same communities in which the clients reside. As such, the use of paraprofessional home visitors is hypothesized to promote trust and rapport between home visitors and clients. Professional home visitors include nurses and social workers who conduct home visits. They are hypothesized to promote positive maternal and child outcomes, in part, due to the clients' willingness to have a trusted professional providing information and support. Although specific HV models vary somewhat in their specific intervention approach, these programs generally involve regular visits to pregnant and recently delivered women. Core HV services typically include (a) preparation for childbirth and having a young child in the home, (b) provision of emotional and tangible (e.g., diapers and formula) social support, (c) discussion about infant and young child development, and (d) referrals to community resources for social and health services.

HV has been shown to produce improved outcomes for mothers and young children in areas such as prevention of child abuse and neglect, maternal health, child development and school readiness, family economic self-sufficiency, and positive parenting practices. A meta-analysis of 60 HV programs conducted by Sweet and Appelbaum (2004) concluded that children of women in HV programs tended to exhibit more favorable outcomes than control group children, with no differences found between programs using professional compared with paraprofessional home

S. D. Tandon (✉)
Feinberg School of Medicine, Northwestern University, Chicago IL, USA
e-mail: dtandon@northwestern.edu

L. Roggman, N. Cardia (eds.), *Home Visitation Programs*,
DOI 10.1007/978-3-319-17984-1_8

visitors. Although HV programs have been shown to be effective in promoting maternal and child health outcomes, at the same time there is growing recognition that a "one size fits all" model of HV is not likely to meet the diverse needs of HV clients and, therefore, will not result in equally favorable outcomes across HV clients.

A growing body of research has illustrated that psychosocial risk factors—in particular, maternal depression, substance abuse, and intimate partner violence—are prevalent among HV clients (Ammerman et al., 2009; Chazen-Cohen et al., 2007; Ferguson et al., 2006). However, these psychosocial risks are often not identified or are poorly addressed by HV programs (Duggan et al., 2007; Tandon, Parillo, Jenkins, and Duggan, 2005). Moreover, the presence of these psychosocial risk factors may limit clients' engagement in their HV programs as well as complicate the development of a working relationship between a client and her home visitor. These psychosocial risk factors are also likely to contribute to HV programs' limited effectiveness in improving outcomes for women enrolled in these programs. For example, Duggan, Berlin, Cassidy, Burrell, and Tandon (2009) found that maternal depression moderates the impact of HV on maternal and child health outcomes. Similarly, Eckenrode et al. (2000) demonstrated that while HV reduced child maltreatment rates for women exposed to fewer incidents of intimate partner violence, HV programs did not have an effect on child maltreatment among those with greater exposure to partner violence. As such, HV programs require specific strategies and approaches for addressing psychosocial risk factors among their clients.

This chapter has three objectives. Each of these objectives attempts to provide HV programs with concrete approaches for addressing psychosocial risks among their clients. First, this chapter will provide recommendations for HV programs to identify psychosocial risks among their clients. Second, it will provide specific examples of approaches to enhance home visitors' capacity to address psychosocial risks among their clients. Third, it will provide recommendations on ways to augment existing HV program models to address psychosocial risk factors.

Identification of Psychosocial Risk Factors by Home Visitation Programs

Screening is an important initial step in addressing psychosocial risks in perinatal women. Effective screening can help HV programs detect women who are affected by these risk factors, facilitating HV programs' ability to make appropriate referrals to outside resources and to discuss the risk factors during the course of home visits. A handful of studies have demonstrated the feasibility of screening for psychosocial risk factors among pregnant and recently delivered women in primary care clinics and OB/GYN clinics (Baisch, Carey, Conway, & Mounts, 2010; Chaudron, Szilagyi, Kitzman, Wadkins, & Conwell, 2004; Miller, Shade, & Vasireddy, 2009; Olson et al., 2005; Segre, O'Hara, Arndt, & Beck, 2010). Despite these findings establishing the feasibility of conducting screening during the perinatal period in primary care and OB/GYN clinics, a relatively small percentage of perinatal women actually are screened for psychosocial risks (Goodman & Tyer-Viola, 2010; Kelly, Zatzick, & Anders, 2001; Marcus, Flynn, Blow, & Barry, 2003). This lack of systematic screening for psychosocial risk factors in primary care and OB/GYN clinics suggests that other settings serving perinatal women, such as HV, are important venues for identifying women who could benefit from services and supports to address these common concerns.

Most HV program models call for systematic assessments to be completed with pregnant or recently delivered women to determine program eligibility and assess client risk and protective factors. As part of this assessment process, many HV programs screen for some psychosocial risk factors. However, not all programs require screening for depression, substance abuse, and intimate partner violence. Additionally, many programs use screening tools that do not have established validity with perinatal populations, calling into question their utility. A final concern related to HV programs' current screening practices is the lack of clarity on how ongoing assessment for psychosocial risks should be conducted. For example, due to the episodic nature of depression, a client may not need mental health services at the time of initial screening, but may develop subclinical or clinical depression in subsequent weeks and months. Relying solely on screening at the time of enrollment would likely not identify this client as needing mental health services.

To promote more effective identification of maternal depression, substance abuse, and intimate partner violence among women enrolled in HV programs, HV programs should focus attention to three interrelated issues:

1. Systematically screen newly enrolling clients

Given the prevalence of maternal depression, substance abuse, and intimate partner violence among HV clients, HV programs should systematically screen all newly enrolling clients for these three psychosocial risk factors. Making psychosocial risk screening part of the routine assessment process used by HV programs is important to eliminate subjectivity or "educated guessing" on the part of those conducting assessments. Equally important, systematic screening can minimize any stigmatization that clients may feel; if all clients are being screened using the same tools and protocols, screening will not be viewed as a "special" service for a segment of HV clients, but as ongoing and accepted activities that are part of the HV program's standard operating procedures.

To conduct systematic screening for maternal depression, substance abuse, and intimate partner violence among newly enrolling clients, HV programs need to identify the point in the enrollment process when screening will be conducted and who will be conducting the screening. For some HV programs, screening is conducted by an intake assessment worker, while other programs have a home visitor administer screening tools to clients that will become part of his/her caseload. Regardless of who conducts the screening, HV programs should provide training on the use of each screening tool. This includes not only instruction on how to administer and score a screening tool, but also on appropriate language and protocol for discussing the results of the screening. In some cases, the individual conducting the screening will refer clients with a "positive" screen to a resource within or outside the HV program for further assessment, while in other programs, this individual will let the client know that results of the screen will be discussed with her at a later point in time. Regardless of the specific process used by a HV program, the individual conducting the screening needs to discuss the screening process and screening results in a nonjudgmental and supportive manner.

2. Use well-established screening tools for psychosocial risks

To effectively screen for psychosocial risks, HV programs should use screening tools that are reliable and valid for a perinatal population. Additionally, to minimize burden on HV enrollees, screening tools should ideally be brief. Fortunately, such screening tools exist and reviews of these tools are available to guide HV programs in their selection (Boyd, Le, & Somberg, 2005; Burns, Gray, & Smith, 2010; Nelson, Bougatson, & Blazina, 2012). In relation to maternal depression, Boyd et al. (2005) recommend the use of the Edinburgh Postnatal Depression Scale (EPDS; Cox, Holden, & Sagovsky, 1987), with the Beck Depression Inventory (BDI-II, Beck, Steer, & Brown, 1996) and the Postpartum Depression Screening Scale (PDSS; Beck & Gable, 2000) was also highlighted as appropriate tools for perinatal depression screening. Although not reviewed by Boyd et al. (2005), the Patent Health Questionnaire 2-item and 9-item scales (Kroenke, Spitzer, & Williams, 2001, 2003) are also increasingly used in primary care and OB/GYN settings and are brief, no-cost measures. For intimate partner violence, a review by Nelson et al. (2012) highlighted several tools with high diagnostic accuracy, including several brief screeners such as the 4-item HITS scale (Chen, Rovi, Vega, Jacobs, & Johnson, 2005) and 3-item Partner Violence Screen (PVS; Houry et al., 2004). Substance abuse screening should encompass both alcohol and drug use with some tools recommended for assessing alcohol use, such as the T-ACE (Sokol, Martier, & Ager, 1989) or TWEAK (Russell, 1994), while others such as the 4P's Plus (Chasnoff et al., 2005) assesses both alcohol and drug use.

3. Develop a plan for ongoing screening

It is also recommended that HV programs conduct ongoing screening for psychosocial risk factors rather than just one screening at the time of client enrollment. Some psychosocial risks that were not present at the time of initial screening may arise later in pregnancy or the postpartum period. For example, many women will eliminate alcohol and drug use during pregnancy out of concern for the health of their baby; however, some women—particularly those living in highly stressful environments—may begin to use alcohol or drugs after delivery as a way to cope with the stressors of parenting. Another reason to conduct repeated psychosocial risk screening relates to the nature of the relationship between HV clients and the HV program. Some clients may not be comfortable endorsing psychosocial screening questions upon enrollment in a HV program because of limited rapport with the program. As trust develops over the course of time thanks to the intensive home visitor–client relationship, a client may be more likely to disclose and discuss sensitive topics such as depression, substance use, or partner violence.

One example of ongoing screening for intimate partner violence in the USA comes from the Multonomah County Health Department (MCHD) in Portland, Oregon. Home visiting services are provided by MCHD, and women are screened for intimate partner violence during the prenatal period and at least once postpartum. In addition, clients are screened for intimate partner violence when significant life changes occur, such as a relationship change or job change. To facilitate ongoing screening for psychosocial risks, HV programs should consider developing automated reminders for home visitors to conduct screenings at predetermined time intervals and/or in conjunction with key client milestones (e.g., relationship change and after delivery). These reminders can be programmed into the management information systems used by HV programs and, therefore, minimize the likelihood that HV programs will forget when to conduct follow-up assessments.

Enhancing Home Visitors' Capacity to Address Psychosocial Risks Among Their Clients

Another notable challenge facing HV programs is their ability to effectively provide needed services and supports, should screening identify one or more psychosocial risks. Several studies have shown that HV programs frequently do not respond to maternal depression, substance use, or intimate partner violence (Duggan et al., 2004, 2007; Tandon et al., 2005). While there are several reasons that contribute to HV programs' lack of response to these psychosocial risks, one factor is home visitors' limited attention to these risk factors during the course of home visits. In a qualitative study conducted with paraprofessional home visitors working in a low-income urban environment in the USA, Tandon et al. (2005) found that home visitors desired more training on when and how to initiate conversations about mental health, substance abuse, and intimate partner violence during the course of home visits. Home visitors in this study also pointed out that their training on psychosocial risk factors was largely focused on knowledge acquisition, with little attention placed on developing skills to introduce and discuss psychosocial risks with clients. A focus group study by Eddy, Kilburn, Chang, Bullock, and Sharps (2008) found similar findings when asking home visitors to discuss challenges to addressing intimate partner violence—specifically, that home visitors felt they lacked knowledge on when and how to address intimate partner violence within the context of a typical home visit. In response to these identified gaps in home visitors' capacity to address clients' psychosocial risks, three recommendations are provided for HV programs:

1. Be explicit in defining when and how psychosocial risks are to be addressed and ensure that home visitors understand their roles

The field of implementation science seeks to understand the behavior of healthcare providers—both professional and paraprofessional—as a key variable related to the implementation of interventions, services, and programs. Central to implementation science is the recognition that healthcare settings, such as HV programs, need to have service delivery models that clearly and coherently describe how services are to be delivered. In the absence of clear service models, programs may not be implemented as model developers intended.

HV programs need to clearly specify when and how psychosocial risks are to be addressed by home visitors during the course of regular home visits. This starts with clearly presenting, in written program manuals, how psychosocial risks should be discussed. For example, if home visitors are required to check in about one or more psychosocial risks during a particular home visit, this should be specified in the HV program's standard operating procedures. Further, if there are specific questions or activities that the home visitor should use to initiate conversation, these should also be provided in HV program manuals. There should also be explicit instructions regarding how to address psychosocial risks if clients appear resistant to discussing these topics with home visitors, or if there are environmental factors that preclude home visitors from discussing psychosocial risks. For example, a home visitor should have clear instructions on how to engage in conversations about intimate partner violence if a client's partner is within earshot.

There also needs to be clarity in HV program models on how home visitors should discuss clients' psychosocial needs if clients have pressing housing, financial, or emergency needs for which clients give greater priority. This is particularly important given the strengths-based approach used by home visiting programs that attempts to "meet the client where she is." Moreover, it should be emphasized to home visitors that addressing psychosocial risk factors is not inconsistent with a strengths-based approach for working with clients, but rather that addressing psychosocial risks is a key variable that affects a HV program's ability to affect its intended maternal and child health outcomes.

2. Acknowledge and address home visitors' attitudes and beliefs toward psychosocial risks

One of the frequently highlighted strengths of paraprofessional HV programs is their recruitment and training of home visitors who are from the same geographic communities as the clients the program serves (Wasik, 1993). By hiring individuals indigenous to the communities in which HV is conducted, paraprofessional HV programs are hypothesized to facilitate greater trust and rapport between clients and home visitors. While previous research has validated the notion that paraprofessional home visitors are able to effectively establish trust and rapport with their clients, it is also important to critically examine areas in which paraprofessional home visitors may require additional training, guidance, and support. Specifically, home visitors' perceptions of mental health as stigmatizing is an understudied, and potentially important, variable impeding HV clients' receipt of needed services of psychosocial risks. To that end, Musik and Scott (1990) note that HV programs need to provide opportunities for staff to reflect on their own attitudes that may influence the manner in which they deliver services to families.

3. Assure that initial and ongoing training and supervision are available and adequate to develop and maintain staff skills in addressing MH, IPV, SA, and to assure that these skills are used

Again drawing on the field of implementation science, training and supervision of home visitors are key components of HV programs' implementation systems. In the same way, HV programs need to have clear and coherent program models that guide service delivery, HV programs also should have training and supervision that effectively prepare home visitors to meet the varied needs of their clients. Evidence-based HV programs will typically include an initial orientation and training for newly hired home visitors. Also common among evidence-based HV programs is the provision of ongoing training to home visitors across a range of topics deemed relevant to improving maternal and child health outcomes. HV programs also provide ongoing supervision to home visitors, typically in the form of weekly one-on-one meetings between an individual home visitor and a program supervisor. Despite the presence of initial and ongoing training and supervision for home visitors, it has been posited that HV programs need to place increasing value and priority on these aspects of their implementation system rather than viewing them simply as an administrative procedure to ensure that home visitors are completing assigned tasks (Wasik, 1993). Several strategies are described below that may enhance home visitors' acquisition and use of knowledge and approaches to address clients' psychosocial risk factors.

One promising strategy for improving home visitors' ability to identify and respond to clients' psychosocial risk factors is the use of reflective supervision. Defined as "the process of examining, with someone else, the thoughts, feelings, actions, and reactions evoked in the course of working closely with young children and their families" (Eggbeer, Mann, & Seibel, 2008), reflective supervision has been increasingly turned to within child and family services as a promising model for enhancing staff members' self-efficacy and autonomy. At its core, reflective supervision emphasizes the creation of a staff–supervisor relationship rather than a hierarchy in which supervisors give directives to staff. Moreover, staff strengths are emphasized while their limitations are considered in the context of partnerships with supervisors to create joint responsibility for addressing clients' needs.

Several key stages of reflective supervision have been clearly articulated (Parlakian, 2001). The initial stage is typically referred to as the planning stage, with an emphasis on developing a regular time for the supervisor and staff member to meet free from interruption. This regularity is important in relation to the home visitors' ability to address psychosocial risk factors in their clients. For example, behavior change related to substance abuse or partner violence is often understood using the transtheoretical or "stages of change" model (Prochaska & DiClemente, 1983) in which an individual moves from a precontemplation (i.e., not yet acknowledging that there is a problem) or contemplation phase (i.e., acknowledging that there is a problem but not being ready or sure of wanting to make a change) to action (i.e., changing behavior). This process may be a lengthy one, in which an individual may encounter a relapse back to an earlier stage. Additionally, throughout the process of moving toward action, an individual needs to gain confidence that they can make and maintain their behavior change. A home visitor working with a client contemplating behavior change is likely to need ongoing support from a clinical or program supervisor, which can be facilitated by the regularity of reflective supervision.

Another stage of the reflective supervision process focuses on information gathering as an approach to most accurately and comprehensively address a situation a staff member may be addressing with a client. Central to information gathering is the use of active listening and open-ended questions by the supervisor to support the development of greater insight and clarification on the part of the staff member. For example, in the context of a reflective supervision session in which a client with possible depressive symptoms is being discussed, the supervisor may ask the staff member an open-ended question such as "Help me understand what you are seeing with your client…" or "Tell me about what you are experiencing when you visited your client…." These open-ended questions can help the home visitor reflect on his/her experiences working with the client. Additionally, when reflecting on these experiences, reflective supervision encourages staff to freely express their challenges and possible solutions. In the example of a client with possible depressive symptoms, a reflective supervision process could facilitate a home visitors' discussion of barriers to getting the client to talk about the stressors in her life contributing to her emotional state. This, in turn, could generate a conversation between the home visitor and his/her supervisor on strategies that could be used to gather this information.

A second strategy to improve home visitors' identification and response to clients' psychosocial risk factors is the use of coaching to develop home visitors' skills. Stokes and Baer (1977) argue that a "train and hope" approach does not appear to generate high-quality program implementation. Fixsen, Naoom, Blase, Friedman, and Wallace (2005) expand on this assertion, claiming that while training is necessary to promote high-quality program implementation, a simultaneous focus on coaching staff on how to use knowledge and skills is essential. Coaching is conducted by an experienced individual who is able to draw on his/her previous experience to provide guidance and support to staff member. Spouse (2001) identified three main functions of coaching that go beyond traditional supervision: (1) teaching during service delivery, (2) assessment and feedback, and (3) provision of emotional support. A meta-analysis by Joyce and Showers (2002) illustrated that the strongest effects on teachers' implementation of knowledge in classroom settings were generated when teachers received not only intensive training (i.e., practice and feedback) but also coaching.

Fixsen et al. (2005) note that one of the reasons coaching is essential is due to the inherent limitations on staff training. Training for new staff is limited, in that it can only develop entry-level knowledge and skills whereas ongoing staff training is largely constrained by time demands. Thus, although staff—such as home visitors—typically receive initial and ongoing training as part of their job, this training typically focuses on knowledge procurement and lacks the ability to practice skills and receive feedback and support. As noted earlier, many home visitors—particularly those who are paraprofessionals—may have attitudes and beliefs toward psychosocial risk factors that influence their handling of these issues with clients. Spouse (2001) notes that coaching can help staff if they experience discomfort or stress in handling a certain situation during a client interaction, largely through the provision of emotional support. As an example, a home visitor who has had an experience with intimate partner violence—either personally or through contact with a friend or family member—may experience discomfort discussing this issue because of feelings this topic conjure up. While a coach may not be able to completely alleviate the discomfort felt by the home visitor, the coach could provide strategies for setting appropriate boundaries for the home visitor such that the home visitor is able to initiate conversation and make an appropriate referral within or outside the program while not engaging in conversations that are too uncomfortable.

The SafeCare home visiting program is an evidence-based structured behavioral skills training program for parents in child protective services (CPS) for child neglect (Lutzker & Bigelow, 2002). As part of a randomized cluster experiment, Chaffin, Hecht, Bard, Silovsky, and Beasley (2012) demonstrated that the use of coached home visitors yielded some advantages over uncoached home visitors, particularly when working with diverse home visiting clients that fell outside typical program inclusion criteria. In this study, individuals who were employed as home visitors in the SafeCare program and nominated as credible and influential by their peers, were trained to serve as coaches using a developmental consultation model (Stoltenberg & McNeill, 2010). Coaches were also given additional, more extensive training on the SafeCare model. Coaches accompanied home visitors on a home visit at least once per month, used fidelity checklists to facilitate the coaching process, and met regularly with study investigators and SafeCare developers to receive guidance on their role as coaches.

Another innovative training tool for home visitors is the use of "simulated" or "standardized" clients trained to play the role of a home visiting client to which home visitors deliver a home visit. Initially used by commercial marketing firms, the use of standardized clients has been increasingly used in recent years as a training tool for physicians, nurses, and other health-care professionals. In the context of HV, standardized clients can allow home visitors to practice the use of skills and approaches for discussing an array of relevant topics, including psychosocial risk factors.

Put into practice, home visitors could be told that as part of their training they will be asked to practice responding to clients' psychosocial needs in the course of a mock, or simulated, home visit. During this mock home visit, the standardized clients would "present" to the home visitor a situation involving one or more psychosocial risk factors—e.g., maternal depression, substance use, or partner violence. To ensure that the simulated clients are trained to produce a situation as reproducible to a real home visit as possible, prior to using a standardized client approach HV programs should generate insights from HV clients, home visitors, and supervisors on common ways in which psychosocial risks are brought up during the course of a home visit. Home visitors could be asked to practice certain skills related to addressing psychosocial risk factors during an interaction with a standardized clients; these skills could vary depending on home visitor characteristics and prior training. For example, a paraprofessional home visitor relatively new to a HV program may need to practice skills related to better understanding the severity and period of time the risk factor has been present, so that the home visitor could provide that information to a clinical supervisor who could determine whether more intensive services are needed. In contrast, a more seasoned home visitor may benefit from a standardized client session in which she is asked to encourage a reticent home visiting client to follow through on a mental health, substance abuse, or intimate partner violence referral.

The use of standardized clients can provide HV programs with a training approach that allows home visitors to practice skills and approaches related to addressing psychosocial risk factors in a setting as close to the real situation as possible. As home visitors are not working with actual clients, they may be more willing to use skills, approaches, and language that they are hesitant to use in an actual home visit for fear of how clients may respond. As a training and teaching tool, the standardized client interaction can be observed by a home visiting program supervisor who can provide immediate feedback to the home visitor on strengths and limitations of the interaction. One of the unique aspects of a standardized client approach is that the individual playing the role of standardized client can also provide feedback to the home visitor. This feedback can focus on several aspects of the home visitors' approach, including but not limited to the ability to establish rapport, body language, choice of words or phrases, and empathy.

Although not focused on addressing psychosocial risks, Bryans and colleagues (Bryans, 2004; Bryans & McIntosh, 2007) undertook a study that used standardized clients in the context of nurse HV program. They note that the rationale for their work emanated from the lack of evidence on how different experiential learning approaches could be used to develop the expertise of home visitors. This study used audio- and video-recorded simulations and analyzed the nature of home visitor–client interactions. Along these lines, HV programs should consider partnerships with researchers who have expertise in the area of physician–client communication. For example, there has been considerable work done in the past two decades on the development of methods to analyze medical encounters and the training of health-care providers to enhance their communication skills (Roter & Larson, 2002).

Augmenting HV Program Models to Address Psychosocial Risk Factors

The strategies described in the previous section—reflective supervision, coaching, and standardized clients—are potentially useful in enhancing home visitors' skills and self-efficacy to respond to clients' psychosocial risk factors. For some clients, home visitor support and guidance may adequately address their needs related to a particular psychosocial risk. For example, some home visiting clients may have chronically stressful lives and exhibit mild depressive symptoms, but regular home visitor contact may be sufficient to provide necessary support to effectively cope with these stressors and monitor clients' mental health. However, many HV clients require additional supports and services beyond what well-trained and supervised home visitors can provide during the course of regular home visits. This section describes two specific strategies for more effectively responding to home visiting clients' psychosocial risk factors.

1. Improve systematic monitoring of client referrals

Although some HV programs have on-site mental health, substance abuse, or intimate partner violence services, a majority of the programs refer women to outside mental health, social service, or healthcare organizations when clients require more intensive services related to these issues. Effective screening for psychosocial risks, as described earlier, may help in improving identification of clients with greatest need for these additional supports and services. However, screening for psychosocial risk factors comes with an ethical responsibility to appropriately provide services to women with identified needs. Unfortunately, many HV programs do not have standardized protocols for referring clients to outside agencies for mental health, substance abuse, or intimate partner violence services. As a result, some women identified as needing services may not be referred in a timely fashion. Moreover, many HV programs do not have standard operating procedures for monitoring clients' receipt of services once referred to an outside agency to address a psychosocial risk factor. This limits home visitors' ability to ensure clients' follow-up with an outside agency. It also inhibits home visitors' capacity to reinforce any key messages provided by an outside agency.

One promising example of how HV can effectively refer and monitor clients for the psychosocial risk factor of maternal depression comes from the Ohio Department of Health's Help-Me-Grow statewide HV program. This HV program, implemented at the county level, throughout the state, works in close collaboration with the state's mental health agency—the Ohio Department of Mental Health. Help-Me-Grow home visitors administer a depression screener—the EPDS (Cox et al., 1987)—to new mothers with infants ages 4–20 weeks. Home visitors enter the EPDS score and demographic data into a web-based data system that automatically scores the EPDS and prompts the home visitor to make a referral for women scoring above the commonly accepted EPDS cutoff for clinically significant depressive symptoms. The web-based data system can email a copy of the EPDS and other pertinent demographic information about the client to an outside mental health agency, or the referral information can be printed and subsequently mailed or faxed by the HV program to the mental health agency. Once a referral is made, the database automatically prompts a designated individual at the HV program to contact the mental health agency at 30 and 90 days to see if an appointment was made and whether it was kept.

Although having formal protocols for initiating and monitoring referrals is critical, another important variable related to strengthening HV programs' referral and monitoring process is the relationship between home visitors and outside agencies to which clients are referred. An example from the field of nursing (Garcia et al., 2012) illustrates how nurses screening for intimate partner violence received staff in-service trainings during which representatives from community-based agencies to which clients would be referred for intimate partner violence came to the nursing clinic to meet nursing staff, present their services, and allow nurses to ask questions of agency providers and build rapport. Through the process of bringing these community-based agencies to the obstetrics clinic, nurses' comfort level with the outside agencies was heightened, thereby enhancing the likelihood that they would make referrals and follow-up with the outside agency about their clients.

2. Augment existing home visiting services

Even with more systematic HV referral and monitoring procedures for psychosocial risks and better relationships between HV programs and outside community agencies, many HV clients may still refrain from initiating or engaging in services provided by an outside agency due to stigma, fear, or practical barriers such as transportation, childcare, or inconvenient hours. In response to these barriers, there are a growing number of approaches being developed and tested that integrate psychosocial risk treatment and prevention interventions into HV. Ammerman et al. (2011) have developed a depression treatment that is delivered in the home to HV clients experiencing major depressive disorder. This intervention—In-Home Cognitive Behavioral Therapy (IH-CBT)—is manualized and provides cognitive-behavioral therapy sessions in the home of HV clients. Home visitors are utilized to facilitate relationships between the master's degree-level therapist providing IH-CBT and the HV client. Findings from a recently completed clinical trial indicate that HV clients receiving IH-CBT had lower rates of major depressive disorder posttreatment and at a 3-month follow-up. Another mental health enhancement done in HV by Beeber et al. (2010) with newly immigrated Latinas in North Carolina used interpersonal psychotherapy delivered by psychiatric nurses and a Spanish interpreter. Findings from a randomized control trial (RCT) found significant reductions in depressive symptoms 1 month post-intervention.

A program of research conducted by Tandon, Mendelson, Kemp, Leis, and Perry (2011) has focused on prevention of perinatal depression among HV clients through the identification of women at risk for developing major depressive disorder and implementation of a group-based cognitive-behavioral intervention led by a clinical psychologist. In this intervention, home visitors reinforced key content intervention content and encouraged completion of "personal projects" during one-on-one home visits with clients between group sessions. Findings from a recently completed RCT indicated that depressive symptoms declined at a significantly greater rate for intervention participants than women receiving only HV services between baseline and 1 week, 3 months, and 6 months post-intervention. Efforts to integrate intimate partner violence interventions into HV are also being developed and tested. The Domestic Violence Enhanced Home Visitation (DOVE) study is focused on training nurse home visitors to more effectively screen for, and assist, women who have experienced intimate partner violence (Bullock & Sharps, 2011). Currently, an experimental study is being conducted in three different settings to determine the effectiveness of the intervention on outcomes including level of danger, adopted safety behaviors, use of intimate partner violence resources, mental health, and parenting stress.

Summary and Future Directions

This chapter has outlined several key challenges to HV programs' identification and response to clients' psychosocial risk factors. Simultaneously, it has provided several concrete strategies and approaches that HV programs can use to enhance their capacity to respond to these risk factors. Given the prevalence of maternal depression, substance abuse, and intimate partner violence among low-income perinatal women—including those in HV—it is imperative that HV programs strive to address these risk factors in a multifaceted manner. It is important to point out the potential adverse events associated with screening for, and responding to, psychosocial risks, including psychological distress, family disruption, and in most dire cases, potential removal of a child from a mother's care. Therefore, the approaches outlined in this chapter should be carefully reviewed and understood by HV programs prior to their adoption, with appropriate measures in place for dealing with potential adverse events. The psychosocial risk factors presented in this chapter also need to be considered as interrelated phenomena given their comorbidity.

As referenced throughout this chapter, an implementation science framework highlights the multiple levers that need to be attended to when attempting to respond to HV clients' psychosocial risk factors. Program models need to clearly highlight the roles and responsibilities of home visitors in addressing psychosocial risk factors; implementation systems need to provide appropriate and varied supports for home visitors, such as coaching and reflective supervision; and community agencies who provide off-site services for psychosocial risk factors need to be meaningfully and systematically linked with HV programs. Implicit in the approaches and strategies outlined in this chapter is the importance of ensuring buy-in by HV program staff—e.g., home visitors, clinical supervisors, and executive directors. Organizational culture is another important component of an implementation science framework that is likely to influence HV programs' success in effectively and efficiently addressing psychosocial risk factors among their clients.

A final point is to acknowledge the important role that research plays in developing the evidence base for approaches and strategies to address psychosocial risk factors in HV. While many studies have empirically tested various HV program enhancements, it is critical that future enhancements be carefully examined to determine whether and how they should be replicated. Future implementation of the approaches found in this chapter and other relevant approaches should also strive to examine not only participant outcomes associated with enhancements but also the cost-effectiveness of the enhancements and feasibility and acceptability of their implementation.

References

Ammerman, R. T., Putnam, F. W., Altaya, M., Chen, L., Holleb, L., Stevens, J., Short, J., & Van Ginkel, J. B. (2009). Changes in depressive symptoms in first time mothers in home visitation. *Child Abuse & Neglect, 33,* 127–138.

Ammerman, R. T., Putnam, F. W., Stevens, J., Bosse, N. R., Short, J.A., Bodley, A. L., & Van Ginkel, J. B. (2011). An open trial of in-home CBT for depressed mothers in home visitation. *Maternal and Child Health Journal, 15,* 1333–1341.

Baisch, M. J., Carey, L. K., Conway, A. E., & Mounts, K. O. (2010). Perinatal depression: A health marketing campaign to improve screening. *Nursing for Women's Health, 14,* 20–33.

Beck, C. T., & Gable, R. K. (2000). Postpartum depression screening scale: Development and psychometric testing. *Nursing Research, 49,* 272–282.

Beck, A. T., Steer, R. A., & Brown, G. K. (1996). *Manual for beck depression inventory-II*. San Antonio: Psychological Corporation.

Beeber, L. S., Holditch-Davis, D., Perreira, K., Schwartz, T., Lewis, V., Blanchard, H., Anuso, R., & Goldman, B. (2010). Short-term in-home intervention reduces depressive symptoms in early head start Latina mothers of infants and toddlers. *Research in Nursing and Health, 33,* 60–76.

Boyd, R. C., Le, H. N., & Somberg, R. (2005). Review of screening instruments for postpartum depression. *Archives of Women's Mental Health, 8,* 141–155.

Bryans, A. (2004). Examining health visiting expertise: Combining simulation, interview and observation. *Journal of Advanced Nursing, 47,* 623–630.

Bryans, A., & McIntosh, J. (2007). An ecological, information-based approach to the study of expertise: Illustrative findings from a study of UK health-visiting practice. *Learning in Health and Social Care, 6,* 44–58.

Bullock, L., & Sharps, P. (2011). Domestic violence within the context of home visiting: Eight lessons learned from the DOVE intervention. *Prevention and Health Practice*. http://www.futureswithoutviolence.org/health/ejournal/2011/04/domestic-violence-within-the-context-of-home-visitingeight-lessons-from-the-dove-intervention/. Accessed 12 Nov 2012.

Burns, E., Gray, R., & Smith, L. (2010). Brief screening questionnaires to identify problem drinking during pregnancy: A systematic review. *Addiction, 105,* 610–614.

Chaffin, M., Hecht, D., Bard, D., Silovsky, J., & Beasley, W. (2012). A statewide trial of the SafeCare home-based services model with parents in Child Protective Services. *Pediatrics, 129,* 509–515.

Chasnoff, I. J., McGourty, R. F., Bailey, G. W., Hutchins, E., Lightfoot, S. O., Pawson, L. L., Fahey, C., May, B., Brodie, P., McCulley, L., & Campbell, J. (2005). The 4P's plus screen for substance use in pregnancy: Clinical applications and outcomes. *Journal of Perinatalogy, 25*(6), 368–374.

Chaudron, L. H., Szilagyi, P. G., Kitzman, H. J., Wadkins, H. I., & Conwell, Y. (2004). Detection of postpartum depressive symptoms by screening at well-child visits. *Pediatrics, 113,* 551–558.

Chazen-Cohen, R., Ayoub, C., Pan, B. A., Roggman, L., Raikes, H., McKelvey, L., & Hart, A. (2007). It takes time: Impacts of early head start that lead to reductions in maternal depression two years later. *Infant Mental Health Journal, 28,* 151–170.

Chen, P. H., Rovi, S., Vega, M., Jacobs, A., & Johnson, M. S. (2005). Screening for domestic violence in a predominantly Hispanic clinical setting. *Family Practice, 22,* 617–623.

Cox, J., Holden, J., & Sagovsky, R. (1987). Detection of postnatal depression: Development of the 10-item Edinburgh Postnatal Depression Scale. *British Journal of Psychiatry, 150,* 782–786.

Duggan, A. K., Fuddy, L., Burrell, L., Higman, S. M., McFarlane, E., Windham, A., et al. (2004). Randomized trial of a statewide home visiting program to prevent child abuse: Impact in reducing parental risk factors. *Child Abuse and Neglect, 28,* 623–643.

Duggan, A. K., Caldera, D., Rodriguez, K., Burrell, L., Rohde, C., & Crowne, S. (2007). Impact of a statewide home visiting program to prevent child abuse. *Child Abuse and Neglect, 31,* 801–827.

Duggan, A. K., Berlin, L. J., Cassidy, J., Burrell, L., & Tandon, S. D. (2009). Examining maternal depression and attachment insecurity as moderators of the impacts of home visiting for at-risk mothers and infants. *Journal of Consulting and Clinical Psychology, 77,* 788–799.

Eckenrode, J., Ganzel, B., Henderson, C., Smith, E., Olds, D., Powers, J., Cole, R., Kitzman, H., & Sidora, K. (2000). Preventing child abuse and neglect with a program of nurse home visitation: The limiting effects of domestic violence. *Journal of the American Medical Association, 284,* 1385–1391.

Eddy, T., Kilburn, E., Chang, C., Bullock, L., & Sharps, P. (2008). Facilitators and barriers for implementing home visit interventions to address intimate partner violence: Town and gown partnerships. *Nursing Clinics of North America, 43,* 419–435.

Eggbeer, L., Mann, T. & Seibel, N. (2007). Reflective supervision: Past, present, and future. *ZERO TO THREE, 28*(2).

Fergusson, D. M., Grant, H., Horwood, L. J., & Ridder, E. M. (2006). Randomized trial of the Early Start program of home visitation: Parent and family outcomes. *Pediatrics,* 117(3), 781–786. doi:10.1542/peds.2005-1517.

Fixsen, D., Naoom, S., Blase, K., Friedman, R., & Wallace, F. (2005). *Implementation research: A synthesis of the literature*. Tampa: University of South Florida, Louis de la Parte Florida Mental Health Institute, The National Implementation Research Network.

Garcia, L., Coker, A., Williams, C., Clear, E., Jennings, N., Hansen, W., McFarlane, J., & Ferguson, J. (2012). *Lessons learned in implementing a psychosocial screener in a high-risk obstetrics clinic. Prevention and health practice.* http://www.futureswithoutviolence.org/health/ejournal/2012/02/lessons-learned-in-implementing-a-psychosocial-screener-in-a-high-risk-obstetrics-clinic. Accessed 12 Nov 2002.

Goodman, J. H., & Tyer-Viola, L. (2010). Detection, treatment, and referral of perinatal depression and anxiety by obstetrical providers. *Journal of Women's Health, 19,* 477–490.

Houry, D., Feldhaus, K., PeeryB., Abbott, J., Lowenstein, S. R., al-Bataa-de-Montero, S., et al. (2004). A positive domestic violence screen predicts future domestic violence. *Journal of Interpersonal Violence, 19,* 955–66.

Joyce, B., & Showers, B. (2002). *Student achievement through staff development* (3rd ed.). Alexandria: Association for Supervision and Curriculum Development.

Kelly, R., Zatzick, D., & Anders, T. (2001). The detection and treatment of psychiatric disorders and substance use among pregnant women cared for in obstetrics. *American Journal of Psychiatry, 158,* 213–219.

Kroenke, K., Spitzer, R., & Williams, J. (2001). The PHQ-9: Validity of a brief depression severity measure. *Journal of General Internal Medicine, 16,* 606–613.

Kroenke, K., Spitzer, R., & Williams, J. (2003). The patient health quesitonnaire-2: Validity of a two-item depression screener. *Medical Care, 41,* 1284–1292.

Lutzker, J. R., & Bigelow, K. M. (2002). *Reducing child maltreatment: A guidebook for parent services*. New York: Guilford Press.

Marcus, S. M., Flynn, H. A., Blow, F. C., & Barry, K. L., 2003. Depressive symptoms among pregnant women screened in obstetrics settings. *Journal of Women's Health, 12,* 373–380.

Miller, L., Shade, M., & Vasireddy, V. (2009). Beyond screening: Assessment of perinatal depression in a perinatal care setting. *Archive of Women's Mental Health, 12,* 329–334.

Musik, J. S., & Stott, F. M. (1990). Paraprofessionals, parenting, and child development: Understanding the problems and seeking solutions. In S. J. Meisels & J. P. Shonkoff (Eds.), *Handbook of early childhood intervention* (pp. 651–667). Cambridge: Cambridge University Press.

Nelson, H., Bougatson, C., & Blazina, I. (2012). Screening women for intimate partner violence: A systematic review to update the U.S. preventive services task force recommendation. *Annals of Internal Medicine, 156,* 796–808.

Olson, A., Dietrich, A. J., Prazar, G., Hurley, J., Tuddenham, A., Hedberg, V., & Napinsky, D. A. (2005). Two approaches to maternal depression screening during well child visits. *Journal of Developmental and Behavioral Pediatrics, 26,* 169–176.

Parlakian, R. (2001). *Look, listen, and learn: Reflective supervision and relationship-based work.* Washington, DC: Zero To Three

Prochaska, J., & DiClemente, C. (1983). Stages and processes of self-change of smoking: Toward an integrative model of change. *Journal of Consulting and Clinical Psychology, 51,* 390–395.

Roter, D., & Larson, S. (2002). The roter interaction analysis system (RIAS): Utility and flexibility for analysis of medical interactions. *Patient Education and Counseling, 46,* 243–251.

Russell, M. (1994). New assessment tools for drinking in pregnancy: T-ACE, TWEAK, and others. *Alcohol Health and Research World, 18*(1), 55–61.

Segre, L. S., O'Hara, M. W., Arndt, S., & Beck, C. T. (2010). Nursing care for postpartum depression, part 1: Do nurses think they should offer both screening and counseling? *American Journal of Maternal and Child Nursing, 35,* 220–225.

Sokol, R. J., Martier, S. S., & Ager, J. W. (1989). The T-ACE question: Practical prenatal detection of risk-drinking. *American Journal of Obstetrics and Gynecology, 160,* 863–871.

Spouse, J. (2001). Bridging theory and practice in the supervisory relationship: A sociocultural perspective. Journal of Advanced Nursing, 33(4), 512–522.

Stokes, T., & Baer, D. (1977). An implicit technology of generalization. *Journal of Applied Behavior Analysis, 10,* 349–367.

Stoltenberg, C.D., & McNeill, B. W. (2010). Counseling and psychotherapy: Investigating practice from scientific, cultural, and historical perspectives. In C. D. Stoltenberg, B. W. McNeill, & U. Delworth (Eds.), *IDM supervision: An integrative developmental model for supervising counselors and therapists* (3rd ed.). New York: Routledge/Taylor & Francis Group.

Sweet, M., & Appelbaum, M. (2004). Is home visiting an effective strategy? A meta-analytic review of home visiting programs for families with young children. *Child Development, 75,* 1435–1456.

Tandon, S. D., Parillo, K. M., Jenkins, C. J., & Duggan, A. K. (2005). Home visitors' recognition of and response to malleable risk factors among low-income pregnant and parenting women. *Maternal and Child Health Journal, 9,* 273–283.

Tandon, S. D., Mendelson, T., Kemp, K., Leis, J., & Perry, D. (2011). Preventing perinatal depression in low-income home visiting clients: A randomized controlled trial. *Journal of Consulting & Clinical Psychology, 79,* 707–712.

Wasik, B. (1993). Staffing issues for home visiting programs. *The Future of Children, 3,* 140–157.

S. Darius Tandon is an associate professor at the Northwestern University Feinberg School of Medicine where he is also the associate director of their Center for Community Health. He is interested in understanding how to address psychosocial risk factors, particularly maternal depression, among women using early childhood intervention programs. Much of his recent work involves the integration of a cognitive-behavioral stress management intervention into early childhood programs with the aim of preventing the onset and worsening of depression.

Chapter 9
Considerations on the Implementation, Innovation, and Improvement of Evidence-Based Home Visiting Programs

Mark S. Innocenti

Home visiting as an approach to deliver services to at-risk young children and families, particularly mothers, has grown in visibility and acceptance. Reviews of research on home visiting have found evidence supporting home visiting (Kahn & Moore, 2008; Nievar, Van Egeren, & Pollard, 2010; Sweet & Applebaum, 2004). Home visiting has been endorsed by groups such as the PEW Charitable Trusts (2010) and the Coalition for Evidence-Based Policy (2009). Support for home visiting can also be found in the business community (Bartik, 2011; Institute for a Competitive Workforce, 2010; ReadyNation, n.d.; Rolnick & Grunewald, 2003).

Home visiting has long been used as an approach to provide services to young children and their families (Roberts, Wasik, Casto, & Ramey, 1991). The use of government funds to support home visiting varies across countries (Nievar et al., 2010). In the USA, federal funds have supported home visiting through programs such as Early Head Start, services for children with disabilities (through Part C of the Individuals with Disabilities Education Act, PL 101–476), and programs through health departments for newborn children. However, until recently, there has not been specific federal funding for home visiting to at-risk families; this has recently changed. In 2010, the US Congress established the Maternal, Infant, and Early Childhood Home Visiting (MIECHV) program administered by the Health Resources and Services Administration (HRSA) and the Administration for Children and Families (ACF) of the US Department of Health and Human Services. The MIECHV funds grants to states to help at-risk families voluntarily receive home visits from qualified staff to improve maternal and child health, child development, school readiness, economic self-sufficiency, and prevent child abuse. Eligible families are defined in the law as families who reside in at-risk communities. This pro-

M. S. Innocenti (✉)
Center for Persons with Disabilities, Emma Eccles Jones College of Education and Human Services, Utah State University, Logan, UT 84322-6580, USA
e-mail: Mark.innocenti@usu.edu

L. Roggman, N. Cardia (eds.), *Home Visitation Programs*,
DOI 10.1007/978-3-319-17984-1_9

gram opens the door to home visiting for families previously unable to receive these services.

The MIECHV program comes with some restrictions. With some limited exceptions, the programs implemented must be evidence-based and programs that meet evidence-based criteria have been identified, along with a process for programs to meet these criteria as new evidence becomes available. The MIECHV program has also identified outcome benchmarks that all programs in all states must meet. These benchmarks are in the following areas:

- Improved maternal and newborn health
- Prevention of child injuries, child abuse, neglect, or maltreatment, and reduction of emergency department visits
- Improvement in school readiness and achievement
- Reduction in crime or domestic violence
- Improvements in family economic self-sufficiency
- Improvements in the coordination and referrals for other community resources and supports

These benchmarks represent worthy areas in which to achieve outcomes.

Underlying this positive legislation, a tension exists between research and policy. Although meta-analyses of the research have identified positive outcomes from home visiting, the magnitude of the outcomes is small to moderate, and the same program when implemented in different communities can yield different results (Astuto & Allen, 2009; Azzi-Lessing, 2011; Daro, 2006; Nievar et al., 2010). States are working to expand existing home visiting programs while some in the research community want to see the development of more focused programs that better match target families with interventions for specific outcomes (Azzi-Lessing, 2011; Daro, 2006; Nievar et al., 2010). These two directions for moving the field forward, state expansion and research specificity, are not mutually exclusive. However, those expanding home visiting in states need to be aware of the limitations identified by research, whereas the researchers need to be sensitive to the political climate to not derail the positive gains made in providing more services to at-risk families.

This chapter focuses on this tension between policy, research and practice, and the innovations needed when implementing programs to reduce this tension primarily by examining how existing programs that work with at-risk families can incorporate innovative aspects as they expand. The questions addressed include:

1. What is the evidence for home visiting?
2. How does the evidence affect practice in the USA?
3. What is the role of innovation within evidence-based home visiting?
4. How can innovation be supported?

The goal of this chapter is to provide solutions that can ensure that our programs meet required outcomes, for most families, most of the time.

What Is the Evidence for Home Visiting?

Evidence-Based Practice

The words "evidence-based practice" are used in many fields these days, from medicine to psychology, to education, and to almost every field that uses research in some way to make decisions about what to do with people whether this be in some treatment, intervention, or classroom. Most people have some familiarity with evidence-based practice, but in my opinion, most people are not really clear on what this means. Experts alternatively talk about evidence-based practice, evidence-based programs, research-based activities, recommended practices, and the list goes on. However, these terms are not interchangeable and their misunderstanding and misuse comes from, in many cases, the experts themselves.

The basic principles behind evidence-based practice, first, are that decisions about what we do as practitioners are based on research studies, typically quantitative research, and second, that the research has been rated along some quality criteria. The first principle indicates the need for more than one study. Science is the accumulation of research on a given topic. One study with a positive finding is good, but if this study is the only one of ten studies that has this finding, then we must ask whether this finding is true or just a random finding. Evidence accumulates from many studies consistently finding the same outcomes.

The second principle is harder to understand for those who are not researchers. This principle is: Not all research is equal. Research studies vary in quality, where quality is in the design of the study. Some research is better able to reduce factors, referred to as threats, that limit our ability to say that A caused B (causality). Research that was conducted by a famous researcher or that was printed in a prestigious research journal does not make it high-quality research (although it may be). All research is designed to help us answer questions and increase knowledge. Research quality, however, comes from factors such as how subjects for the study were identified and assigned to groups, how well we know and document what happened to subjects during the intervention, how outcomes were measured, and how we take care of factors that may provide alternative explanations for findings. Evidence-based practice requires that a group of experts has gone through a research study and rated the quality of the research; some studies will reach the desired criteria, others will not.

At a practical level, this means that one study with one positive finding is never enough to make a practice or program evidence based. Similarly, a handful of poor-quality studies that find the same outcome (although promising) do not make for an evidence-based practice. On the other hand, once a practice is deemed evidence based, one high-quality study that does not get the same outcome does not take away the designation of evidence-based practice. The message for us as consumers of research is that a designation of evidence-based practice must be based on many high-quality studies all of which agree that the intervention (program, curriculum, etc.) under examination caused the same outcome.

At one level this is very simple. Different professional organizations and federal agencies have been identifying criteria on which research can be judged to define practices as evidence-based practices. The complicated part is that these organizations and agencies do not all use the same criteria and/or do not look at the same outcomes. My recommendation is that practitioners need to refer to the agencies that fund their programs and the organizations to which they belong, for recommendations on evidence-based practice.[1]

Evidence-Based Practice in Home Visiting

As part of the MIECHV program, the law requires that 75 % of the available funds must be used for home visiting programs with evidence of effectiveness based on rigorous evaluation research: They must be evidence-based programs. In preparation for the implementation of the MIECHV program in the USA, an interagency workgroup from the US Department of Health and Human Service contracted with Mathematica Policy Research to review the home visiting research literature and assess the evidence of effectiveness for home visiting program models for women (and pregnant women) with children from birth through age 5. This review, begun in 2009, was called the Home Visiting Evidence of Effectiveness (HomVEE)[2]. Program models identified by HomVEE are the ones from which states must select programs.

HomVEE conducted a rigorous review process to identify relevant home visiting research. They focused on studies that examined outcomes in: (a) maternal health; (b) child health; (c) child development and school readiness; (d) reductions in child maltreatment; (e) reductions in juvenile delinquency, family violence, or crime; (f) positive parenting practices; (g) family economic factors; and (h) linkages and referrals. HomVEE used an evidence-based criteria developed by the US Department of Health and Human Service where identified studies for each program model had to meet one of these primary criteria: (a) at least one high- or moderate-quality impact study of the model finds favorable, statistically significant impacts in two or more identified outcome domains or (b) at least two high- or moderate-quality impact studies of the model using unique study samples find one or more favorable, statistically significant impacts in the same domain.[3]

---

[1] For more information on evidence-based practice, there are many books on different topic areas (e.g., Buysse & Wesley, 2006). An easy primer on the topic is provided by Child Trends (Metz, Espiritu, & Moore, 2007). Websites that link to the evidence-based practice criteria and findings for different organizations may be more helpful. The National Early Childhood Technical Assistance Center, for example, has a page with links to early childhood organizations (http://www.nectac.org/topics/evbased/evbased.asp#practices) and the Metz and colleagues' article also has links.

[2] Information on the process and outcomes from HomVEE can be found at the following website: http://homvee.acf.hhs.gov/document.aspx?rid=5&sid=20&mid=2.

[3] More detail on this process can be found at: http://homvee.acf.hhs.gov/document.aspx?rid=4&sid=19.

HomVEE published an executive summary of this process and findings in 2010 and then an updated executive summary in 2014 (Avellar et al., 2014; Paulsell, Avellar, Sama Martin, & Del Grosso, 2010). As this is an active, ongoing process, program models continue to be added. Seventeen home visiting program models were identified as evidenced based in the most recent summary (2014). Interested readers need to check the HomVEE website on a regular basis. The 17 program models identified as evidence-based practice are: Child First, Durham Connects/Family Connects, Early Head Start—Home Visiting (EHS), Early Intervention Program (EIP), Early Start (New Zealand), Family Check-Up, Family Spirit, Healthy Families America (HFA), Healthy Steps, Home Instruction of Parents of Preschool Youngsters (HIPPY), Maternal Early Childhood Sustained Home Visiting, Minding the Baby, Nurse Family Partnership (NFP), Oklahoma Community-Based Family Resource and Support (CBFRS), Parents as Teachers (PAT), Play and Learning Strategies (PALS) Infant, and SafeCare Augmented. Table 9.1 presents information on the outcome areas by program models for which evidence was established for those models as reported in the 2014 summary and updated in June 2015 from the HomVEE website. Program models may have had multiple positive outcomes in a single outcome area but these are not reported here (see Avellar et al., 2014, for more details).

The areas of greatest impact for the evidence-based models are in positive parenting practices (12 models) and child development and school readiness (11 models). Health outcomes were found in some models for children (eight models) and mothers (nine models). Six models found reductions in child maltreatment. The remaining outcomes were found in five or fewer programs. To be fair, not all programs measured all outcomes.

The results of the HomVEE review are positive. As of 2014, 17 program models were identified as evidence-based practice. Each of these program models has requirements for training people, for supervision, and for how the program is put into practice. These fidelity requirements were included in the process for identifying program models as evidence-based practice and are needed so that we can see that programs who use these models are actually implementing the models as designed.

From a practice perspective, however, concerns were also identified. No program model , except HFA, found outcomes in all MIECHV-required outcome areas. Remember that all outcomes are required as part of MIECHV. Some program models did not find lasting program effects after the program ended. For most program models, findings were not replicated in all studies reviewed or were not replicated for all positive outcome impacts. Some of the program models found findings that were unfavorable or ambiguous in some studies as compared with outcomes that were found favorable in other studies.

The findings from the HomVEE review provide practitioners with a place to begin. The review allows the selection of program models for implementation that find outcomes in desired areas using quality research designs. However, this review also makes it clear that none of these program models are effective all the time, for all of the required outcomes. It raises questions about what the field needs as it

Table 9.1 Domains with positive impacts as identified by the HomVEE review

Home visiting program	Child development	Parenting practices	Child health	Maternal health	Economic self-sufficiency	Child maltreatment	Violence and crime	Linkages and referrals
Child First	x			x		x		x
Durham Connects		x	x	x				x
Early Head Start—Home Visiting	x	x			x			x
EIP			x		x			
Early Start (New Zealand)	x	x	x			x		
Family Check-Up	x	x		x				
Family Spirit	x			x				
Healthy Families America	x	x	x	x	x	x	x	x
Healthy Steps		x	x					
HIPPY	x	x						
Maternal Early Childhood Sustained Home Visiting		x	x	x				
Minding the Baby			x	x				
Nurse Family Partnership	x	x	x	x	x	x	x	
Oklahoma CBFRS		x		x				
Parents as Teachers	x	x			x	x		
PALS Infant	x							
SafeCare Augmented	x	x		x		x		x

EIP Early Intervention Program, *HIPPY* Home Instruction of Parents of Preschool Youngsters, *CBFRS* Community-Based Family Resource and Support, *PALS* Play and Learning Strategies moves forward with implementing these program models. It raises questions about what we should expect from the program models we implement as we move forward. The reality is that we do not know which program model would work best for any particular family in any particular place, for any particular outcome. The question becomes "How do we plan our services knowing this reality?"

Innovation in Home Visiting

The HomVEE review highlights not only positive home visiting program models[4] and outcomes but also areas of concern. These concerns are amplified, for example, when the requirements for receiving funding (in the USA) require that programs demonstrate outcomes in multiple areas, outcome areas for which some program models have established no evidence or mixed evidence. Other concerns also exist. Many of these program models were developed for use in urban areas. Can these program models be successfully adapted to rural areas; would distance technology be effective? The program models have been conducted primarily with low-income Euro- and African American families. Will these program models be effective for new immigrants, for indigenous peoples (cf. Chaffin, Bard, Bigfoot, & Maher, 2012)? Most evidence-based practice models were developed with an earlier generation of parents. Will these program models work with young parents who expect more technologically based materials? There is an ongoing concern about the correct dosage of intervention (Roggman, Cook, Peterson, & Raikes, 2008) because the frequency of home visits seems to be a critical variable to success (Nievar et al., 2010). Beyond the frequency of visits, the length of time families' stay in a program is a question. Research shows the people receive about half of the home visits expected according to program model designs (Paulsell, 2010; Riley, Brady, Goldberg, Jacobs, & Easterbrooks, 2008). These are only some of the many issues to be considered. Azzi-Lessing (2011) provides a detailed overview of many more critical issues for home visiting programs to consider. Given the funds required to implement the evidence-based home visiting program models as they are currently structured, the question may be: How can we innovate and still remain true to our evidence-based program model?

Before innovation can occur, programs need to have a strong "theory of change" or logic model (Raikes et al., 2014; Roggman, Boyce, & Innocenti, 2008). There are many resources available on the Internet that discusses how to develop a logic model.[5] At a basic level, a logic model includes program inputs, program outputs, and program outcomes. Figure 9.1 presents a very basic home visiting logic model. The

---

[4] The term "program models" has been used to indicate the programs being implemented are evidence-based models. From this point, programs will be defined as the implementation of a program model.

[5] For example, see http://www.wkkf.org/knowledge-center/resources/2006/02/WK-Kellogg-Foundation-Logic-Model-Development-Guide.aspx for a guide developed by the W. K. Kellogg Foundation.

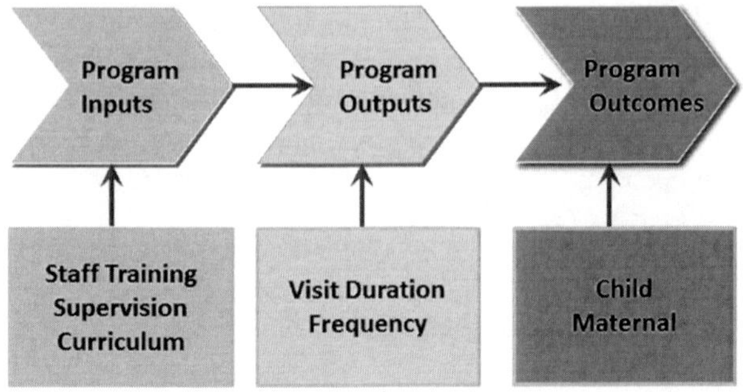

Fig. 9.1 Basic theory of change diagram

program inputs are the program model fidelity components. This includes the people hired as practitioners, the training they receive, the supervision they receive, the curriculum used, the plan for the frequency and duration of visits, and other similar program fidelity concerns. Each evidence-based program model in the HomVEE review identified fidelity components and those would be included here.

Program outputs have traditionally been aspects of service delivery. They include whether the home visits are occurring as regularly or for as long as they are intended. They also include information on whether the curriculum (if there is one) and/or the plan for working with the family are followed.

The program outcomes are those areas in which the program should have impacts.Most HomVEE program models demonstrated impacts in child development and school readiness, so these would be outcomes. Many program models had impacts on other outcomes and those would be included here. All areas where a program claims it should have outcomes would be included. It is important that each of the components—inputs, outputs, and outcomes—be measured. Only by measuring each of the components can a program have evidence that what they do leads to the outcomes they want. All of the evidence-based program models have a logic model but these may not address the MIECHV requirements and it is good practice for individual programs to develop/adapt the logic model in their program.

Figure 9.2 brings innovation into the logic model. This model shows an example of an additional layer of potential innovative components added to the basic logic model. These added innovations are not a comprehensive list, and not all innovations would happen at the same time; Fig. 9.2 is merely an illustrative example. Innovative inputs might include new types of training to impact new target outcomes. These inputs might include new ways of looking at families that could enhance existing process, such as identifying family factors to guide individualization, or new procedures to begin implementing, such as a continuous quality improvement (CQI) process.

Innovation at the output level may require that different aspects of services be examined to incorporate new strategies or deliver new content. Some recent advances in practice would suggest looking at the quality of what happened during the visit, the processes and practices (Design Options for Home Visiting Evaluation [DOHVE], 2012; Innocenti & Roggman, 2011; Paulsell, Boller, Hallgren, & Mraz Esposito, 2010), and this could take the form of new home visiting strategies to implement.

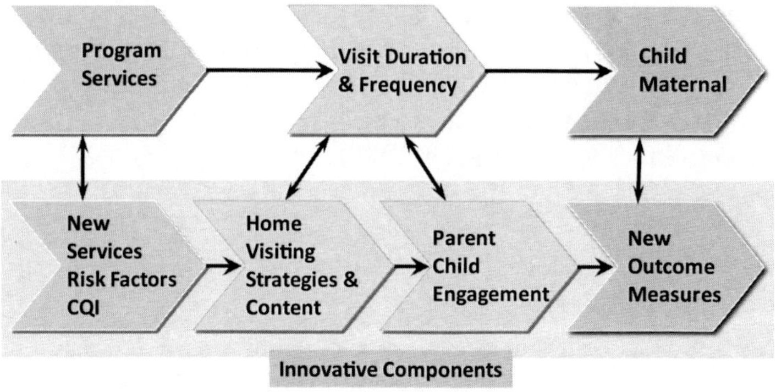

Fig. 9.2 Basic theory of change including process and innovation

The Home Visiting Rating Scale (HOVRS; Roggman, Cook, Jump Norman et al., 2008) would be an example of a tool that measures home visitor practices during a home visit. The DOHVE and Paulsell et al. (2010) papers identify other new tools to consider. New types of content, related to new outcomes, may need to be delivered during home visits. Figure 9.2 also shows outputs related to engagement in the home visit; the importance of engagement, at the parent and child levels, has been emphasized (Azzi-Lessing, 2011; Nievar et al., 2010; Paulsell, 2012).

The eight benchmark outcomes identified by MIECHV include outcomes that not all program models measured as a part of research underlying their evidence base. In program models for which these outcomes have not been tested in high-quality research, these new outcomes are innovative. For example, in the HomVEE review (Avellar et al., 2014), few of the evidence-based program models demonstrated impacts on reductions in family violence. Family violence would be an innovative outcome and, if included, would require a fresh look at the relation of innovative inputs and outputs to affect this outcome.

This approach to innovation is flexible and responsive to the need for change, whether it is to meet new benchmark outcomes or to be sure that the program is meeting outcomes for specific groups the program serves (e.g., families with toxic stress). Each program needs to use its current logic model and adapt it as innovation is needed. Each component needs to be measurable in a way that the program can use the information to respond and make changes to inputs and outputs, and those are then reflected in outcomes. The next section provides more information on what is needed not only to put innovation into practice but also to ensure that evidence-based programs continue to be driven by evidence.

From Innovation to Practice

The people who work in home visiting programs work hard. It is difficult work, and in too many places, people are not paid well for this work. The need to innovate cannot be considered a luxury, but a necessity, especially in an environment where having evidence is not only helpful but also required. Innovation requires extra time for staff and program resources. Infrastructure both for and within programs is needed. Four areas that require consideration to make implementation effective and innovation part of ongoing practice are: implementation science, data-informed practice, supervision and coaching, and CQI.

Implementation Science

Evidence-based practice has helped identify program models that have successful outcomes. Identifying program models is only the first step. The next step, which has been happening in the USA, is wide-scale implementation of the program models. Adopting an evidence-based program model and obtaining the requisite training required by the model developer does not ensure that the program will have the desired outcomes (Durlak & DuPre, 2008). An already established evidence-based program model that expands to a new city or county may not be effective or effective in the same way when implemented elsewhere (Azzi-Lessing, 2011; Paulsell et al., 2010).

Implementation of evidence-based program models is a practice in its own right. Fixsen, Naoom, Blasé, Frideman, and Wallace (2005) conducted a comprehensive review of the research literature on the implementation of programs from diverse fields of practice (including agriculture, business, child welfare, medicine, and others) and found that the implementation of evidence-based practice programs did not always go as intended. Just because a program has been proven effective does not mean that it can be adopted by others and successfully implemented. Fixsen and colleagues identified factors that lead to more successful implementation. This field of research has been called implementation science. Implementation science (or implementation research) is the scientific study of methods to promote the successful transition of programs from evidence-based practice to routine practice while maintaining the same outcomes. Implementation science examines the conditions that impact changes at the practice, organization, and system levels (Blasé et al., 2010).[6]

Implementation science has identified six implementation drivers (see Metz, Blasé, & Bowie, 2007). These six drivers or components were identified in research where successful implementation of programs occurred. These are:

1. Staff recruitment and selection
2. Preservice or inservice training
3. Coaching, mentoring, and supervision
4. Internal management support
5. Systems-level partnerships
6. Staff and program evaluation

These drivers have recently been grouped into competency drivers (1–3 above), organizational drivers (4–6 above), and leadership drivers (technical and adaptive).

[6] Fixsen and colleagues operate the National Implementation Resarch Network (http://nirn.fpg.unc.edu/), which has useful resources.

Fixsen (2014) provides evidence that when the implementation drivers are used effectively, evidence-based programs can be implemented with 80% fidelity in 3 years. This compares to 17 years of implementation with only 14% fidelity for evidence-based programs that do not use the implementation drivers.

All of the HomVEE-identified evidence-based practice programs have requirements for staff recruitment and for required training. Each of the program models has identified the minimum requirements for staff. Most program models also have required training and practice criteria for a program to be considered as having fidelity to the model. Most program models require supervision. All require some type of evaluation, and some come with data collection and reporting requirements. These components are implementation drivers and need to be included in the logic model for a new program just beginning to implement an evidence-based program model.

Although some of the HomVEE evidence-based program models have national offices which oversee the general fidelity of the program, these offices do not necessarily work as part of a system. Each individual program is not necessarily linked to other similar programs within a state or region. One of the potential strengths of the MIECHV system is that it is administered at the state level (in the USA), which immediately puts home visiting into a larger system. This state system can help support the implementation drivers that facilitate implementation of the models and benefit all programs. This not only includes the implementation drivers that may be available as part of the model but also the implementation drivers that need to be included as the program implements the model in a new setting. The state system can help each home visiting program consider the implementation drivers specific to their model. Ongoing training may be needed to build skills to promote outcomes that are now required but were not emphasized in research by the program model developers. For example, the competency drivers of coaching, mentoring, and supervision may be considered in the model but the programs may need additional technical assistance and resources to make these happen so that model fidelity is achieved. These drivers may be especially critical as home visiting programs innovate. The infrastructure needs to include ongoing data collection to support internal management. The state may assist programs to implement organizational drivers, especially when each state has its own data reporting requirements. For effective implementation, drivers need to occur as long as the program exists and they need to be regular activities. Strong implementation science practices support the innovation process. Some key implementation drivers the state can facilitate to establish model fidelity are discussed in more detail below.

Data Availability

An organizational driver that supports staff and program evaluation is having data available for regular review—data-informed practice. Information about the key components of the program's logic model is of paramount importance. A system is needed to provide an efficient way for staff to enter information into a data management system as it is collected. This system can build on the data management system that program models may already use. Most of the evidence-based program models require some level of data collection; some already have extensive data collection systems. The data management system must be logical and easy to use for both the home visitor who enters the data from each visit and to the program managers who review the data.

The implementation of the MIECHV program is driving the development of data management systems in participating states. National consultants are providing services to develop these systems and some states are hiring local consultants to design systems for local use. One example is Utah, where in-state consultants developed a data management system. The development of this system began before MIECHV funding as part of another project examining the effect of home visiting programs and then evolved to add MIECHV data requirements. In their State Health Department, Utah has an Office of Home Visiting that has oversight for MIECHV. Like many states, Utah has a mix of evidence-based home visiting program models being implemented and must be responsive to the needs of each program. The data system developers worked collaboratively with the state and program staff to identify needed data components. The process next included multiple field tests to get feedback on the system and make changes as needed. When new MIECHV benchmark requirements were added, a similar process was completed. Program staff and the state built a data management system useful to all.

After the data system is in place, staff must be trained to regularly input the data and to regularly use the resulting information. The data entry process itself needs to be monitored as a goal until data entry becomes routine. Program managers use these data to evaluate how services are provided, how parents engage in home visits, and how outcome variables are affected. This information can be used to examine the effectiveness of the current logic model, as long as the logic model components have been identified, defined, and measured. If innovative components are added, these data will help programs understand the impacts of innovation. Supervisors must regularly access the data and use it to guide supervision. The process needs to be internally monitored to ensure it continues to be useful.

Developing a useful data management system takes funding and time for staff to learn and use. The Utah example demonstrates one benefit of being in a system such as MIECHV. This is a system driver for implementation.

Supervision and Coaching

Implementation research competency drivers identify professional development, including ongoing coaching and supervisory support, as critical to successful implementation. Our review of the current literature specific to professional development for home visitors finds few relevant articles on supervision, except for the outcome of improving retention of staff, an import outcome with both program fidelity and cost implications. Home visitors who were given supervision and consultation had lower levels of emotional exhaustion and burnout, two variables found to negatively impact fidelity and retention (Aarons, Fettes, Flores, & Sommerfeld, 2009; Aarons, Sommerfeld, Hecht, Silovsky, & Chaffin, 2009).

Much of the supervision literature for home visiting focuses on the practice of reflective supervision (Heller & Gilkerson, 2011). However, Innocenti and Roggman (2011) found limited research support for reflective supervision and suggested that there is a need to move beyond reflective supervision to developmental supervision, an approach which maintains reflective supervision while building practices suggested by recent reviews of the adult learning literature (Dunst & Trivette, 2009). This proposed approach to supervision includes supervision practices similar to coaching and incorporates the use of measurement tools to provide information on implemented home visiting quality to the supervisor and home visitor (see Design Options for Home Visiting Evaluation [DOHVE], 2012; Paulsell et al., 2010; Roggman, Cook, Jump Norman et al., 2008).

A recent meta-analysis of the adult learning literature has clearly identified that better outcomes result when the training process includes strategies that more actively involve the learner in using, processing, and evaluating the mastery of newly acquired skills (Dunst & Trivette, 2009). Coaching is an approach that makes use of these strategies. Research shows that coaching is an effective adult learning strategy to improve existing abilities, develop new skills, and gain a deeper understanding of practices (Hanft, Rush, & Shelden, 2004). Coaching supports the learner in identifying what works, what might need to be done differently, and what level of support is needed from the coach (Rush & Shelden, 2011). Coaching has been used successfully for working with parents who have a child with disabilities (Janssen, Riksen-Walraven, Dijk, & Ruijssenaars, 2010). Results from randomized controlled trial studies of professional development interventions, primarily in educational settings that included coaching, revealed small but significant effects on children's learning, with somewhat larger effects on intervention practices (e.g., Bierman, Nix, Greenberg, Blair, & Domitrovich, 2008; Powell, Diamond, Burchinal, & Koehler, 2010; Wasik, Bond, & Hindman, 2006). These results suggest that coaching should provide a positive mechanism for changing practitioner behavior to align with evidence-based home visiting practices that lead to desired outcomes.

A point for consideration is the job descriptions of supervisor and coach. Supervisors typically have a power differential in respect to the practitioner in that supervisors not only provide supervision but also typically have the power to make decisions on job advancement and payment. This can be a disincentive to practitioners to discuss weaknesses in practice. Coaches, in contrast, are typically advanced peers who do not have a role in making position recommendations. Although it can be more expensive, dedicated coaches are recommended; this is a recommended practice although not a research-based recommendation.

Implementation science is clear that supervision and coaching are competency drivers for successful program replication. Although research on training for home visiting program staff is growing (Whitaker et al., 2012), research on best practices in coaching and supervision for home visiting need continued study.

Continuous Quality Improvement

CQI brings together the implementation drivers to ensure model fidelity and incorporate innovation. CQI has been described as the process of identifying, describing, and analyzing strengths and problems, and then testing, implementing, learning from, and revising solutions. CQI uses the data collected by the program, data that measures outcomes and implementation practices, to identify what the program is doing well and where it needs improvement. All program staff are involved in looking at the data to answer the question of where the program needs to improve and based upon the program logic model, what the program needs to change. The CQI process needs to occur in an atmosphere where the activities and performance of staff are discussed in a nonthreatening manner. The goal is to improve—not to blame—and this requires a network of good strengths-based relationships among program staff (similar to what we want to see between the home visitors and parents). Staff identify potential solutions and these are implemented quickly; the process is action oriented. As part of the process, staff members determine how to collect information on the solution they identify. CQI may require the collection of new data on inputs, process, outputs, or outcomes depending on the focus of the CQI process. The CQI process needs to be a part of regular meetings, at least monthly. At these meetings the program data are reviewed and immediate changes can be made to the process. This process is cyclical in that it does not stop until the initial concern is resolved and once resolved, the new solution becomes a potential area for more CQI. The goal is to develop a program that emphasizes quality as defined by meeting the program goals. Ammerman, Putnam, Margolis, and Van Ginkel (2009) provided a clear description on the practice of CQI and examples of its implementation in child abuse prevention programs.

The CQI process is logical and straightforward (Langley et al., 2009). The process begins by asking some basic questions about the program's aims, measures, and ideas. The aims question is: What are we trying to accomplish? The measures question is: How will we know change is an improvement? The ideas question is: What change can we make that will result in that improvement? Once these questions are answered, the CQI process uses a plan-do-study-act (PDSA) cycle where all steps are written down. The "plan" is the decision on what needs to change. The "do" is implementing the changes identified. The "study" is looking at your measures to monitor and analyze the impact of your changes. The "act" is revising and standardizing the changes. The cycle is then repeated for the new "act." Ammerman and colleagues (2009) provided information on this process from a human services perspective (see also Bickman & Nosser, 1999). Websites by groups such as the Casey Foundation, the Center for Institutional Effectiveness, and the Institute for Healthcare Improvement have information to help better understand the process.

Earlier, we discussed the example of innovation for a program with a strong evidence base for achieving child development outcomes being required to also focus on decreasing intimate partner violence, an area not supported by prior research on that program model. The CQI process could help drive this innovation. This program would set a goal of decreasing intimate partner violence. The program, as what it would "do," decides to provide specialized training to staff on intimate partner violence. This program could measure that this training occurred, which staff members attended, and what staff learned about certain skills or techniques from the training. The program could then examine changes in their intimate partner violence outcome from before to after this training, the "study" part of the cycle. The program would then need to "act" on what it had learned.

Continuing with this example, imagine that the program finds that this training has no effect on the intimate partner violence outcome. The next strategy (plan) may be to have the home visitor provide specific information during a home visit to mothers on how to respond to intimate partner violence. This could be implemented for all program participants or only for mothers who respond in certain ways on a regularly used measure or who express concerns to the home visitor about intimate partner violence (do). The program would not only continue to measure the training the staff receive but also add onto that a measure that indicates whether the parents received the specific information. This measure could be as simple as the home visitor reporting that the specific information was provided to each parent. The program would continue to monitor changes in intimate partner violence outcomes (study). The information obtained would lead to decisions on what to do next (act). The program might continue this approach or try something else. The cycle continues until the program has achieved the desired outcome. Once the desired outcome has been met, the program will continue to monitor it, while identifying the next outcome for the CQI process. This CQI process can be a strong driver of innovation and quality.

Conclusions

Research has demonstrated the effectiveness of home visiting. The practice of home visiting has received support from groups that vary from those focused on societal outcomes to those focused on business outcomes. Governments in different countries have responded and are supporting home visiting. This support provides the opportunity to expand home visiting and potentially result in more families and children who have better outcomes. However, with this support also come added pressures. Evidence-based home visiting programs are being asked to expand and work with new groups of people or to focus on additional outcomes, people and outcomes on which the original program may not have been evaluated or may not have demonstrated effectiveness. Programs need to work to establish evidence for these new groups if home visiting is to continue receiving funding and support. Even in situations in which funding and support are secure, programs should collect data to monitor quality and ensure desired outcomes are being met.

This chapter provided information on the expansion of home visiting in the USA and the pressures that result from this expansion. These pressures require that programs become more comfortable with innovation and adopt practices that will help lead to successful innovation. These practices need to be supported, through funding and infrastructure development, by governments and other agencies who oversee the expansion of home visiting programs and by the programs themselves, if these programs are to continue to be effective.

This chapter has identified some of the practices that should help home visiting programs as they move forward with expansion and innovation. These practices only represent some of the steps that may be required. There may be other practices not yet anticipated or different practices needed for different systems. The goal of this chapter was to provide ideas for consideration. Just as home visiting programs need to report the data on outcomes, systems research is needed to determine what practices are necessary for successful expansion.

The final goal of these practices is that we gain a better understanding of which programs and program activities work best for which families and for which outcomes. Providing home visiting programs with data and the supports needed to use the data on a regular basis allows those in the field to better address the needs of those they serve. This process needs to occur in an environment that continues to support research within and across different home visiting programs. At the same time, support is needed for developing new programs and for programs that are establishing their evidence base. New programs bring with them innovations that help improve the entire home visiting field. These are some of the challenges that need to be met to continue to help those who can benefit from home visiting.

References

Aarons, G. A., Sommerfeld, D. H., Hecht, D. B., Silovsky, J. F., & Chaffin, M. J. (2009). The impact of evidence-based practice implementation and fidelity monitoring on staff turnover: Evidence for a protective effect. *Journal of Consulting & Clinical Psychology, 77,* 270–280.

Aarons, G. A., Fettes, D. L., Flores, L. E., & Sommerfeld, D. H. (2009). Evidence-based practice implementation and staff emotional exhaustion in children's services. *Behavior Research & Therapy, 47,* 954–960.

Ammerman, R. T., Putnam, F. W., Margolis, P. A., & Van Ginkel, J. B. (2009). Quality improvement in child abuse prevention programs. In K. A. Dodge & D. L. Coleman (Eds.), *Preventing child maltreatment: Community approaches* (pp. 121–138). New York: Guilford.

Astuto, J., & Allen, L. (2009). Home-visitation and young children: An approach worth investing in? *Social Policy Reports*, *23*(4), 1–21. http://www.srcd.org/index.php?option=comcontent&task=view&id=232&Itemid=550.

Avellar, S., Paulsell, D., Sama-Miller, E., Del Grosso, P., Akers, L., & Kleinman, R. (2014). *Home visiting evidence of effectiveness review: Executive summary*. Washington, DC: Office of Planning, Research and Evaluation, Administration for Children and Families, U.S. Department of Health and Human Services. http://homvee.acf.hhs.gov/HomVEE_Executive_Summary_2014-59.pdf.

Azzi-Lessing, L. (2011). Home visitation programs: Critical issues and future directions. *Early Childhood Research Quarterly, 26,* 387–398.

Bartik, T. (2011). *Investing in kids: Early childhood programs and local economic development.* Kalamazoo: Upjohn Institute for Employment Research.

Bickman, L., & Nosser, K. (1999). Meeting the challenges in the delivery of child and adolescent mental health services in the next millennium: The continuous quality improvement approach. *Applied & Preventive Psychology, 8,* 247–255.

Bierman, K. L., Nix, R. L., Greenberg, M. T., Blair, C., & Domitrovich, C. E. (2008). Executive functions and school readiness intervention: Impact, moderation, and mediation in the Head Start REDI program. *Development & Psychopathology, 20,* 821–843.

Blasé, K. A., Fixsen, D. L., Duda, M. A., Metz, A. J., Naoom, S. F., & Van Dyke, M. K. (2010, April). *Implementing and sustaining evidence-based programs: Have we got a sporting chance*? Paper presented at the Blueprints for Violence Prevention, San Antonio.

Buysse, V., & Wesley, P. W. (2006). *Evidence-based practice in the early childhood field.* Washington, DC: ZERO TO THREE.

Chaffin, M., Bard, D., Bigfoot, D. S., & Maher, E. J. (2012). Is a structured, manualized, evidence-based treatment protocol culturally competent and equivalently effective among American Indian parents in child welfare? *Child Maltreatment, 17,* 242–252.

Coalition for Evidence-Based Policy. (2009). *Early childhood home visitation program models: An objective summary of the evidence about which are effective.* Washington, DC: Coalition for Evidence-Based Policy. http://coalition4evidence.org/wp-content/uploads/2011/07/Update-Evidence-on-home-visitn-4.23.09.pdf.

Daro, D. (2006). *Home-visitation: Assessing progress, managing expectations.* Chicago: Ounce of Prevention Fund and Chapin Hall Center for Children at the University of Chicago.

Design Options for Home Visiting Evaluation. (2012). *Overview of observational measurement instruments available for home visiting. Design Options for Home Visiting Evaluation: Home visit observation brief.* Washington, DC: Design Options for Home Visiting Evaluation. http://www.mdrc.org/.

Dunst, C. J., & Trivette, C. M. (2009). Let's be PALS: An evidence-based approach to professional development. *Infants & Young Children, 22,* 164–176.

Durlak, J. A., & DuPre, E. P. (2008). Implementation matters: A review of research on the influence of implementation on program outcomes and the factors affecting implementation. *American Journal of Community Psychology, 41,* 327–350.

Fixsen, D. L. (2014). *Scaling an effective intervention: How to build implementation capacity, replicate with fidelity, and produce consistent outcomes.* Baltimore: Social Solutions. http://www.socialsolutions.com/wp-content/uploads/2014/10/10142014_ScalingEffectively_PerformWell-Webinar.pdf.

Fixsen, D. L., Naoom, S. F., Blasé, K. A., Frideman, R. M., & Wallace, F. (2005). *Implementation research: A synthesis of the literature (FMHI Publication #231).* Tampa: University of South Florida, Louis de la Parte Florida Mental Health Institute. The National Implementation Research Network.

Hanft, B. E., Rush, D. D., & Shelden, M. L. L. (2004). *Coaching families and colleagues in early childhood.* Baltimore: Brookes.

Heller, S. S., & Gilkerson, L. (2011). *A practical guide to reflective supervision.* Washington, DC: ZERO TO THREE.

Innocenti, M. S., & Roggman, L. A. (2011, December). *Beyond reflective supervision: Using tools to improve the supervision process in home visiting.* Paper presented at the ZERO TO THREE National Training Institute. National Harbor, MD.

Institute for a Competitive Workforce. (2010). *Why business should support early childhood education.* Washington, DC: US Chamber of Commerce, Institute for a Competitive Workforce.

Janssen, M. J., Riksen-Walraven, J. M., van Dijk, J. P., & Ruijssenaars, W. A. J. J. (2010). Interaction coaching with mothers of children with congenital deaf-blindness at home: Applying the diagnostic intervention model. *Journal of Visual Impairment & Blindness, 104,* 15–29.

Kahn, J., & Moore, K. A. (2008). *What works for home visiting programs: Lessons from experimental evaluations of programs and interventions. Child Trends Fact Sheet (#2010).* Washington, DC: Child Trends.

Langley, G. J., Moen, R., Nolan, K. M., Nolan, T. W., Norman, C. L., & Provost, L. P. (2009). *The improvement guide: A practical approach to enhancing organizational performance.* San Francisco: Jossey-Bass.

Metz, A. J., Blasé, K., & Bowie, L. (2007). *Implementing evidence-based practices: Six drivers of success.* Washington, DC: Child Trends.

Metz, A. J., Espiritu, R., & Moore, K. A. (2007). What is evidence-based practice? *Child Trends, 14,* 1–5.

Nievar, M. A., Van Egeren, L. A., & Pollard, S. (2010). A meta-analysis of home visiting programs: Moderators of improvements in maternal behavior. *Infant Mental Health Journal, 31,* 499–520.

Paulsell, D. (2012). Replicating and scaling up evidence-based home visiting programs: The role of implementation research. *Encyclopedia on Early Childhood Development.* http://www.childencyclopedia.com/pages/PDF/synthesis-home_visiting_programs.pdf.

Paulsell, D., Boller, K., Hallgren, K., & Mraz Esposito, A. (2010). Assessing home visit quality: Dosage, content, and relationships. *Zero to Three, 30*(6), 16–21.

Paulsell, D., Avellar, S., Sama Martin, E., & Del Grosso, P. (2010). *Home visiting evidence of effectiveness review: Executive summary.* Washington, DC: US Department of Health and Human Services, Administration for Children and Families, Office of Planning, Research and Evaluation.

PEW Charitable Trusts (2010). *The case for home visiting.* Washington, DC: PEW Charitable Trusts.

Powell, D. R., Diamond, K. E., Burchinal, M. R., & Koehler, M. J. (2010). Effects of an early literacy professional development intervention on Head Start teachers and children. *Journal of Educational Psychology, 102,* 299–312.

Raikes, H. H., Roggman, L. A., Peterson, C. A., Brooks-Gunn, J., Chazan-Cohen, R., Zhang, X., & Schiffman, R. F. (2014). Theories of change and outcomes in home-based Early Head Start programs. *Early Childhood Research Quarterly, 29,* 574–585.

ReadyNation. (n.d.). *Business case for early childhood investments.* http://www.readynation.org/uploads/20120409_ReadyNationBusinessCaseLowRes.pdf.

Riley, S., Brady, A. E., Goldberg, J., Jacobs, F., & Easterbrooks, M. A. (2008). Once the door closes: Understanding the parent-provider relationship. *Children & Youth Services Review, 30,* 597–612.

Roberts, R. N., Wasik, B. H., Casto, G., & Ramey, C. T. (1991). Family support in the home: Programs, policy and social change. *American Psychologist, 46,* 131–137.

Roggman, L. A., Cook, G. A., Peterson, C. A., & Raikes, H. H. (2008). Who drops out of Early Head Start home visiting programs? *Early Education & Development, 19,* 1–26.

Roggman, L. A., Cook, G. A., & Jump Norman, V. K., Christiansen, K., Boyce, L. K., & Innocenti, M. S. (2008). Home Visit Rating Scales. In L. A. Roggman, L. K. Boyce, & M. S. Innocenti (Eds.), *Developmental parenting: A guide for early childhood practitioners* (pp. 209–217). Baltimore: Brookes.

Roggman, L. A., Boyce, L. K., & Innocenti, M. S. (2008). *Developmental parenting: A guide for early childhood practitioner.* Baltimore: Brookes.

Rolnick, A., & Grunewald, R. (2003). *Early childhood development: Economic development with a high public return.* http://www.minneapolisfed.org/publicationspapers/studies/earlychild/abc-part2.pdf.

Rush, D. D., & Shelden, M. L. L. (2011). *The early childhood coaching handbook.* Baltimore: Brookes.

Sweet, M., & Applebaum, M. I. (2004). Is home visiting an effective strategy? A meta-analytic review of home visiting programs for families with young children. *Child Development, 75,* 1435–1456.

Wasik, B. A., Bond, M. A., & Hindman, A. (2006). The effects of a language and literacy intervention on Head Start children and teachers. *Journal of Educational Psychology, 98,* 63–74.

Whitaker, D. J., Ryan, K. A., Wild, R. C., Self-Brown, S., Lutzker, J. R., Shanley, J. R., Edwards, A. M., McFry, E. A., Moseley, C. N., & Hodges, A. E. (2012). Initial implementation indicators from a state wide rollout of SafeCare within a child welfare system. *Child Maltreatment, 17,* 96–101.

Mark S. Innocenti (USA): Associate professor of psychology at Utah State University and director of the Research and Evaluation Division of the Center for Persons with Disabilities, a university center of excellence for the development of people with disabilities. He has over 30 years of multidisciplinary work with children at risk and with disabilities and their families, and has coordinated a series of research projects, including a 10-year longitudinal study on the effects and costs of early intervention with children with disabilities and a study of early literacy and bilingual early language support. His current research focuses on developing strategies and evaluation assessments for home visitation programs and in evaluating preschool education as a means of preventing later special education.

Part III
Home Visiting Programs Outside the USA

Chapter 10
Home Visitation Programs for Early Child Development: Experiences in Latin America and the Caribbean

Nancy Cardia, Renato Alves, Aline Gomes, and Alder Mourão

Research on child development over the past decades has consistently highlighted the importance of early childhood for the quality of life over a person's life span (Engle et al., 2007; Irwin, Siddiqi, & Hertzman, 2007; Shore, 2003; Shonkoff, 2010). The promotion of good conditions for early child development has significant and lifelong effects on brain development, physical and mental health, emotional development, and learning (Hertzman, 2000; Mustard, 2010; Shonkoff & Phillips, 2000).

It has been demonstrated that good care in the first years of life: (a) lowers mortality rates and morbidity (accidents and injuries) during childhood and promotes better health during adult life (Dreyer, 2011; Grantham-McGregor et al., 2007; Power, Hypponen, & Smith, 2005); (b) improves emotional well-being and capabilities to cope with stress and frustration (Gunnar & Davis, 2003 and Armus et al., 2012); (c) promotes learning, resulting in smoother school progression, with lower school retention and abandonment rates; and (d) improves overall health conditions (Barker, 1994; Engle et al., 2007; Irwin et al., 2007; Power & Hertzman, 1997), thus promoting children's welfare and the development to their full potential. Benefits from investing in this stage of life are not limited to the individual but bear fruits to society as well (Alderman, 2011; Karoly, Kilburn, & Cannon, 2005; Korfmacher, 2005; Mercy & Saul, 2009; Olds, 1988; Young, 2007). A study carried out by the World Bank (Heckman, 2006) concluded that for each dollar invested in early child development programs, at least US$7 are saved in future costs in health, education, social welfare programs, and the criminal system. Furthermore, providing adequate care and support during early childhood builds the foundations for every aspect of subsequent development and can compensate social inequalities. Moreover, public policies targeted at this stage of life can be important tools to prevent intergenera-

N. Cardia (✉) · R. Alves · A. Gomes · A. Mourão
Center for the Study of Violence, University of São Paulo, São Paulo, Brazil
e-mail: ncardia@usp.br

R. Alves
e-mail: ralves@usp.br

L. Roggman, N. Cardia (eds.), *Home Visitation Programs*,
DOI 10.1007/978-3-319-17984-1_10

tional cycles of poverty, strengthening families, their children, and the communities they live in.

Since 1989, when the United Nations General Assembly adopted the Convention on the Rights of the Child (CRC), currently endorsed by 192 countries, a new perspective has emerged, explicitly recognizing children as social actors and active holders of their own rights. The CRC constitutes a unique instrument for the defense of children's rights to survival, development, and protection. The convention alerts the signatory countries of their duties regarding the development of comprehensive policies on health, nutrition, care, and education, particularly for the youngest children, pointing out their special developmental needs. However, despite this movement and the proven economic and social benefits of investments in early childhood programs, the youngest children are still neglected. According to the UNESCO 2006 report, almost half the countries in the world do not have formal programs specifically for children under 3 years of age, particularly for the most vulnerable among them, for whom access to public policies is badly needed.

In this chapter, we present some currently implemented programs and policies in Latin American countries that focus their intervention mainly on improving the quality of children's lives during early childhood (Table 10.1). To identify experiences in Latin America, we conducted an Internet search focused especially on official government's sites[1]. For this search, the names of the countries were combined with the following keywords: home visiting, early childhood, and child development.

Though most programs are quite recent and are not yet national policies universally applied, their presence in numerous Latin American countries indicate that early child development is beginning to gain a visibility and relevance that previously did not exist. This is no minor achievement as until very recently it appeared that promoting a child's development consisted only of reducing infant mortality by securing prenatal care and reducing child mortality by ensuring inoculations. The need for special care for children and their caregivers to promote healthy development with interventions is a new concept. Also new is the idea that this intervention has to follow the child's development from conception to at least the age of 5 years and that numerous families need external support over time to successfully cover this period.

The dissemination of information about effective programs to help families and children, at this stage of development, is growing, and the number of programs that include some form of home visitation grows as well. Still, some challenges remain such as heterogeneous population growth rates, from comparatively higher birth rates in rural areas and peripheries of urban centers, combined with higher rates of adolescent pregnancy compared with other age groups. These conditions demand

[1] Limitations of sources used in the program: It is important to keep in mind that online information was a major source for this work. Governmental, academic, and NGO's websites do not cover all experiences in place at a moment; for those they do report, not all information needed is provided. We expect that more information is provided about the experiences that for some reason are deemed to be more successful.

Table 10.1 Programs for pregnant women and families with infants and children in Latin America and the Caribbean

Name	Location and coverage level	Initial year	Target group	Main purposes	Method	Professionals' profile	Number of families per professional
Chile Crece Contigo	Chile/national	2007	Pregnant women and under 4-year-old children (HV)	To monitor, protect, and grant full support to children and their families, favoring their adequate development	HV; TV, radio, Internet, phone calls	Health professionals	
Canelones Crece Contigo	Canelones/state	2008	Pregnant women and under 4-year-old children (HV)	Support families so they can contribute to their children's growth and development	HVi	Multi-professional technicians	
Uruguay Crece Contigo	Uruguay/national	2012	Pregnant women and under 4-year-old children (HV)	To guarantee care and protection to pregnant women and children, favoring adequate childhood development	HVi, sensitizing campaigns	Multi-professional technicians	
Educa a Tu Hijo	Cuba/national	1993	Pregnant women and under 6-year-old children (not attending day care program)	To attain maximum development level according to each child's potential; to provide educational opportunities for children who are not attending the formal educational system	HVi (children from birth to 2 years old) and groups	Professionals (monitors) and lay trained people (performers)	6 children/visitor
Crescendo com Nuestros Hijos	Ecuador/national	1997	Under 6-year-old children (HV)	To contribute to the development of the child's intellectual, linguistic, socio-affective and psychomotor potential	HVi (children from birth to 2 years old) and groups	Trained lay people from the community	60 families/visitor
Niños y Niñas Educándose en Comunidad	Oaxaca (Mexico)/state	2007	Under 6-year-old children (indigenous area)	To prepare the family to bring up their children and promote their development since early childhood	HVi (children from birth to 2 years old) and groups	Trained community volunteers	15 families

Table 10.1 (continued)

Name	Location and coverage level	Initial year	Target group	Main purposes	Method	Professionals' profile	Number of families per professional
De la Mano Edúcame	Guatemala/ 12 states	2002	Pregnant women and under 6-year-old children	To offer an alternative access to knowledge to children who were not included in the preschool system	HVi (children from birth to 2 years old) and groups	Trained community volunteers	15–20 families/ visitor
Hogares Comunitarios de Bienestar	Colombia/ national	1986	Children from 6 months to 6 years old (HV)	To attain minimum levels of health, nutrition and both cognitive and psychosocial development	Community mothers	Trained mothers from the community	12–14 children/ community mother
Família, Mujer e Infancia	Colombia/ national	1991	Pregnant women and mothers of children from birth to 2 years old	To support and strengthen families in the promotion of their children's development	HVi and group meetings	Community education agent	12–15 women/ agent
Primeros Años	Argentina/ national	2003	Children from birth to 4 years old (including indigenous people)	To strengthen families as protagonists in providing attention and care to their children	Family groups	Community lay people trained (mediators)	
Cuna Más	Peru/national	2012	Children from birth to 3 years old (HV)	To promote children's cognitive, social, physical and emotional development	HVi (weekly) and groups (fortnightly)	Community lay people (trained mediators) and multidisciplinary technicians	
Kallpa Wawa	Bolivia/ 22 communities	2001	*Quechua* families with children from birth to 3 years old	To improve parental skills to enable parents to promote a healthy and stimulating ambiance for their children's development	HVi and workshops	Development promoters trained	

Table 10.1 (continued)

Name	Location and coverage level	Initial year	Target group	Main purposes	Method	Professionals' profile	Number of families per professional
Nutrición y Protección Social	Honduras/ national	2006	Pregnant women and children from birth to 2 years old	To offer early stimulation for learning and cognitive development	Monthly group meetings and HVi (some cases)	Volunteer monitors from the community trained	25 children/visitor
Madres Guias	Honduras/ national	1992	Pregnant women and children from birth to 4–6 years old (HV)	To guide families on the promotion of their children's development	HVi, groups, radio	Volunteer mothers from the community trained	
The Roving Caregivers	Jamaica (Clarendon, St. Catherine, Manchester)	1992	Children from 3 months to 3 years old (not attending day care programs)	To improve parental skills in order to enable parents to contribute in positive manners to their children's development	HVi (weekly)	Youngsters recently graduated in high school	30 families/visitor
Primeira Infância Melhor	Rio Grande do Sul/state	2003	Pregnant women and children from birth to 6 years old (not attending day care programs)	To empower parents to stimulate and promote the child's physical, intellectual, social and affective skills	HVi (children from birth to 2 years old) and groups	Community lay people trained	25 families/visitor
Mãe Coruja Pernambucana	Pernambuco/ state	2007	Pregnant women and children from birth to 5 years old (HV)	To reduce maternal and infant morbidity and mortality rates and to strengthen positive mother–child bonds	Assistance at *Mãe Coruja Spaces*	Health technicians	
Mãe Curitibana	Curitiba-PR/ municipal	1999	Pregnant women and children from birth to 5 years old (HV)	To increase adhesion of both pregnant women and mothers to medical care and health services recommendations for prevention of health risks	Monitoring at health centers	Health technicians	

Table 10.1 (continued)

Name	Location and coverage level	Initial year	Target group	Main purposes	Method	Professionals' profile	Number of families per professional
Capital Criança	Florianópo-lis-SC/ municipal	1997	Pregnant women and children from birth to 10 years old	To reduce maternal and infant morbidity and mortality	Monitoring at the mater-nity ward/ afterbirth HV	Health technicians	
Estratégia Trevo de Quatro Folhas	Sobral-CE/ municipal	2001	Pregnant women and children from birth to 2 years old	To reduce maternal and infant morbidity and mortality and to offer social and nutritional support	HVi	Health techni-cians/women from the community	
Mãe Paulistana	São Paulo-SP/ municipal	2006	Pregnant women and children from birth to 1 year old	To reduce maternal mortality, premature deliveries and prob-lems during the perinatal period, and to encourage breast-feeding	Monitoring at health centers	Health technicians	
Cegonha Carioca	Rio de Janeiro/ municipal	2001	Pregnant women	To reduce maternal and infant mortality and foster submission to prenatal exams	Monitoring at health centers	Health technicians	
Primeira Infância Completa	Rio de Janeiro/ municipal	2009	Children from 6 months to 3 years old (not attending a day care program)	To focus on the education of children who failed to obtain places in day care centers	Day care centers on Saturdays from 9 am to 5 pm/School	Education technicians	
Asinhas da Florestania	Acre/state	2009	Children from 4 to 5 years old, living in rural areas	To stimulate the child's devel-opment in order to minimize disadvantages in comparison to children who had the opportu-nity to attend preschool	HVi (twice a week)	Persons attending or already gradu-ated in upper high school	

HVi home visitation intervention, *HV* high vulnerability

that programs be tailored to specific needs of each community. The lack of a universal model of intervention as well as the costs of such programs can be serious obstacles for governments to invest in such programs. Disseminating information about successful, low-budget programs can be a way to improve their adoption as public policy by different governments.

Knowledge about and experiences with home visitation interventions are rare in Latin America, even though home visitation has been employed for over a century in many countries in the Northern hemisphere, and their results have evidenced positive and long-term effects on the life of children and parents assisted by these services (Cardia, 2006; Cardone, Gilkerson, & Welchsler, 2008; Kemp et al., 2011; Korfmacher, Green, Spellmann, & Thornburg, 2007; Olds et al., 1997; Sandler, Schoenfelder, Wolchik, & MacKinnon, 2011; Wasik & Bryant, 2001), including better health and development indicators (Lee et al., 2009; Love et al., 2005; Mitchell-Herzfeld, Izzo, Greene, Lee, & Lowenfels, 2005; Olds et al., 2004), as well as the prevention of violence against children (Guterman, 2001; MacMillan et al., 2005; Pinheiro, 2006; Rodriguez, Dumont, Mitchell-Herzfeld, Walden, & Greene, 2010; Sandler et al., 2011). Among several current home visitation initiatives in Latin America, we highlight the program *Infância Saudável* (Healthy Childhood), carried out by the *Núcleo de Estudos da Violência* (Center for the Study of Violence) of the University of São Paulo (NEV-USP) because it focuses on adolescent mothers (a most at-risk group) and uses paraprofessional home visitors (a more affordable alternative).

Experiences in Latin American and Caribbean Countries

Latin America is tracing the first steps to consolidate public policies to promote early child development, particularly by policies that demand the cooperation/integration of multiple actors such as family, community, public services, and different institutions (Araújo et al., 2013). In the most economically developed countries, such interventions often require the assistance of multiple professionals such as health practitioners, education experts, social services professionals, and psychologists. This presence of various professionals does not seem to be frequently found in programs to foster early child development in Latin America and Caribbean countries. Still some policies for the promotion of early childhood development stand out.

Chile

A good example of promotion of early childhood development is that of *Chile Crece Contigo*[2] (Chile Develops with You), a program first implemented in 2006 and then

[2] http://www.crececontigo.gob.cl.

in 2009, incorporated into the country's social protection system, thus becoming a national policy. Through this policy, several initiatives, benefits, and programs targeted at children and families involving different sectors were organized as a support network to promote child development. The objective of *Chile Crece Contigo* is to monitor, protect, and support every child and his/her family through universal interventions ranging from the initial prenatal appointments up to the child's entry in the school system, around age 4. Although aimed at universal assistance, the program also has an individual component to assist the more vulnerable families. The program is complemented by radio and TV broadcasts of educational content for parents provided by experts on child development. A website can be accessed for information and downloading. Parents can also receive assistance and guidance through phone calls.

Uruguay

Inspired by the Chilean program, two programs were developed in Uruguay. In 2008, a program for the promotion of child development, modeled after the Chilean one, was implemented by the Province of Canelones, and after the original it was named *Canelones Crece Contigo* (Canelones Develops with You). This program is coordinated by the *Dirección de Desarrollo y Cohesión Social de la Intendencia de Canelones* (Development and Social Cohesion Directory of the Canelones Administration). According to the website, *Banco de Buenas Prácticas* (BBP)[3], its objective is to help families foster their children's growth and development. The program targets mothers with children up to 4 years of age and pregnant women, living in areas of high social and economic vulnerability. According to BBP, to improve results and meet their goals, Canelones Crece Contigo *adapts home visitation strategies to the actual needs of the families involved.*

In this model of intervention, an interdisciplinary team is engaged in the fieldwork to assess the family's needs. After this initial assessment, the families are referred to different programs and social projects that can best attend to their needs. To be implemented, this program requires that local services promoting early child development be connected as a network. The first results have been so promising that in 2012 the federal government adopted the Canelones version as a national program aimed at the full protection of children from zero onwards—*Uruguay Crece Contigo*[4] (Uruguay Develops with You). This program is now coordinated by the *Oficina de Planeamiento y Presupuesto (OPP) da Presidência da República* (Planning and Financial Administration Office of the Presidency of the Republic).

According to the OPP report[5], the program targets women in similar conditions to those in Canelones: pregnant women and/or mothers of children under 4 years,

[3] http://www.bancodebuenaspracticas.org/proyecto.php?idp=71.

[4] http://www.crececontigo.opp.gub.uy/.

[5] http://www.mides.gub.uy/innovaportal/file/22416/1/uruguay+crece+contigo+-+sintesis.pdf.

living in vulnerable circumstances, whether from social, economic, housing, or environmental risks. The program monitors child development and assists families by providing basic information about health issues, child development, and housing conditions (e.g., sanitation, security, and prevention of accidents). The program also involves strengthening local institutional capacity. Home visitation is one of the strategies employed by the program.

Cuba

Another important national public policy is the program *Educa a Tu Hijo*[6] (Bring-up your Child), by the *Centro de Referencia Latinoamerica para la Educación Preescolar* (CELEP—Latin American Reference Center for Preschool Education), in Cuba. This program resulted from an experimental research carried out between 1982 and 1992, aimed at the identification of alternatives to improve educational results of children living in remote rural areas, who did not have access to day care centers, that is to preschool (Gómez, 2011).

According to Gómez (2011), the methods developed in this study produced such promising results that, in 1993, the Ministry of Education adopted this model in a preschool education program. The program's coverage was extended from birth to 5 years of age. This was the root of the "Social Program of Educational Attention" named *Educa a tu Hijo*.

The program starts during pregnancy, with prenatal monitoring by health professionals. From birth until the child is 2 years old, the families receive home visits once or twice a week by a trained professional. At this stage, the objective of the home visit is to inform the mother about specific aspects of the development of the child and teach the mother techniques she can use to safely stimulate the child's development at each stage.

From the age of 2 until the child is 6 years old, contacts with the families are made through group work. Groups of parents and children from different families living in the same region are brought together for activities. Parents and children perform collective activities, and parents are informed about how they can stimulate their children's social development and communication skills. Similarly to the home visits, the groups meet once or twice a week. Home visitors may be health, education, culture, or sports professionals, or lay people from the same community who have received home visits themselves and were later trained to dispense the program. Lay candidates for the position of home visitors are selected, trained, and permanently monitored by the program. The children/visitor ratio is of six children per home visitor (Gómez, 2011). The program is currently operating in all 14 Cuban provinces and in the special municipality of *Isla de la Juventud* (Youth Island), involving families living in rural, urban, and mountain areas.

---

[6] http://www.ecured.cu/index.php/Educa_a_tu_Hijo.

The *Educa su Hijo* format has influenced a number of Latin American programs designed to promote child development such as the Ecuadorian program *Creciendo con Nuestros Hijos* (Growing up with our Children), the Guatemalan program *De la Mano Edúcame* (You Teach Me by your Hand), the Mexican program *Niños y Niñas Educándose en Comunidad* (Boys and Girls Brought up in Community), and the Brazilian program *Primeira Infância Melhor* (Improved Early Childhood). This influence was reported in a special report for UNICEF: *La contextualización del modelo de atención educativa no institucional Cubano "Educa a tu Hijo" en países latinoamericanos* (Gómez, 2011). We have relied on this study to present the information on Ecuador, Guatemala, and Mexico.

Ecuador

The Ecuadorian program *Crescendo con Nuestros Hijos*[7] (Growing up with our Children) was launched in 1997 under the responsibility of the Ministry of Economic and Social Inclusion[8]. The program targets families with children under 6 years of age, living in poverty. The program targets parents or caregivers, enabling them to educate and stimulate their child's development through different activities. The activities are designed to contribute to the development of the child's intellectual, socioaffective, and psychomotor potential. The methodology includes home visits to families with children from 0 to 2 years old, and for group work for families with older children. Home visitors are recruited in the local community. After initial training, they receive supplementary monthly training by program supervisors. Each home visitor is responsible for 60 families (Gómez, 2011).

Guatemala

In Guatemala, the Ministry of Education, in partnership with international institutions such as UNICEF, implemented a nonformal educational program called *De la Mano Edúcame*[9] (You Teach Me by your Hand) between 2002 and 2008. The main purpose was to offer alternative access to education for children not assisted by the official preschool educational system. The program trained and guided families on how to implement at-home activities to promote their children's development. Pregnant women and families with children under 2 years of age were the target of this program.

The program combined home visits and group activities, at a community school, for children from 2 to 6 years old. During the meetings, families received informa-

[7] http://www.oei.es/inicial/ecuadorne.htm#4.

[8] http://www.inclusion.gob.ec/.

[9] http://www.mineduc.gob.gt/portal/contenido/menu_lateral/sistema_educativo/educacion_preescolar/index2.html.

tion about how to care for their child's health and on how to promote the child's intellectual, physical, and emotional development. The program also tried to reinforce attitudes and values conducive to promoting the child's healthy development. Follow-up was performed by volunteer women from the community, trained and supervised by teachers from the public education system and by university education students. Each volunteer was in charge of 15–20 families (Gómez, 2011).

According to the Ministry of Education, in 2008 the program was operating in 20 communities of 12 provinces, assisting 3025 children per year. The program was interrupted when a new administration came into power.

Mexico

The program *Niños y Niñas Educándose en Comunidad* (NyNEC; Boys and Girls Brought up in Community) developed by Unidad de Proyectos Estratégicos[10] (Unit for Strategic Projects) of the State Institute for Public Education of Oaxaca, Mexico (UPE) was also inspired by the *Educa tu Hijo*. This Oaxaca state program has been in place since 2007.

NyNEC aims to prepare families to educate and stimulate the development of their children beginning in early childhood. The program targets both family and community's education. The program is designed for families with children between birth to 6 years of age. The strategy adopted combines home visits for families with children under 2 years of age and group work with families with children between 2 and 6 years (Gómez, 2011).

NyNEC differs from other programs that focus on early child development in that it includes a local school component. Although NyNEC is not a formal educational program, local schools are encouraged to discuss strategies and to help plan activities and train professionals working with the families. Another characteristic of this program is that the population reached by the program is mostly that of indigenous Mexicans. The program was developed after consultations with local families and community leaders to ensure that the contents and actions were in tune with the local culture characteristics and practices. Finally, the NyNEC program is dispensed by volunteer home visitors, most of them are members of the local community; each home visitor is in charge of 15 families (Gómez, 2011).

Colombia

In 1986 in Colombia, the National Council for Economic and Social Policies created the program *Hogares Comunitarios de Bienestar*[11] (*HCB*—Welfare Com-

[10] http://www.ieepo.oaxaca.gob.mx/node/36.

[11] http://www.icbf.gov.co/portal/page/portal/PrimeraInfanciaICBF/Serviciosdeatencion/modalidadesdeeducacioninicial/Modalidad Comunitaria.

munity Homes), under the responsibility of the Instituto Colombiano de Bienestar Familiar[12] (ICBF—Colombian Institute for Family Welfare). According to Quintero-Velasquez (2011), the HCB program targets children from the age of 6 months to 6 years, in families living in extreme poverty, in both rural and urban regions. Unlike other programs that use home visitors, the strategy here is to use "community mothers." Women are chosen by the community and authorized by ICBF to care for children in their own homes (the "surrogate" mother's home) 5 days per week. Martínez and Tello (2009) point out that to qualify as a community mother, a women must have children of her own and at least 9 years of schooling. After being selected by the community, she is trained by the National Learning Service (SENA) and is paid around US$3.50 (approximately 37 % of a daily minimum wage per child assisted).

To accommodate the children, the community mother's house is upgraded by the ICBF to ensure the safety and adequacy of the house to the children's needs. Each community mother is provided with funds to feed the child as well as for materials to be used to teach the children (US$14.50 monthly per child). The ICBF requires each community mother to limit her work load to between 12 and 14 children. The community mothers are expected to ensure that the children under their care are healthy, well nourished, and developing accordingly to what is expected for the age group (Bernal et al., 2009; Martínez & Tello, 2009).

Children attending the HCB are also registered in the community's health programs and are inoculated according to the immunization calendar. Their parents, in turn, are engaged in local family schools linked to health services. In this setting, the families are informed about the stages of child development and taught how to encourage their children's development. Families also receive instructions about regular schooling processes and means to strengthen their relationships with their children, with other families, and in the community. In 2008 in Colombia, there were 61,500 HCBs, serving approximately 780,000 children (Martínez & Tello, 2009).

Created in 1991, another Colombian initiative under the responsibility of ICBF is the program *Familia, Mujer y Infancia*[13] (*FAMI*—Family, Women, and Childhood). FAMI works directly with pregnant women and mothers in highly vulnerable contexts, offering them guidance on how to promote their children's development. Guidance is provided through home visits and groups. The intervention starts during the pregnancy and lasts until the child is 2 years old. During home visits and group work, activities related to child development are carried out with the families by a community educational agent, who also delivers a package of food or nutrition supplements, ensuring that each child is given at least 25 % of the proteins and calories required in daily diet (Mantilla, Sánchez, & Torrado, 2007).

FAMI educational agents are selected according to the following criteria: to be under 55 years of age, to have at least 9 years of schooling, to live in the area where

[12] http://www.icbf.gov.co/portal/page/portal/PortalICBF.

[13] http://www.icbf.gov.co/portal/page/portal/PrimeraInfanciaICBF/Serviciosdeatencion/modalidadesdeeducacioninicial/Modalidad Familiar.

the program is developed, and to be a respected member of the community. Each educational agent provides support for 12–15 women.

The program seeks to improve parenting skills by providing support and strengthening families bonds; helping to stimulate the child's socialization; teaching non-violent practices for conflict resolution; encouraging positive attitudes to care and discipline the child; preventing and protecting the child from accidents, mistreatment, neglect, and abandonment; and encouraging families to develop a lifestyle that contributes to improving the quality of family life, and thus increasing their capacity to invest in their children's development (Mantilla et al., 2007). At the local level, FAMI is dispensed by a local organization (e.g., NGO, community association, parents association, and universities) selected by ICFB. Resources are provided by the state to the local organization so they can select, train, supervise, and pay educational agents for their services. Local organizations are also responsible for the distribution of food supplements and for the establishment of a local support network.

Argentina

In Argentina, the national program for child development called *Primeros Años*[14] (Early Years) has been in place since 2003 under the coordination of *Consejo Nacional de Coordinación de Políticas Sociales* (CNCPS –National Council for the Coordination of Social Policies). This coordination involves bringing together resources and policies coming from different ministries such as Social Development, Educational, Health, Labor and Social Security, and Justice and Human Rights.

According to report of CNCPS[15], the program's main purpose is to strengthen the role of families in providing attention and care to children from birth to 4 years of age. The program also aims to enhance community participation and to sensitize the different political and organizational levels to the importance of promoting good conditions for early child development. To achieve this, goal partnerships are formed with provinces and municipalities to set up intersectoral committees, to add resources, and to plan and implement joint efforts to promote child development.

In the Argentinian territory, the program develops activities to help parents solve problems, ensure the child's health and good nutrition as well as a safe and healthy environment, and ensure the child's access to education and to the protections of human rights. Care is also taken to promote the parents' own education with adult literacy training, preparing them for the labor market, and/or improving their income-generating skills.

The intervention is implemented by women living in the same district or area, selected according to their experience in community work and/or sensitivity to and commitment to improving conditions for children. There is a preliminary training,

[14] http://www.primerosanios.gov.ar/.

[15] http://www.primerosanios.gov.ar/descargas/publicaciones/informes/informe2009.pdf.

when the main aspects of the program are presented and discussed, followed by actual training on different aspects of child development, community participation, and management, in addition to specific themes, such as health prevention on specific risks of Aedes aegypti or the H1N1 virus epidemics.

The strategy to deliver the program *Primeros Años* is that of group work with families. Differently from other programs, families may start contact with the "mediators" or be contacted by them to participate. The group work strategy was selected to promote the exchange of experience between participant families about their everyday experiences as well as to encourage families to think about such experiences, meanwhile strengthening bonds between them. Participating families are also expected to become local resources for the promotion of child development. Groups meet at the local district's community facilities (e.g., health centers, community centers, schools, and churches).

One of the challenges faced by *Primeros Años* was to include Native Argentinian families. To assist these populations, the program had community leaders, anthropologists, and bilingual teachers from the various Native Argentinian communities as advisors. The advisors also guided the selection and training of the mediators who were to work with their communities. By 2011, the program was operating in 23 provinces, covering 232 Argentinean communities, involving 11,339 mediators, and assisting 554,272 families.

Peru

Peru has a national program for early childhood under development: *Cuna Más*[16] (Cradle More), coordinated by the Ministry of Development and Social Inclusion (MDIS). Launched in 2012, the program targets children from birth to the age of three, living in either rural or urban areas evaluated as poor or extremely poor.

The program's main purpose is to promote the children's cognitive, social, physical, and emotional development. The program works with families to strengthen emotional bonds, promote the exchange of experiences between caregivers and their children, offer guidance on care and educational and developmental stimulation practices, promote families' access to other public services and programs, monitor the child's development and overall health, as well as identify risk factors in the household and in the neighborhood.

Cuna Más consists of a 1 h weekly home visit to individual families combined with group work that takes place every fortnight for one and a half hours. The objective of the group work is to promote socialization, inform parents, and promote the exchange of experiences between participating families regarding child development.

Home visits are carried out by the local mediators—that is, by persons from the same community who are selected, trained, and supervised by a technical team.

[16] http://www.cunamas.gob.pe/.

Group meetings are managed by the program's consultants (with college degrees in education, pedagogy, psychology, health, or social sciences) and take place at *Cuna Más* centers or in other locations available in the community, where work with the families can be properly supervised.

Bolivia

In Bolivia, with financial support from a Swedish Committee, UNICEF has implemented a pilot project named *Kallpa Wawa*[17] (Strengthening the Child) to enhance parental abilities among *Quechua* families. This type of intervention by UNICEF with this Native Bolivian group is part of a broader set of initiatives to reduce poverty in the Andean region.

The project was launched in 1997 and was implemented in cities such as Cochabamba and Potosí. *Kallpa Wawa* targeted families with children from birth to 3 years old. The project's purpose was to inform, train, and support families to offer a safe, healthy, and psychological stimulating environment for their children's development.

The training process combined literacy (in both their mother language and Spanish) for at least one of the parents—usually the mother—and practical guidance regarding the promotion of child development. Training was offered for parents in workshops and in home visits carried out by development promoters, under the supervision of municipal civil servants (Vegas & Santibáñez, 2010).

According to Narayan (2005), the program, between 1997 and 2001, assisted more than 11,000 *Quechua* families, and 1500 participants were selected among them and trained to work as development promoters in 22 communities. However, despite its quite promising results over several years, *Kallpa Wawa* was discontinued in 2001.

The lack of continuity in interventions to foster healthy child development has been highlighted by many authors as a key problem in the field. Vargas-Barón (2009) observes that the lack of sustained support by governments, donors, and sources of financial support are the main obstacles to sustain and expand pilot projects, particularly when there is large dependency on foreign donors that usually provide support only for short periods.

Honduras

In Honduras, the project *Nutrición y Protección Social*[18] (Social Nutrition and Protection) has been implemented since 2006 by the Ministry of Health and by the

[17] http://www.unicef.org/bolivia/spanish/local_development_1966.htm.

[18] http://www.sdp.gob.hn/sitio/index.php?option=com_content&view=article&id=29&Itemid=182.

Programa de Asignación Familiar da Presidência da República (Family Grant Program of the Presidency of the Republic). According to Vargas-Barón (2009), this project is part of a previous initiative, the strategy *Atención Integral a la Niñez en la Comunidad* (AIN-C—Full Attention to Children in the Community), which has been operating since 1991 to prevent infant and child mortality and malnutrition.

Nutrición y Protección Social focuses on children from vulnerable families as identified by AIN-C, that is, families living below the poverty line or in extreme poverty in rural areas, with high rates of malnutrition and infant mortality. The program ensures nutritional health and promotes psychosocial development by stimulating the children's learning and cognitive development (Vargas-Barón, 2009).

To improve overall conditions for this group of children, the program monitors pregnant women during the pregnancy and after the birth until the children are 2 years old. The intervention teams include professionals from health areas as well as the monitors who carry out the intervention. The professionals are in charge of supervising the monitors while in the field. Both professionals and monitors receive an initial 1-week training followed by ongoing monthly training (Schaetzel, Griffiths, Del Rosso, & Plowman, 2008). Monitors are community volunteers trained to guide and help families in the promotion of their children's development. They deliver the program's content and follow the families' and children's progress over time.

Two follow-up strategies are employed, and the most important is the monthly meeting, usually carried out at a local community center. When cases require further attention (e.g., when the child has no weight gain or indicates developmental deficits) or when the family finds it difficult to attend the meetings, the home visiting strategy is adopted. Home visits are also used to register new families in the program and to follow-up with them after the child's birth (Schaetzel et al., 2008).

According to data presented by Fiedler (2003), each team was composed of three volunteer monitors, in charge of approximately 25 children each. In 2003, the program was operating in 1800 communities, covering 24 out of 42 health districts in Honduras. The average yearly cost was US$6.82 per child.

Vegas and Santibáñez (2010) reported the results of an evaluation of the program, carried out in 2008, comparing data for children who took part in the program (intervention group) with data for those who did not (control group). The results suggested a significant impact on feeding, caregiving practices, and children's nutritional conditions for those participating in the program. The impact was larger among the poorest families and among those whose attendance to the program was more regular. Among participant mothers, the mean duration of exclusive breastfeeding was 1.5 months longer than among nonparticipant mothers. Participant children presented larger immunization coverage, and at 23 months of age, the percentage of children who were still receiving iron and vitamin A supplementation was also larger among them.

Another Honduran program is *Madres Guias* (Guiding Mothers), supported by the Christian Fund for Childhood. The program was launched in 1992, aiming to guide families on different actions to promote their children's development (Vegas & Santibáñez, 2010). The program is meant to monitor families living in areas evaluated as below the poverty line, with high mortality and malnutrition rates, from pregnancy to the child's fourth or sixth year of life (Spiker & Gaylor, 2012).

This program is also delivered by community volunteers such as local women *(Madres Guias)* are selected and trained to monitor the families. One of the requisites to qualify is to have children of their own. According to Yánez and Yánez (2006), the work starts with periodical home visits, but when the children enter preschool, the meetings move from home to a local community center. Besides monitoring families, the program also uses the radio to broadcast messages about childcare and development.

According to Vegas and Santibáñez (2010), evaluations reveal that the program has effects on health care, the control of childhood typical diseases, the reduction of malnutrition, children's readiness for school, and the mothers' self-esteem and confidence to face challenges posed by their children's development with positive attitudes.

Jamaica

The program *The Roving Caregivers*[19] (RCP), launched in 1992 in Jamaica, with the financial support of UNICEF and the Bernard Van Leer Foundation, stands out among Caribbean countries. Under the responsibility of the NGO *Rural Family Support Organization* (RuFanSo), the program was initially implemented in the administrative region (parish) of Clarendon, and was later expanded to the St. Catherine and Manchester regions. According to Jones, Brown, and Brown (2011), RCP targeted poor children living in rural areas who did not attend day care centers. The program's aim was to enhance those parental abilities that contribute to their children's development.

Home visitation was the strategy adopted by RCP. Families received weekly 45–60 min home visits. To carry out that work, the program selected, hired, and trained youngsters from the community who had just completed high school, to act as home visitors—the "Rovers" (Jules, 2010). According to McDonald (2000), the home visitors' training took place in two stages. The first one occurred before they started working and consisted of 1-week training. The second one was carried out through continued training meetings, held every fortnight and lasting a full day, during which the different processes related to the home visits were discussed. Besides the training, home visitors were supervised by the program's professionals in weekly meetings in the communities that were visited.

Roopnarine and Hossain (2007) report that home visitors performed activities with the parents aimed at strengthening parent–child bonds, developing positive parental abilities, and teaching activities that parents could perform with the children to stimulate their social and cognitive development. A further concern of RCP was to develop positive beliefs and practices regarding child education. The children's

[19] http://www.unicef.org/infobycountry/jamaica_36354.html.

follow-up started at 3 months of age and continued until the end of the third year of life. The home visitor/child ratio was 1/30 (Jones et al., 2011).

From 2002 to 2004, RCP had attended approximately 2500 children (Jones et al., 2011). In 2004, the program was evaluated comparing participant children (intervention group) with nonparticipant children (control group). Including mothers and children from both groups, 131 individuals participated in the evaluation. The groups were evaluated at two time points: at the start of the intervention and after a year. Results showed that the intervention group presented better results as to both children's development and mothers' knowledge about their children's development and education. Participating children presented better scores in performance scales and in motor coordination of eyes and hands—important abilities for the schooling process ahead. According to this evaluation, the program had more impact on participant mothers' knowledge about child development than on their educational practices.

The RCP cost-benefit relation was also evaluated. For each dollar invested, the return varied from US$438.00 to 470.00. Unfortunately, the program was discontinued due to lack of financial resources, which again highlights the need to find more sustainable financial sources to guarantee the continuity of programs targeted at this population segment.

Brazil

Various strategies are being designed in Brazil to promote child development. However, none is universal, and the majority have been in place for a few years and represent local initiatives to promote some aspect of early childhood. Still it is possible to detect a growing interest by the federal government to invest in home visiting programs aimed at the development of children, and some steps in that direction seem to be in progress.

In 1983 started the first intervention that used home visitation to improve children's well-being by reducing mortality and malnutrition: the *Pastoral da Criança*[20] (The Pastoral for Children), part of the National Conference of Bishops in Brazil (CNBB). In this program, volunteers visit families every month to develop simple, inexpensive, and easily replicable educational practices and train the families in childcare and actions to prevent/treat dehydration and prevent malnutrition. This initiative resulted in a major reduction in infant and child mortality and in the development of various strategies easily transferred to caregivers.

More recently, in 1994, the Ministry of Health through the *Programa Saúde da Família*[21] (PSF—The Family Health Program), in a partnership with municipalities, implemented a major program with home visitation by community health agents to

[20] http://www.pastoraldacrianca.org.br/.

[21] http://dab.saude.gov.br/portaldab/ape_esf.php.

monitor how health services' recommendations are being put into practice and to identify needs for exams and specialized follow-up.

Another program by the federal government, again by the Ministry of Health, is the *Estratégia Brasileirinhos e Brasileirinhas Saudáveis—Primeiros Passos para o Desenvolvimento Nacional*[22] (Strategy Healthy Brazilian Children—First Steps to National Development). Starting in 2008, this policy integrates the promotion of and the attention to mother–child health issues. The age group served is that of children from birth to 5 years of age. The aim of the program is to guarantee quality of life for every Brazilian child from birth, by stimulating their physical, emotional, cognitive, and social competencies and abilities. This strategy was first experimentally implemented in five towns in different states of the country. It is a transversal policy, encompassing collaborative actions between the Ministries of Education, Social Development and Hunger, and Justice, under the leadership of the Ministry of Health.

In 2011, the Ministry of Health launched a new strategy entitled *Rede Cegonha*[23] (The Stork Network). This program is based on humanization principles of the Unified Health System (SUS)[24]. It involves a new model of attention at childbirth and of follow-up to:

- Broaden the access of pregnant women to better prenatal care
- Ensure basic conditions for prenatal visits and for child delivery, such as promoting a good interaction between the pregnant woman and the staff at a reference unit for delivery assistance and ensuring that the mother's right to choose a companion during delivery procedures is respected
- Ensure safe delivery procedures using best practices
- Secure good-quality health care for children from birth to 24 months
- Secure access to reproductive planning.

Income supplementation programs are also part of some governmental initiatives. In 2012, the program *Brasil Carinhoso*[25] (Caring Brazil) announced its objective to provide care for around 2 million families with children under 6 years of age. The program is part of the *Bolsa Família* (Family Grant) providing income supplement to families living in extreme poverty, defined as monthly income of under R$70—approximately US$35. *Bolsa Família* is a direct income transfer program, regulated by Act 10.836, as of January 9, 2004, which benefits families living in poverty and extreme poverty all over the country. The families' commitment is to keep their children in school and to seek regular health checks for the child (measuring and weighing the child, maintaining the inoculation schedule, etc.). The program aims to reduce poverty in the short and long term, enhance the families' autonomy, and promote social inclusion. The project also aimed to increase day care centers in all

[22] http://portal.saude.gov.br/portal/saude/odm_saude/visualizar_texto.cfm?idtxt=35139.

[23] http://portal.saude.gov.br/portal/saude/Gestor/visualizar_texto.cfm?idtxt=37082.

[24] To know more about these principles: http://bvsms.saude.gov.br/bvs/publicacoes/humaniza_sus_marco_teorico.pdf.

[25] http://www.mds.gov.br/brasilsemmiseria/brasil-carinhoso.

Brazilian states and improve health services and facilities to provide for families with young children.

Some state and municipal early child development initiatives are older and more consolidated than those at the national level, as mentioned previously. One example is the program *Primeira Infância Melhor*[26] (PIM—Improved Early Childhood). Operating since 2003 in the Rio Grande do Sul state, it is a state government program for the promotion of child development.

PIM is based on the Cuban model *Educa a tu Hijo*, described previously. This program has a socio-educational focus, that is, it teaches parents to stimulate and promote the children's physical, intellectual, social, and emotional abilities, taking into account the different development stages. This is done through the provision of information as well as by teaching parents how to stimulate their child. The program uses two forms of delivery (1) individual—weekly home visits to families with children from birth to 35 months of life, living in very vulnerable contexts and having no access to day care and preschool and (2) group work—targeting families with children between 3 and 6 years old with meetings at local community centers. Pregnant women are visited at home every fortnight and take part in monthly group meetings. The home visitor, a professional with either secondary or university education, works with and provides guidance to up to 25 families. Home visitors are the central actors in this program. They are in charge of the weekly home visits to families, planning, demonstrating, and evaluating the activities. A continued training program of monitoring and supervision by a monitor or a consultant from the Secretariat involved (health, education, or social services) provides support for home visitors.

PIM's main objective has been to promote the child's full development. This demanded an interdisciplinary approach and an intersectoral strategy. The program brings together professionals from different state and municipal secretariats: education, culture, work, and social and health development, integrating different levels of the administration—state and municipal, securing commitments from all levels involved.

Another program in Brazil is *Mãe Coruja Pernambucana*[27] (The *Pernambucan* Mother Owl), created in 2007 by the Health Secretariat of the State of Pernambuco. Its objectives include the reduction in maternal and infant morbidity and mortality, and the establishment and strengthening of positive bonds between mother, child, and family. Similarly to PIM, it is delivered through an intersectoral set of actions that include state and local administrations and civil society.

Municipalities with child mortality rates above 25/1000 born alive children were initially chosen to take part in the program. Municipalities, mothers, and children in the most vulnerable conditions were identified and enrolled in the program and monitored from pregnancy to the child's fifth year of life. By 2012, the program had assisted 66,000 pregnant women in 56 % of Pernambuco's state municipalities.

---

[26] http://www.pim.saude.rs.gov.br/a_PIM/php/index.php.

[27] http://maecorujape.blogspot.com.br/.

The earliest municipal-level programs for child development are *Capital Criança* (Child Capital), launched in 1997, and *Mãe Curitibana* (The *Curitibana* Mother), launched in 1999. *Capital Criança*[28] was first implemented in Florianópolis (state of Santa Catarina), with the purpose of reducing maternal and infant mortality and morbidity. This program covers the period from pregnancy to the child's tenth year of life. The delivery of the program involves collaborations between health centers, maternity wards, policlinics, and other health services. In addition, to secure and reinforce relationships established during the prenatal care period and to ensure adherence to this assistance, the program has a continued follow-up at maternity wards. During this period and until they are discharged, mother and child are visited daily by one of the program's professionals. During those visits, the child receives immunizations and a developmental evaluation, and the mother receives practical information about breast-feeding and neonatal care. On being discharged from the hospital, the mother receives a bag that includes educational material, medication for the umbilical cord and the blisters, and a thermometer.

While the child is still in the maternity ward should nurses or doctors identify risk factors, one of the nurses visits the child at home during the first 15 days of life, and afterwards a physician or a nurse make monthly home visits until risk is minimized. Results show that since the program was introduced, the rate of infant mortality decreased from 19.6/1000 born alive (1996), to 8.8/1000 born alive (2011).

Mãe Curitibana[29] program was designed to improve the quality of the assistance offered to mothers and neonates by public health services. The purpose of the program requires the adherence of pregnant women and mothers to care visits and to the guidance provided to prevent health risks.

Follow-up visits enable routine evaluations to be carried out on risks for the pregnant woman, the mother, or the baby, and whether it is necessary to refer them to other services. To avoid mismatches or losses in the process, the health service network was reorganized. A further specificity of this program is that it tries to include the presence of fathers as well as that of mothers whenever possible. This presence is encouraged at all stages and activities covered by the program. From 1999 to 2011, approximately 200,000 women and their babies were assisted in the program.

A number of municipalities in Brazil have adapted *Mãe Curitibana* models. One example is the *Estratégia Trevo de Quatro Folhas*[30] (The Four-leafed Clover Strategy) in Sobral, state of Ceará. Created in 2001, this program seeks to reduce maternal and infant mortality through a follow-up focused on four different time points: pregnancy, delivery, puerperal period, and follow-up until the child is 2 years old. Besides the basic actions recommended by the Ministry of Health, this one offers pregnant women and new mothers a different social support service and, when necessary, food supplies. The social support service offers home visits by one of the program's professionals to provide guidance on pregnancy, baby care, and self-care, as well as help with domestic tasks while the new mothers are not able to perform

[28] http://www.pmf.sc.gov.br/entidades/saude/index.php?cms=capital+crianca&menu=6.

[29] http://www.maecuritibana.com.br/.

[30] http://atencaobasica.org.br/relato/2512.

these. Women are selected in the local community, trained, and incorporated into the program to deliver the services to the pregnant women and/or new mothers.

In 2010, the program's team included 5 nurses, 3 nursing assistants, 1 social service professional, 1 psychologist, and 79 follow-up visitors. From 2002 to 2010, the program assisted 3316 women. Results indicate a reduction by more than half in the rate of infant mortality from 30/1000 born alive in 2001 to 14/1000 born alive in 2010.

The program *Rede de Proteção à Mãe Paulistana*[31] (Protection Network for *Paulistana* Mothers), known as *Mãe Paulistana*, was launched in the city of São Paulo in 2006. The program's aim is to reduce infant mortality and premature deliveries, prevent perinatal asphyxia and congenital infections, particularly AIDS and syphilis, and encourage breast-feeding.

Also according to the Municipal Secretariat of Health, besides direct care for the mother and child, this program has demanded the integration of Basic Health Units (UBS) with clinics and hospital facilities so that patient flow from prenatal to natal to postnatal care ensures that the newborn baby is continually followed-up by the different health services involved. Another characteristic of the program is the adoption of procedures to improve the care by providing psychological support to the new mothers or the pregnant women.

Mãe Paulistana offers prospective mothers the following support:

a. At least seven prenatal appointments
b. All routine clinical care and medical exams at each stage of the pregnancy
c. Immunization, medication (if needed), and nutritional supplements
d. Free transport for pregnant women to the clinic/health facility appointments
e. Room available at a public maternity ward for the delivery
f. Acquainting the pregnant mother with the maternity ward before the delivery
g. A basic trousseau for the new born
h. Follow-up for the mother and the baby during the postnatal period and for the first year of the child's life

To participate in the program, pregnant women register for prenatal care in one of the UBS of the city. From 2006 to 2011, *Mãe Paulistana* assisted 669,798 pregnant women, performing 4,081,480 clinical consultations, 5,105,054 exams, 642,138 ultrasonography exams, and 653,562 deliveries. The system includes a network of 436 UBSs, 23 specialized clinics, and 37 maternity wards.

More recently, in 2011, Rio de Janeiro city launched the program *Cegonha Carioca*[32] (The *Carioca* Stork) to reduce maternal and infant mortality and encourage prenatal exams. *Cegonha Carioca* expects that during the past 3 months of pregnancy, participants should pay a visit to the maternity ward where delivery is to take place to be acquainted with the premises and its functioning and to clear up any doubts about the hospitalization and the delivery. The program allows a pregnant woman to bring a companion of her choice for the visit to the maternity ward, if she

[31] http://ww2.prefeitura.sp.gov.br/secretarias/saude/mae_paulistana/.

[32] http://www.rio.rj.gov.br/web/sms/cegonha-carioca.

wishes to. At the end of the visit, the mother receives a small trousseau for the future baby. Another important aspect of the program is to guarantee ambulance service to the hospital for delivery. *Cegonha Carioca* does not yet cover all the city's regions, but data provided by the program show that in 1 year of operation, the program reached at least 21,000 women.

Primeira Infância Completa[33] (PIC—Good Childhood) is a program that started in 2009 in the city of Rio de Janeiro. Unlike the programs previously presented, mostly implemented and coordinated by Secretariats of Health, PIC was an initiative by the Secretariat of Education (SME), which develops the program in partnership with the Secretariats of Health, Civil Defense, and Social Welfare.

The purpose of PIC is to assist children from 6 months to 3 years of age waiting for proper placement in day care centers, providing them with 1 day a week of care in public day care centers. This care is provided on Saturdays, when day care centers are closed for their regular clientele. PIC also aims to work with the children's parents having developed what is called *Escola de Pais* (The School for Parents). This is an information-dispensing activity. For 1 h, at the end of their children's stay in the day care center, parents receive information about their children's health and development as well as the opportunity to resolve doubts about their children's progress.

PIC was integrated to the income supplementation program of the city, the *Cartão Família Carioca*[34] (The *Carioca* Family Card) in 2011. Through this program, economically vulnerable families enrolled in the PIC program receive income supplementation. In 2011, the PIC program was operating in 52 municipal day care centers, reaching at least 5000 children in all regions of the city, and by 2012 was present in 100 day care centers.

Another project that seeks to improve readiness of children for school is in the state of Acre—*Asinhas da Florestania* (Little Wings of Florestania). This is a state-level program designed by the State Secretariat of Education (SEE) of Acre, with the help of the World Bank and implemented in partnership with municipal governments. *Asinhas* is part of a larger project named *Asas da Florestania*[35] (Wings of the Florestania), with the goal to improve the quality of education in physically difficult to reach rural communities, areas that are to be environmentally preserved in the Amazon region.

Asas da Florestania was created in 2005 to promote middle-level schooling to children in such rural areas. In 2008, it was expanded to include secondary schools, and in 2009, to promote childhood education with *Asinhas da Florestania*[36]. The program targets children aged 4 and 5 years living in rural areas far away from formal teaching centers. To reduce their disadvantages when compared to children

---

[33] http://www.rio.rj.gov.br/web/sme/exibeconteudo?article-id=131779.

[34] http://www.rio.rj.gov.br/dlstatic/10112/124978/DLFE-236796.pdf/cartao_familia_carioca2.pdf.

[35] http://www.dialogosfederativos.gov.br/wp-content/uploads/2012/08/descric3a7c3a3o-da-iniciativa19.pdf.

[36] http://see.ac.gov.br/portal/index.php?option=com_content&view=article&id=92:a-educacao-que-da-asas&catid=1:noticias&Itemid=320.

attending regular city school, *Asinhas da Floresta* provides two weekly home visits by educational agents to stimulate the child's development, based on activities guided by the National Curriculum for Childhood Education. Home visitors are selected from the local population to ensure their access to the children assisted. Requirements for the position of educational agent, or home visitor, are to have completed secondary school and to live locally. According to the SEE, in 2011, the program was operating in most of the state's municipalities, assisting 2400 children in more than 260 communities.

Program *Infância Saudável* (The Healthy Childhood Program)

Given the volume of evidence about the gains from investing in early child development, the *Núcleo de Estudos da Violência* (Center for Studies on Violence) of the University of São Paulo (NEV-USP) invested in developing a methodology of home visitation to promote development. Of particular interest was the combination of the promotion of development and the gains in terms of the prevention of a variety of problems later in life, including violent victimization as well as offending, by preventing violence against the children assisted. Since the literature shows that the most vulnerable group is that of children born of adolescent parents, this age group was chosen for the experimental program. Adolescent parents were chosen also because of the situation of a "child" (according to the United Nations' definition, childhood goes from 0 to 18 years) mothering (or fathering) a child.

Adolescent mothers were chosen after an exploratory study, carried out by NEV-USP in the city of São Paulo, revealed the lack of public programs for adolescent mothers during the pregnancy and the first years of the child's life as well as their concentration in the most precarious social economic conditions (Gwatkin et al., 2007). Thus, most children born from adolescent mothers start life in unfavorable developmental conditions, with their mothers having little social support or education and living in overcrowded households in stressful contexts. Adolescent parents in contexts of high social vulnerability often have difficulties accessing traditional assistance networks, and their children suffer as result. However, research indicates that children living in socially and economically unfavorable conditions, but having access to investment programs in early childhood, may acquire lifelong developmental gains (Korfmacher, 2005; Korfmacher & Marchi, 2002). Investments in these children are thus one of the pathways to break up the perverse cycle of vulnerability.

The program was designed in 2006, in partnership with the World Health Organization (WHO), the Pan-American Health Organization (PAHO), and an International and National Advisory Committee[37] that monitored the development of the

[37] Maria Sallum—Instituto da Saúde/Secretaria de Estado de Saúde de São Paulo; Pâmela Ximena/OPAS Brasil; Simone de Assis—CLAVES/Fiocruz; Alberto Concha-Eastman—OPAS/Washington; Alexander Butchart—OMS/Genebra; Alexandra Guedes—OPAS/Washington; Christopher

program, providing technical and scientific oversight. *Infância Saudável* promotes child development by emphasizing access to rights; helping families circumvent obstacles in their access to public policies and services; teaching caregivers how to prevent accidents, negligence, abuse, maltreatment, and violence; informing them about the stages of child development; and teaching them simple means to stimulate their children. Paraprofessionals carry out home visits during the pregnancy and until the child is 2 years old.

Paraprofessional home visitors have the following profile: mothers living in the community where the intervention was carried out, having completed secondary school education, and aged between 30 and 40 years old. The choice of local paraprofessionals was guided by the need for some proximity between the home visitor and the adolescent mother and to reduce loss of time with transportation across the city. Home visits take place once a week lasting on average 50 min and involving three parts:

1. *Review of what was discussed in the previous meeting:* checking for doubts, asking about attempts to put into practice recommendations and/or solutions to problems raised, identifying difficulties, and identifying solutions
2. *Theme discussion:* presenting the theme to the adolescent in each home visit that has been selected and discussed during supervision meetings and takes into account needs identified, the stage of pregnancy or the child development, and the programs' aims
3. *Suggestions for the following week:* whenever possible, translating issues raised by the mother into practical solutions, identifying behaviors that can be adopted, role-playing to practice new behaviors, and encouraging the mother to experiment in the interval between home visits

Home visits contribute to the establishment of a climate of trust, in which the mother can express her beliefs, insecurities, and doubts regarding herself, her child's development, the assistance recommended and received, the orientation provided by public services, how to educate her child, or how to access her rights. In the case of adolescent mothers, this climate may allow them to voice values and expectations that guide their actions regarding motherhood.

Several strategies are used to approach and develop all themes. Among them are:

a. *Presenting and discussing information:* The information presented during the home visit takes into account the stage of pregnancy or the child's development, the knowledge already mastered by the mother, the services and social support networks she resorts to, her perceptions about herself and her child, and the home visitor's observations.
b. *Talking about difficulties and obstacles:* Once the information is presented, this is followed by a discussion on how to put it into practice. At that point, close

---

Mitkon—OMS/Genebra; Joanne Klevens—CDC/Washington; Jon Korfmacher—Erikson Institute/Chicago; Magdalena Cerda—University of Michigan; and Rosario Valdez—Instituto de Salud Publica de Mexico.

attention is given to difficulties and obstacles hindering the practice. This gives an opportunity to plan together strategies to overcome such difficulties.

c. *Anticipating scenarios:* Discussing future situations related to the child's development allows the adolescent mother to feel closer to her child's next developmental stages, recognizing what is or is not expected in each stage and preparing herself to cope with potentially stressful situations by anticipating protective measures.
d. *Redundancy:* Key information is presented and discussed in different ways—using folders, videos, role-play, and workshops—in different home visits of the program, thus enhancing the probability of being understood and used.
e. *Watching and doing together:* Whenever possible, the information is put into practice so the adolescent can observe how it can be done. Role-play is also used to increase her confidence.

Monthly group meetings allow adolescent mothers to share experiences, doubts, and achievements, thus favoring integration and mutual support. The group is also useful for reviewing content explored during the home visits.

Home visitors are individually monitored by a supervisor who is in charge of providing information, follow-up, and support for their activities. During supervision, the home visitor reports the home visit, evaluates the adequacy of activities and approach strategies, examines whether they need rethinking, and if so, the next visit and future procedures will be planned. It is also important to analyze the difficulties faced by the home visitor—whether they are related to the home visitation process, to interferences by the family or parent or her own difficulties, or to the supervisor's difficulties.

Since 2009, the experimental program has been implemented in a very violent and deprived area of the city of São Paulo: Jardim Angela. Between 2009 and 2012, 72 adolescents and their children were assisted by the program, about half of them before the child was born.

Though a proper external evaluation of the program was not carried out, some results are visible: (a) higher rates of prenatal care, in which adolescents in the program attend medical appointments and clinical examinations at higher rates than nonparticipating ones; (b) higher rates of normal delivery, in which 80 % of pregnant adolescents had a normal delivery, compared with the national average of 54 %, the state average of 59 %, and the municipal average of 58 %; (c) lower rates of premature births; (d) higher rates of birth registration without delay, in which almost all children were immediately registered; (e) higher rates of father's recognition of paternity of the child on the birth certificate; (f) higher rates of contact between the father and the child; (g) continued attendance at appointments by the health services to monitor the child's development, in which the vast majority attended appointments though many complained that the data (measuring and weighing) were not correct (i.e., they could assess whether the health professionals were doing their work well; (h) higher rates of inoculations, in which all children were inoculated at the right age; and (i) no developmental problems identified except in two children born with congenital problems of hydrocephalus and Down's syndrome.

Less successful have been attempts to secure breast-feeding up to child aged 6 months: Only one third of mothers breast-fed the child up to 6 months. The major obstacles were the adolescents' family values. Other problems identified involved poor networking between governmental and nongovernmental organizations[38]. This lack of a comprehensive approach to handle complex, multicausal problems that demand professionals from different areas—social service, law, health, and education—reduces the effectiveness of interventions.

One of the key innovations of this home visitation program was that it informed adolescents of their rights as well as the means to access these rights. Information about services and policies such as *Mãe Paulistana, Bolsa Família*, and training courses were given to the adolescents as well as how to effectively access these. The Brazilian *Estatuto da Criança e do Adolescente* (ECA; The Statute of Child and Adolescent, 1990)[39]. ECA assures pregnant girls the right to study at home from the 8th month of pregnancy on. However, not all schools inform pregnant adolescents, and as a result, many abandon school.

Another obstacle is the attitude of civil servants towards pregnant adolescents; often adolescents reported feeling rejected by health professionals. This reduced their trust in the professionals and increased their reticence to communicate problems or to seek advice. Effects of the rejection of adolescent pregnancy are also identified in the discrimination they report when trying to find a placement for their children in day care centers. They state that the community discriminates against them and does not legitimate their right to day care, presuming they have free time to look after their children.

The choice of paraprofessionals as home visitors has proved a rich and interesting experience. Paraprofessionals have established good bonds with the adolescent parents in the program. Besides the theoretical content that ensured both the quality and the adequacy of the interventions, continued monitoring provided the opportunity for home visitors to express their anxieties. Continued supervision meant that training was also sustained. The use of paraprofessionals from the community also meant that the knowledge they acquired from training was shared with other members of the community, not restricted to the adolescents who were visited. Field observations also suggest that the home visits may have had an impact on other members of the families of the adolescents visited, as they often witnessed role playing or overheard the home visitor instructions. Thus, knowledge was directly or indirectly shared in many ways.

This experiment carried out with such a challenging group has confirmed our initial assumption that adolescent mothers and their children not only need support

---

[38] Main partnerships involved were Sociedade Santos Mártires (SASF, NPJ, Casa Sofia), ONG Social Bom Jesus (SASF II), ARCO Associação Beneficiente, UBS Jardim Aracati.

[39] ECA is recognized as one of the more advanced legislation for the promotion and protection of children's and adolescents' development, though such rights are not always accessible in daily life. A variety of obstacles hinder the effectiveness of legal dispositions: precarious conditions, waiting lists, absence of clear and objective information on the services' operations, absence of qualified professionals, lack of equipment, and so forth.

but also that they are the dyads that stand to gain the most from interventions. We have discovered that this can be done at lower costs but with multiple gains.

Conclusion

This review of programs indicates that although there is a growing trend to promote early childhood, the use of home visitation methodology in Latin America and Caribbean countries and in Brazil specifically is still not as intensive as it would be expected given the existing needs. Nevertheless, there are some long-standing successful home visiting initiatives that serve only those families with the highest vulnerability, as opposed to offering universal programs.

Most programs reviewed were established during the 1990s and early 2000s, and these mainly target the health care of pregnant women and children during their first years of life to reduce maternal death and infant mortality. The review also points to the role that *Educa a tu Hijo* in Cuba and *Chile Crece Contigo* in Chile have played in offering models for other interventions in Latin America. Both programs have encouraged different governments to design similar interventions.

The child development programs presented here also have in common three drawbacks: (a) lack of scale—many interventions are local programs having small impacts, (b) lack of continuity—such interventions need time to mature and produce solid results, and (c) lack of adequate funding—often to reduce costs, unpaid or lowly paid volunteers are used to dispense the intervention. Despite these aspects, since the 2000s, some nationwide initiatives have started in places such as Chile, Brazil, Uruguay, Argentina, and Peru. Though few such initiatives have been evaluated, it is expected that the results of these initiatives, if properly measured and disseminated to the public, will promote greater public awareness and support and hopefully more pressure from the public for sustained public policies for home visiting services to promote children's early health and development.

References

Alderman, H. (2011). *No small matter: The impact of poverty, shocks, and human capital investments in early childhood development*. Washington, DC: World Bank.

Araujo, M. C., López-Boo, F., & Puyana, J. M. (2013). Overview of early childhood development services in Latin America and the Caribbean. http://publications.iadb.org/bitstream/handle/11319/3617/BID_Panorama_ENG%20%28Web%29.pdf?sequence=2. Accessed June 2012.

Argentina, Consejo Nacional de Coordinación de Políticas Sociales (CNCPS). (s/d). El Programa Nacional de Desarrollo Infantil Primeros Años. http://www.primerosanios.gov.ar/index.html. Accessed Oct 2012.

Argentina, Consejo Nacional de Coordinación de Políticas Sociales (CNCPS). (2009). Primeros Años: Informe de actividades 2009. http://www.primerosanios.gov.ar/descargas/publicaciones/informes/informe2009.pdf http://www.primerosanios.gov.ar/index.html. Accessed Oct 2012.

Armus, M., Duhalde, C., Oliver, M., & Woscoboinik, N. (2012). Desarrollo emocional. Clave para la primera infância. 0 a 3. Argentina: UNICEF/Fundación Kaleidos. http://www.unicef.org/argentina/spanish/Desarrollo_emocional_0a3_simples.pdf. Accessed Oct 2012.

Barker, D. J. P. (1994). *Mothers, babies and disease in later life*. London: BMJ Publishing Group.

Bernal, R., Fernández, C., Flórez Nieto, C. E., Garviria, A., Ocampo, P. R., Samper, B., & Sánchez, F. (2009). *Evaluation of the early childhood program Hogares Comunitarios De Bienestar in Colombia*. Bogotá: Centro de Estudios sobre Desarrollo Económico.

Brasil, Ministério da Saúde. Estratégia Brasileirinhos e Brasileirinhas Saudáveis—Primeiros Passos para o Desenvolvimento Nacional. http://portal.saude.gov.br/portal/saude/odm_saude/visualizar_texto.cfm?idtxt=35139. Accessed Oct 2012.

Brasil, Ministério da Saúde. Humaniza SUS: Política Nacional de Humanização. http://bvsms.saude.gov.br/bvs/publicacoes/humaniza_sus_marco_teorico.pdf. Accessed Oct 2012.

Brasil, Ministério da Saúde. Departamento de Atenção Básica. http://dab.saude.gov.br/portaldab/ape_esf.php. Accessed Oct 2012.

Brasil, Ministério da Saúde. Diretrizes Gerais e Operacionais da Rede Cegonha. http://portal.saude.gov.br/portal/saude/Gestor/visualizar_texto.cfm?idtxt=37082. Accessed Oct 2012.

Cardia, N. (2006). *Estado del arte de los programas de prevención de la violencia en jóvenes basados en la promoción del desarrollo*. Washington, DC: OPS.

Cardone, I., Gilkerson, L., & Welchsler, N. (2008). *Teenagers and their babies: A perinatal home visitor's guide*. Washington, DC: ZERO TO THREE.

Chile, Ministerio de Desarrollo Social. Chile Crece Contigo del Sistema de Promoción y Protección Social. http://www.crececontigo.gob.cl/. Accessed Oct 2012.

Colombia, Instituto Colombiano de Bienestar Familiar. Departamento para la Prosperidad Social. http://www.icbf.gov.co/portal/page/portal/PortalICBF. Accessed Oct 2013.

Dreyer, B. P. (2011). Early childhood stimulation in the developing and developed world: If not now, when? *Pediatrics, 127*(5), 975–977.

EcuRed. Programa Educa a tu Hijo. http://www.ecured.cu/index.php/Educa_a_tu_Hijo. Accessed Oct 2012.

Engle, P. L., Black, M. M., Behrman, J. R., Mello, M. C., Gertler, P. J., Kapiriri, L., Martorell, R., & Young, M. E. (2007). Strategies to avoid the loss of developmental potential in more than 200 million children in the developing world. *The Lancet, 369*(9557), 229–242.

Estado do Acre, Secretaria de Educação e Esporte. A Educação que dá Asas. http://see.ac.gov.br/portal/index.php?option=com_content&view=article&id=92:a-educacao-que-da-asas&catid=1:noticias&Itemid=320. Accessed Oct 2012.

Estado do Pernambuco Secretaria de Saúde. Programa Mãe Coruja. http://maecorujape.blogspot.com.br/coruja. Accessed Oct 2012.

Estado do Rio Grande do Sul, Secretaria de Saúde. UNESCO. Programa Primeira Infância Melhor. http://www.pim.saude.rs.gov.br/a_PIM/php/index.php. Accessed Oct 2012.

Fiedler, J. L. (2003). A cost analysis of the Honduras community-based integrated child care program. Washington, DC: International Bank for Reconstruction and Development/World Bank.

Gómez, A. M. S. (2011). La contextualización del modelo de atención educativa no institucional Cubano "Educa a tu Hijo" en países latinoamericanos. UNICEF: Oficina Regional para América Latina y el Caribe. http://primerainfancialac.org/documentos/Educa_a_tu_Hijo_UNICEF_Siverio.pdf. Accessed Oct 2012.

Grantham-McGregor, S., Cheunq, Y. B., Cueto, S., Glewwe, P., Ritcher, L., Strupp, B., & International Child Development Steering Group. (2007). Developmental potential in the first 5 years for children in developing countries. *Lancet, 369*(9555), 60–70.

Guatemala, Ministerio da Educación. Educación Preescolar. Programa De La Mano, Educame. http://www.mineduc.gob.gt/portal/contenido/menu_lateral/sistema_educativo/educacion_preescolar/index2.html. Accessed Oct 2012.

Gunnar, M. R., & Davis E. (2003). Stress and emotion in early childhood. In R. Lerner, M. A. Easterbrooks, & J. Mistry (Orgs.). *Handbook of psychology: Developmental psychology* (Vol. 6, pp. 113–134). Hoboken: Wiley.

Guterman, N. B. (2001). *Stopping child maltreatment before it starts: Emerging horizons in early home visitation services*. Thousand Oaks: Sage.

Gwatkin, R. D., Rutstein, S., Johnson, K., Suliman, E., Wagstaff, A., & Amouzou, A. (2007). *Socio-economic differences in health, nutrition and population within developing countries*. Washington, DC: HNP/Poverty thematic group/World Bank.

Heckman, J. J. (2006). Skill formation and the economics of investing in disadvantaged children. *Science, 312*(5782), 1900–1902.

Hertzman, C. (2000). The case for an early childhood development strategy. *Isuma: Canadian Journal of Policy Research, 1*(2), 11–18.

Honduras, Secretaría de Estado de la Presidencia. Unidad Administradora de Proyectos. Proyecto Nutrición Y Protección Social. http://www.sdp.gob.hn/sitio/index.php?option=com_content&view=article&id=29&Itemid=182. Accessed Oct 2013.

Irwin, L. G., Siddiqi, A., & Hertzman, C. (2007). Early child development: A powerful equalizer. Final report to the WHO Commission on Social Determinants of Health, Geneva.

Jones, J., Brown, A., & Brown, J. (2011). Caring and learning together: A case study of Jamaica. Early Childhood and Family Policy Series, 21. Paris: Unesco/ Section for Basic Education. http://unesdoc.unesco.org/images/0019/001913/191327e.pdf. Accessed Oct 2012.

Jules, D. (2010). Positioning the Roving Caregivers Programme as a Caribbean model. Caribe, Caribbean Child Support Initiative. http://www.globalchilddevelopment.com/sites/default/files/RCP%20Position%20Paper%20REPORT.pdf. Accessed Oct 2012.

Karoly, L. A., Kilburn, M. R., & Cannon, J. S. (2005). *Early childhood interventions: Prove results, future promise*. Santa Monica: RAND Corporation.

Kemp, L., Harris, E., McMahon, C., Matthey, S., Vimpani, G., Anderson, T., Schmied, V., Aslam, H., & Zapart, S. (2011). Child and family outcomes of a long-term nurse home visitation programme: A randomised controlled trial. *Archives of Disease in Childhood, 96*(6), 533–540.

Korfmacher, J. (2005). Teen parents in early childhood interventions. *Zero to Three, 25*(4), 7–13.

Korfmacher J., & Marchi, I. (2002). The helping relationship in a teen parenting program. *Zero to Three, 23*(2), 21–26.

Korfmacher, J., Green, B., Spellmann, M., & Thornburg, K. R. (2007). The helping relationship and program participation in early childhood home visiting. *Infant Mental Health Journal, 28*(5), 450–480.

Lee, E., Mitchell-Herzfeld, S., Lowenfels, A., Greene, R., Dorabawilla, V., & DuMont, K. A. (2009). *Improving birth outcomes through prenatal home visitation: A randomized trial of healthy families New York*. Albany: University at Albany.

Love, J. M., Kisker, E. E., Ross, C., Constantine, J., Boller, K., Chazan-Cohen, R., Brady-Smith, C., Fuligni, A. S., Raikes, H., Brooks-Gunn, J., Tarullo, L. B., Schochet, P. Z., Paulsell, D., & Vogel, C. (2005). The effectiveness of Early Head Start for 3-year-old children and their parents: Lessons for policy and programs. *Developmental Psychology, 41*(6), 885–901.

MacMillan, H. L., Thomas, B. H., Jamieson, E., Walsh, C. A., Boyle, M. H., Shannon, H. S., & Gafni, A. (2005). Effectiveness of home visitation by public-health nurses in prevention of the recurrence of child physical abuse and neglect: A randomized controlled trial. *Lancet, 365*(9473), 1786–1793.

Mantilla, B. P; Sánchez, R. H., & Torrado, P. M. C. (2007). Evaluación Nacional HCB-FAMI: Resumen ejecutivo (Julho 2007). Colombia: Instituto Colombiano de Bienestar Familiar (ICBF). http://proinapsa.uis.edu.co/docsdeinteres/pdf/RESUMEN_EJECUTIVO_final_Evaluacion_FAMI.pdf. Accessed Oct 2012.

Martínez, M., & Tello, E. (2009). Evaluación de impacto del programa Hogares Comunitarios de Bienestar del ICBF. Bogotá: Departamento Nacional de Planeación. http://www.dnp.gov.co/LinkClick.aspx?fileticket=W30Ag1a2h68%3d&tabid=843. Accessed Oct 2012.

McDonald, K. (2000). Elements of quality in early childhood home visiting programmes. Jamaica: UNICEF. http://siteresources.worldbank.org/INTECD/Resources/kerida.htm. Accessed Oct 2012.

Mercy, J. A., & Saul, J. (2009). Creating a healthier future through early interventions for children. *JAMA, 301*(21), 1–3.

Mitchell-Herzfeld, S., Izzo, C., Greene, R., Lee, E., & Lowenfels, A. (2005). *Evaluation of healthy families New York (HFNY): First year program impacts*. New York: New York State Office of Children & Family Services, Center for Human Services Research. http://www.ocfs.state.ny.us/main/reports/HFNY_FirstYearProgramImpacts.pdf. Accessed Oct 2012.

Mustard, J. F. (2010). O Desenvolvimento da Primeira Infância e o Cérebro—a base para a saúde, o aprendizado e o comportamento durante a vida toda. In M. E. Young (Ed.), *Do Desenvolvimento da Primeira Infância ao Desenvolvimento Humano*. (M. Lopes, Trad.) São Paulo: Fundação Maria Cecília Souto Vidigal.

Narayan, O. P. (2005). *Harnessing child development: Children and the right to education*. Deli: Isha Books.

Olds, D. (1988). The prenatal/early infancy project. In R. Price, E. Cowen, R. Lorion, & J. Ramos-Mckay (Eds.), *Fourteen ounces of prevention: A casebook for practitioners*. Washington, DC: American Psychological Association.

Olds, D., Eckenrode, J., Henderson, C. R., Jr., Kitzman, H., Powers, J., Cole, R., Sidora, K., Morris, P., Pettitt, L. M., & Luckey, D. (1997). Long-term effects of home visitation on maternal life course and child abuse and neglect. Fifteen-year follow-up of a randomized trial. *JAMA, 278*(8), 637–643.

Olds, D., Kitzman, H., Cole, R., Robinson, J., Sidora-Arcoleo, K., Luckey, D. W., Henderson, C. R., Hanks, C., Bondy, J., & Holmberg, J. (2004). Effects of nurse home-visiting on maternal life course and child development: Age 6 follow-up results of a randomized trial. *Pediatrics, 114*(6), 1150–1159.

Organización de Estados Iberoamericanos para la Educación, la Ciencia y la Cultura (OEI). Programa Creciendo con Nuestros Hijos. http://www.oei.es/inicial/ecuadorne.htm#4. Accessed Oct 2012.

Pastoral da Criança. Conferência de Bispos do Brasil. http://www.pastoraldacrianca.org.br/. Accessed Oct 2012.

Peru Ministerio de Desarrollo e Inclusion Social. Programa Nacional Cuna Mas. http://www.cunamas.gob.pe/. Accessed Oct 2012.

Pinheiro, P. S. (2006). *World report on violence against children*. Geneva: United Nations.

Power, C., & Hertzman, C. (1997). Social and biological pathways linking early life and adult disease. *British Medical Bulletin, 53*(1), 210–221.

Power, C., Hypponen, E., & Smith, G. D. (2005). Socioeconomic position in childhood and early adult life and risk of mortality: a prospective study of the mothers of the 1958 British birth cohort. *American Journal of Public Health, 95*(8), 1396–1402.

Prefeitura Municipal de Curitiba, Secretaria de Saúde. Programa Mãe Curitibana. http://www.maecuritibana.com.br/. Accessed Oct 2012.

Prefeitura Municipal de Florianópolis, Secretaria de Saúde Programa Capital Infância. http://www.pmf.sc.gov.br/entidades/saude/index.php?cms=capital+crianca&menu=6. Accessed Oct 2012.

Prefeitura Municipal de São Paulo, Secretaria de Saúde Programa Mãe Paulistana. http://ww2.prefeitura.sp.gov.br/secretarias/saude/mae_paulistana/index.asp. Accessed Oct 2012.

Prefeitura Municipal do Rio de Janeiro, Secretaria de Educação. Primeira Infância Completa. http://www.rio.rj.gov.br/web/sme/exibeconteudo?article-id=131779. Accessed Oct 2012.

Quintero-Velasquez, A. M. (2011). Modelos de políticas públicas de Colombia, en beneficio de las familias. *Revista Katálysis, 14*(1), 116–125.

Rodriguez, M. L., Dumont, K., Mitchell-Herzfeld, S. D., Walden, N. J., & Greene, R. (2010). Effects of healthy families New York on the promotion of maternal parenting competencies and the prevention of harsh parenting. *Child Abuse & Neglect, 34*(10), 711–723. doi:10.1016/j.chiabu.2010.03.004.

Roopnarine, J. L., & Hossain, Z. (2007). The Roving Caregiver Program: A family-based early intervention programme for enhancing early childhood development and parenting. *Early Childhood Matters, 109*, 25–29. (The Netherlands: Bernard van Leer Foundation).

Sandler, I. N., Schoenfelder, E. N., Wolchik, S. A., & MacKinnon, D. P. (2011). Long-term impact of prevention programs to promote effective parenting: Lasting effects bust uncertain processes. *Annual Review of Psychology, 62*, 299–329. doi:10.1146/annurev.psych.121208.131619.

Schaetzel, T., Griffiths, M., Del Rosso, J. M., & Plowman, B. (2008). *Evaluation of the AIN-C program in Honduras*. Arlington: Basic Support for Institutionalizing Child Survival (BASICS) for the United States Agency for International Development (USAID).

Shonkoff, J. P. (2010). Building a new biodevelopmental framework to guide the future of early childhood policy. *Child Development, 81*(1), 357–367.

Shonkoff, J. P., Phillips, D. A., & Committee on integrating the science of early childhood development. (2000). *From neurons to neighborhoods: The science of early childhood development*. Washington, DC: National Academy Press.

Shore, A. (2003). *Affect disregulation and disorders of the self*. New York: W. W. Norton & Company.

Spiker, D., & Gaylor, E. (2012). Home visiting programs (prenatal and postnatal)—Synthesis. In R. E. Tremblay, M. Boivin, & R. de V. Peters (Eds.), *Encyclopedia on early childhood development*. Montreal: Centre of Excellence for Early Childhood Development and Strategic Knowledge Cluster on Early Child Development. http://www.child-encyclopedia.com/pages/PDF/home_visiting_programs.pdf. Accessed Oct 2012.

UNESCO. (2006). *EFA global monitoring report. Strong foundations: Early childhood care and education*. Paris: UNESCO.

UNICEF. Experiencias de Desarrollo Infantil Integral en Bolivia. http://www.unicef.org/bolivia/spanish/local_development_1966.htm. Accessed Oct 2013.

UNICEF. 'Roving Caregivers' promote early childhood development at home in Jamaica. http://www.unicef.org/infobycountry/jamaica_36354.html. Accessed Oct 2012.

Uruguay Oficina de Planeamiento y Presupuesto and Presidencia de la República Oriental del Uruguay. Uruguay Crece Contigo. http://www.crececontigo.opp.gub.uy/. Accessed Oct 2012.

Vargas-Barón, E. (2009). *Going to scale: Early childhood development in Latin America*. Washington, DC: The RISE Institute.

Vegas, E., & Santibáñez, L. (2010). *The promise of early childhood development in Latin America and the Caribbean*. Washington, DC: World Bank. http://siteresources.worldbank.org/EDUCATION/Resources/278200-1099079877269/547664-1099079922573/ECD_LAC.pdf. Accessed Oct 2012.

Wasik, B. H., & Bryant, D. M. (2001). *Home visiting: Procedures for helping families*. Thousand Oaks: Sage.

Yánez, A. M., & Yánez, J. L. (2006). Al otro lado de la ventana: Programas internacionales de cuidado y desarrollo infantil para niños en situación de vulnerabilidad social y económica. http://portal.oas.org/LinkClick.aspx?fileticket=XEDraJdb8Vk%3D&tabid=1282&mid=3693. Accessed Oct 2012.

Young, M. E. (Ed.). (2007). *Early child development: From measurement to action*. Washington, DC: World Bank.

Nancy Cardia (Brazil): Professor and deputy coordinator of the Center for the Study of Violence and coordinator of the activities of knowledge transfer. She represented the center as a Collaborating Centre of the World Health Organization (WHO) in the issue of prevention of violence at the Department of Prevention of Violence and Injuries (2004–2014). She has organized the series of books, *Police and Society*, and the series *Human Rights Education*. She was a member of the Editing Committee of the World Report on Violence against Children (The United Nations Secretary-General's Report), author of a book about murders of children in Brazil (WHO/PAHO). She compiled the module of youth violence: causes and prevention for the WHO TEACH-VIP and produced, for the PAHO/GTZ, a study on how to prevent youth violence and promote healthy development. She is general coordinator of the pilot deployment of the program of domestic visitation for adolescent mothers and their children: a program to promote healthy development and prevent violence and is also the coordinator of research on exposure to violence and its impact on attitudes, values, norms regarding violence, human rights, justice, and democracy.

Renato Alves (Brazil): PhD student and master's degree holder in psychology from the University of São Paulo. He holds a degree in psychology from the Methodist University of São Paulo and a degree in social sciences from the University of São Paulo. He is a researcher at the Center for the Study of Violence at the University of São Paulo (NEV/USP) and professor of psychology at the Methodist University of São Paulo.

Aline Gomes (Brazil): Researcher at the Center for the Study of Violence at the University of São Paulo (NEV/USP). She collaborated in the development of a home visiting program for pregnant adolescents and their children to prevent violence and secure a healthy development, being a visitor herself as well as a supervisor for paraprofessional visitors. She has a masters and an MA degree in Psychology as well as a psychologist degree (5-year degree). She was a home visitor and continued as a trainer in the Infância Saudável (a home visitation program). At the Center for the Study of Violence, her research interests are early child development, adolescent pregnancy, and violence prevention.

Alder Mourão (Brazil): Researcher at the Center for the Study of Violence at the University of São Paulo (NEV/USP). He collaborated in the development of a home visiting program to promote healthy early child development as well as to prevent violence for a high-risk group as a visitor and as a supervisor. He has a masters and an MSc in nursing. His research focuses on public and family health, early child development, and violence prevention.

Chapter 11
Home Visiting Interventions to Promote Values That Support School Success

Martha Julia García-Sellers

In the past two decades, public schools in the USA have found themselves challenged to accommodate and educate a significant influx of immigrant children in a classroom. This is not the first time that the schools have been called upon to serve the important function of facilitating the entry of recent immigrant families into the USA; it occurred, for example, in the first decades of the twentieth century (Pedraza, 1996). However, the expectations about school transitions and academic success have changed over the past century. Now there is more acceptance of the notion that growing up bilingual and retaining one's cultural heritage is feasible and perhaps desirable, so long as it does not impede the achievement of educational goals (Bradley, 2011; Soria, 2012; Suarez-Orozco, 2000). Problematically, the resources required to enable nonstandard educational processes are often lacking in public schools.

Recently, a major worry of the public school system is that the high school dropout rates and low performances of Latino immigrant students continue at an alarming rate (Greene & Winters, 2006; Suarez-Orozco & Páez, 2009). This has provoked some specific social policy efforts to support the educational rights of immigrant students, their language, and learning needs. At the community level, initiatives have been undertaken to reach out to recent immigrant families and provide them with resources that can help them become familiar with school requirements and educational expectations.

Academic research on this topic tends to focus on dissecting and explaining Latino children's school performance in the framework of their cultural background and transitional experiences (Calzada, Fernandez, & Cortes, 2010; García & Ozturk, 2011; Haskins & Tienda, 2011; Severns, 2011; Soria, 2012). Less research, regrettably, has been devoted to improving our knowledge about more effective teaching practices for bicultural students (Baker & Peterson, 2010;

M. J. García-Sellers (✉)
Tufts University, Medford, MA, USA
e-mail: mj.garcia.sellers@gmail.com

L. Roggman, N. Cardia (eds.), *Home Visitation Programs*,
DOI 10.1007/978-3-319-17984-1_11

García & Náñez, 2011). Specific studies have focused more often on Latino children's readiness and transitions to school, their process of immigration, family background, the challenge of growing up bilingual, and the different behaviors valued in their home and at school.

Home–School Relations

Over the years, studies have consistently found that parental involvement in children's education is a strong predictor of their academic success (Jeynes, 2005, 2012). While most of these studies have been conducted with US middle-class, nonminority participants, the findings have been assumed to apply generally to the school performance of immigrant students as well. Studies that have focused specifically on home–school relations among Latino immigrant families appear to confirm a lack of parental involvement in their children's education (Jeynes, 2003; Williams & Sánchez, 2012). However, it can be questioned if the findings of "low parental involvement" among Latino immigrants might be a reflection of how cultural values and expectations are understood and expressed.

In the course of interviews we carried out, my students and I have noted school staff statements that Latino parents "don't want to get involved," "don't support their children's education," and "don't encourage their children's academic success." Parents, on the other hand, say (in Spanish) "we came to the US in order to have better educational opportunities for our children." They "want their children to do well at school," and they report that they are helping their children in whatever ways they can. From their own words, it is evident that teachers and parents have different perceptions of parents' involvement in their children's schooling. This observation has proven to be a useful starting point to improve communication and understanding between parents and teachers.

The first thing to be aware of is that "parental involvement" and "school success" have more than one single meaning; what teachers and parents (as well as investigators) understand by these terms can differ significantly. School success might refer to the child's understanding of classroom routines, learning to read, studying independently, obtaining good grades, doing well on standardized tests, behaving properly in the classroom, or regularly attending school to mention a few possibilities. Similarly, depending on one's perspective, parental involvement might imply participation in school-related committees, occasional help in the classroom, chaperoning school field trips or—with regard to tasks pertaining to the child's learning—organizing home routines and activities that foster learning, helping the child with homework, understanding the child's developmental progress, and anticipating their educational needs. When evaluating outcomes from projects that intend to promote parental school involvement or school success, it is necessary to agree on how we define these terms, taking into consideration that parents and teachers as well as researchers and media in general might have different definitions in mind.

The three projects reported here are similar in that they promote home–school connections, focus on parent–teacher communication, and involve Latino families. The projects provide an informative comparison because (a) they were designed in accordance with the salient needs and the predominant cultural values of each site, and consequently, (b) they differed in regard to specific objectives that constituted school success and parental involvement. All three projects relied on a home visiting approach; additionally, they involved school participants and a home–school mediator or liaison.

Home Visiting Approach

Internationally, the home visitation methodology has been widely used for several decades in newborn and follow-up programs, especially those related to preventive maternal and child health. In the USA, home visiting is being used more frequently for research studies and intervention programs relating, for example, to early intervention, early literacy, physical and mental health services, and in particular, programs aiming to prevent violence in the home (Brooks-Gunn, Berlin, & Fuligni, 2000). In the educational realm, with few exceptions, proactively reaching out to families through home visits, even those new to the community with young children, is not a standard practice for the US public schools.

For many parents of children in the US public school system, "parental involvement" denotes the parent–teacher association (PTA or PTO) through which parents discuss school policies, volunteer for school activities, and talk over issues with teachers. The term might also call to their minds open-house meetings with teachers, back to school night, and fundraising—all of which are activities centered on the school. Teachers devote significant time to preparing these school events and often conclude that parental attendance tends to be wanting. Several reasons for low involvement may be cited, for example, parents' work schedules, childcare arrangements, and difficulty of transportation. Latino immigrant parents cite these logistical reasons, but they mention other reasons as well: They feel unfamiliar with the nature of these events and are unsure about their relevance for their children's school achievement. Unlike the US public school system, the public schools of Latin America did not evolve out of community-based schools, and therefore, parents tend to see themselves as recipients of educational services rather than collaborators. And even though the local school may take the initiative to reach out to immigrant families by translating school announcements and flyers into their native languages, school meetings are conducted primarily in English and thus require a higher degree of exertion and self-assurance for Spanish-speaking parents to express themselves.

In contrast to their hesitation to respond to meetings announced publicly by the school, we have found that Latino parents are receptive to social activities and classroom gatherings, especially when the invitation is addressed personally to the family and, even more so, when their own children are involved in a classroom activity or performance. Similarly, they are often willing and pleased to volunteer to participate in research and programs that are conducted through home visits. Parents feel that home visits better fit their schedules and child-care arrangements. Moreover, the inclusion of the whole family is more sociable, and therefore, the format resembles a friendly visit in which the conversation, in Spanish, is less imposing. Whereas a schooling-related home visit to a middle-class Anglo family might be expected to be oriented around addressing issues and resolving problems, for Latino families the personal interaction is important; the home visit itself is significant, and they feel honored to receive a visitor from the school who cares about their child and family. This is especially true for immigrant families (as compared to Latin Americans in their countries of origin), who may feel lonely and misunderstood: Receiving a visitor, especially one who shares their language and culture, lowers the barriers of mistrust and opens their inclination to express themselves. In their own home and in their own language, they feel more confident to ask questions and reveal their doubts and concerns than they would in a one-to-one appointment with a teacher, staff member, or an administrator at school.

As for the students, the home visits have important effects that reach beyond academics but are themselves significant for success at school. Children usually see home and school as two very separate worlds. The home visits provide a concrete way of bridging their school experiences with their family life. While many tend to be reserved (but unquestionably attentive) in the initial visits, they soon become comfortable and over time look forward to the visits as well as the interaction with the home visitor. The children's reaction when they recognize the home visitor at school is one of revelation, delight, and pride in realizing that this person shares their own special knowledge of both school and home. Because the home visitor is an adult with whom they identify, it feels like they are being given permission to make this connection on their own. These perceptions facilitate interventions at school and the child's more comfortable acceptance of parental involvement in their school life.

In summary, home visiting fulfills several important functions in our approach to improving students' academic success by promoting communication between home and school. First, the home visitor bridges the gap between home and school, thereby, enabling parents and children to recognize a connection between the two environments. Building on this connection, parents are more inclined to approach school personnel themselves. Second, the home visitor becomes knowledgeable about the child and family's circumstances at home, knowledge that can be relevant to interpreting behavior and providing guidance at school. Third, as detailed below, the home visit may become the vehicle for intervention to promote learning at home and thereby advance school readiness or reinforce learning that goes on in the classroom.

It is important to emphasize that our approach to home visiting is not "one size fits all." On the contrary, we recognize that the home visiting procedure needs to be adapted to the objectives, circumstances, and cultural context of each project.

Project One: Somerville

The project with Latino immigrants in Somerville began in the mid-1990s. Somerville has long been a gateway city for immigrants to the Boston area, and in the 1990s Latinos composed more than 10% of the population. The public schools, in which Latinos far surpassed 10% in many classrooms, were straining to serve this new population, and, because Tufts University falls partly within Somerville, I found myself advising students and consulting with school staff regarding Latino students and their families.

The design and purpose of what came to be called the "Home-School Connection Program" (H-SCP) evolved from a series of focus groups with members of the Somerville community, longitudinal case studies collected in interviews, and pilot study trials in several classrooms at two elementary schools (García-Sellers, 1997, García-Sellers, 1998). In retrospect, it can be said that conceiving the program from the expressed needs of the community was critical to its success; the program was a response to, and designed in close collaboration with, the needs aired by administrators, teachers, and Latino immigrants who were the parents of young students attending those schools. Administrators were concerned about the needs and low classroom performances of the Latino students and were at a loss in knowing how to reach out to parents. On their part, parents recognized the value of education and expressed a desire to support their children in school, but they also had doubts about when and how to communicate with teachers.

I formed the H-SCP in 1996 as an outgrowth of several years of collaboration between the Eliot-Pearson Child Development Department of Tufts University and public schools in Somerville, Massachusetts. Implementation of the program started in 1996 focusing on six first-to-third-grade classrooms with Spanish-speaking children from Central America immigrant families, funded by a 4-year grant from the W. K. Kellogg Foundation. During the initial stage, information suggested that many of the schools' concerns about Latino children's performance were due, at least in part, to the different educational expectations at home and school. Both parents and teachers wanted the best for the child but were unaware of each other's expectations; there was a communication gap leading to a lack of support for the child's transition from home to school.

After familiarizing ourselves with the situation, we developed a model of school adaptation to depict children's school adaptation, improving the communication between parents and teachers (García-Sellers, 1997, 1998). As illustrated in Fig. 11.1, there is a considerable overlap and continuity of expectations between the home and the school environment for the modal US child.

In contrast, as shown in Fig. 11.2, we encountered several modes of adaptation among the immigrant children and families we were working with. We identified those modes as *Unadapted, Transferred, Adapted,* and *Adapted with Support*. The last of those was the mode that program intervention sought to achieve.

Most children participating in the H-SCP fell into the first three groups. Children in the Unadapted group were unsuccessful in adapting to the classroom routine,

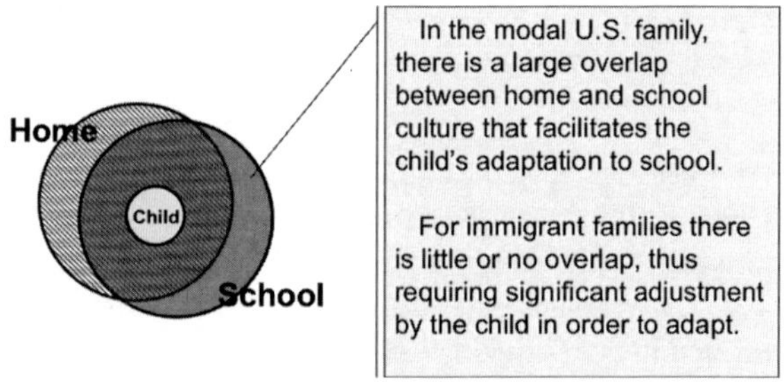

Fig. 11.1 Modal school adaptation

internalizing failure and expressing behaviors and strategies suitable to their homes but not with the classroom. Parents and teachers were worried about their school performance, with no understanding of how to help them. At the same time, neither parents nor teachers took the initiative to discover the children's needs, and school personnel tended to blame the family for children's low performances.

Children in the Transferred group were thriving in the classroom, but at the same time rejecting home values and adopting behaviors that gave them more acceptance from their teacher and satisfied classroom expectations. They refused to speak Spanish at home and their parents sadly reported that they were becoming "Americanized." Unexpectedly, a few parents of children in this group thought the change could be advantageous and encouraged their child to become Americanized to succeed in the US society.

The Adapted group somehow managed to maintain dual sets of behavior: one at home and the other at school. At home, they spoke Spanish and were more compliant and obedient; at school, they made an effort to speak English, were more

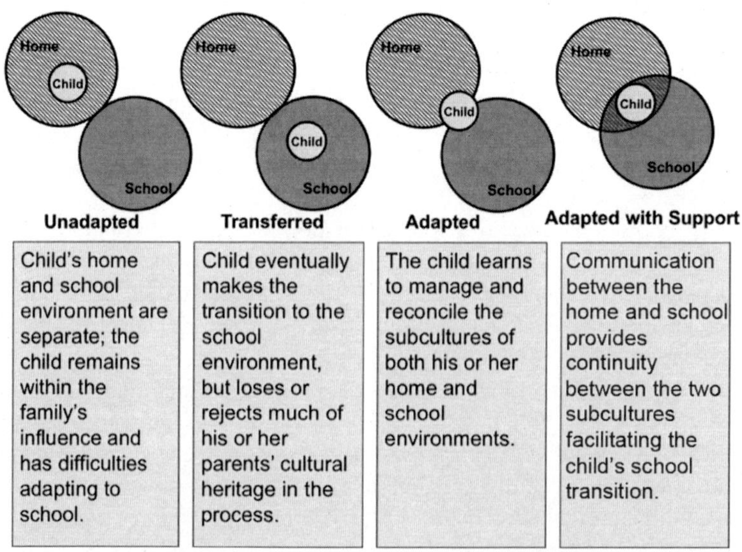

Fig. 11.2 Model of school adaption

independent, and worked hard to fulfill classroom expectations. However, this dual identity tended to be transitory; by third grade, most of them had shifted to Transferred.

The intervention promoted by the H-SCP attempted to move children toward Adapted with Support. The specific objectives of the intervention are: improving communication between parents and children, improving communication between parents and teachers, and encouraging a common understanding of each child's educational needs at home and school. Understanding each child's particular talents and needs serves a foundation for communication; improved communication leads to greater consistency and continuity of expectations at home and school; and finally, consistent expectations and practices at home and school facilitate effective school adaptation for the child. Although often we refer school adaptation as the child's accomplishment, it is suggested here that we understand it as a triangular process among child, parents, and teacher (Brizuela & García-Sellers, 1998).

By design, the program incorporated activities at home and school carried out by trained mediators who were regularly supervised (Parra-Velasco & García-Sellers, 2005). Home visits enabled mediators to familiarize themselves with families: their acquaintance with the neighborhood school and understanding of the educational system, their child rearing practices at home, and their expectations about their children's education. During the home visits, mediators provided frequent guidance and support, seeking ways to promote ongoing communication with classroom teachers and empowering parents to support their child's transition to school and academic work.

With regard to activities in the school, mediators spent time in the child's classroom becoming familiar with the child's character, academic performance, interaction with peers, and ability to adapt. Mediators were also attentive to the teachers' teaching style and how well they understood students' personal attributes. They communicated a supportive attitude toward the teacher. The mediator scheduled regular appointments with the teacher to provide guidance and feedback about each child and his family in order to promote better understanding and appreciation of their characteristics and to facilitate regular communication.

Mediators also scheduled group meetings with parents and teachers, separately and together, to amplify issues and topics that had previously been discussed individually and were pertinent to many of them. When necessary, individual meetings with parents and teachers were scheduled to discuss the specific needs of a particular child.

Intervention followed similar procedures: collection of information and the feedback and guidance offered to teachers and parents was tailored to the circumstances of each child. Families' characteristics varied significantly as did the teachers'. However, over time, teachers began to adopt the methodology themselves and to implement some recommendations spontaneously to different children.

One gratifying outcome of the study was the high level of satisfaction and participation: 100 % of parents volunteered for the program and continued till its conclusion, while teachers expressed high satisfaction in the classroom activities. This led to 4 more years of the program, expanding to 12 kindergarten classrooms for

Spanish transitional bilingual children, English speakers, and special-needs children. The expansion was supported by the Somerville Public Schools as part of the Full Day Kindergarten initiative of the Massachusetts Department of Education.

Evaluation of the H-SCP program identified several important outcomes that confirmed improved communication between parents and teachers. First, children's school attendance increased, as did parents' participation in classroom and school activities. Second, children became engaged in classroom routines and reported back to their parents about school activities. Third, teachers became more knowledgeable of children's family conditions and sometimes applied that awareness to guiding the child in school. Teachers also reported that conversations with parents about grade placement, retention, and special needs evaluations were less tense and more collaborative than in the past. And fourth, from our evaluation in subsequent years, we found that some parents were taking the initiative in advocating for their children's educational needs as they changed grade or school. Likewise, some teachers took it upon themselves to reach out to parents in the absence of the program mediators.

In 2002, voters in Massachusetts approved ballot Question 2 which altered the policy for English learners in public schools. Consequently, the Transitional Bilingual Program ended and with it the H-SCP in Somerville. However, individual teachers who participated in the program continued to carry out some of the activities, including occasional home visits to families. Moreover, Tufts University graduates who were trained in the H-SCP continued to practice activities with parents and teachers working with the students enrolled in Somerville Two-Way Bilingual classrooms that replaced the Transitional Bilingual Program.

Project Two: East Boston

In 2002, the Boston Public Schools' Department of Early Childhood initiated a program called Countdown to Kindergarten to promote school readiness for infants and toddlers. During the second year of the program, more than 50 immigrant families in East Boston, many of them Latinos, expressed interest in the preschool classes. This gave rise to playgroups attended primarily by Spanish-speaking families with children enrolled in three East Boston elementary schools.

The playgroups are offered to children under 3 years of age who attend a preschool classroom two or three times a week for 2 hours accompanied by a parent or caregiver. During their time at school, children and parents participate as a group and individually, in activities such as fine and gross motor games, singing, making crafts, and reading.

I began to collaborate with Countdown to Kindergarten through my students who carried out internships in the program; the program staff, on their part, became interested in what we had accomplished with the H-SCP in Somerville, and this led to conversations about work in partnership. In some ways, the circumstances resembled those in Somerville: They were Latino immigrant families and a similar pattern of adaptation problems existed. However, these children were several years younger and had not yet entered the school system. This presented us with the opportunity to try to improve the learning environment for young children in their homes in anticipation of their entry into the school system.

One observation from the Somerville project was that even though immigrant parents affirmed the importance of education and wanted their children to be successful at school, they tended to believe that there was a clear distinction between what the child should be taught at home and what the child should be taught at school. At home the child learns proper behavior and responsibilities ("*aprender a comportarse bien*"), whereas at school the child learns to read, write, and acquire other academic skills (Calzada, et al. 2010, Livas-Dlott, 2010). In contrast to the prevailing notion in most middle-class American homes, Latino parents did not place particular emphasis on stimulating intellectual curiosity, and it was thought that this might be disadvantageous for Latino immigrant children as they entered the public schools. Even for entering kindergarten, the schools assume a certain level of readiness, and this is consistent with the objectives of Countdown to Kindergarten.

The East Boston project, then, was designed to promote the school adaptation of Latino immigrant children by beginning at an early age to improve their readiness for school.[1] Specifically, we planned to introduce values and practices at home that would promote learning: intellectual curiosity, autonomy, and collaboration. These values are especially esteemed in the USA, tend to be nurtured at home at a very early age (Kagan, 2006), and are considered important for children's educational achievement.

The participants were 20 Latino mothers and their toddlers, averaging 22.8 months of age at the outset of the study and recruited from playgroups in the Countdown to Kindergarten Program in East Boston. All the children had been born in or around Boston and their parents had been living in the USA for at least 6 years, having immigrated predominantly from rural Central America, Mexico, and several South American countries. Spanish was the primary language spoken at home, although some English was spoken to the child in most families.

At the outset of the study, a young woman, a native Spanish speaker, visited each mother–child pair in their home for 1 hour. During this visit, the visitor interviewed mothers about their family characteristics and their child's developmental history. A basket of toys was placed on the floor for the child and they were filmed for 20 min as they played spontaneously.

After this initial home visit, the intervention was carried out with half of the families in 12 sessions over the course of 8 months. The remaining families were maintained for comparison of results in the final assessment.

As mentioned above, our goals for the intervention sessions were to promote the values of intellectual curiosity, autonomy, and collaboration. If successful, what we hoped to observe at the end of the intervention (see Fig. 11.3) was that while accomplishing tasks, the child would become more actively engaged, inquisitive, persevering, and assertive; they would become inventive and talkative while engaged

[1] Funding for this project was provided in part by the Cultural Change Institute at the Fletcher School of Tufts University.

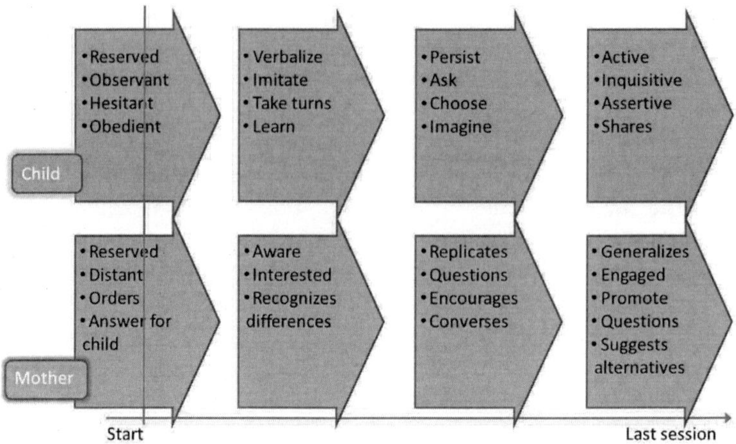

Fig. 11.3 Goals of intervention home visits

in exploratory play. As for the mothers, we intended that they would come to have a better appreciation of their child's developmental potential and learning style and a better understanding of the importance of promoting autonomy and encouraging the use of language while playing. Specifically, we wanted them to become less direct during their interactions, encourage questions, converse, suggest alternatives, and instill a sense of accomplishment when doing a task together with the child.

We found in the initial session that children were generally reserved but observant of the home visitor. The mother, too, was responsive to the home visitor but did not initiate conversation. When the home visitor sought to engage the child, the mother would often answer for the child or instruct the child what to answer. The 12 home visits were designed to progressively involve the mother in encouraging the child's intellectual curiosity, initiative, and collaboration in accomplishing tasks. In the earlier sessions, the mother was expected to observe the home visitor's interaction with the child and then imitate it herself. The home visitor would explain why, for example, she chose to encourage the child's own attempts to solve a problem instead of doing it for the child. In the later sessions, the mother and child were asked to design tasks of their own to show to the home visitor.

As the intervention home visits progressed, children as well as parents showed more familiarity with the content and format of the sessions. After completing the fourth session with all families, the Countdown to Kindergarten coordinator indicated that several mothers had commented to her how much they were learning during the home visits and that they were looking forward to upcoming visits as much as their children were. They related how their children sometimes reenacted with them and their siblings some of the activities they had done with the home visitor.

Mothers reported to the home visitor that their children were asking them to sit with them on the floor and play. Two children even asked their mother to buy a small rug like the one the home visitor brought to each session. They set aside a place to keep all materials given during the sessions and were incorporating other toys they had at home into the activities. Some mothers mentioned that the idea of sitting together on the floor to play was unfamiliar to them and they had felt uncomfortable when they were asked to do so at the playgroup. With practice at home, they were feeling more at ease.

Preliminary results from evaluating the home visits suggest some immediate benefits for the mothers and children who received the home visit intervention. First, attendance to the playgroup classroom activities increased. Children appeared more receptive to the playgroup routine and spent more time playing with their mother or caregivers.

Second, as the sessions progressed, all of the children verbalized more, engaged with the home visitor, and looked forward with anticipation to the next activities. However, only a subset showed consistent improvement in terms of assertiveness, engagement, persistence, sharing, and delayed gratification. The mothers of these children were the ones who increased their speaking to the child, indirectly guiding (in contrast with commands), encouraging, and suggesting efficient strategies when helping their child to do the activities.

Third, some of these same mothers also became more talkative with the home visitor beyond the planned activities of the session. They asked about aspects of their child's development, strengths, and weakness, showing pride in the child's progress and playgroup behavior. Several mothers described activities that they came up with on their own to continue playing with their child after the end of the study, and they asked the home visitor for suggestions about those activities.

In summary, the East Boston project is an example where home visiting was used to carry out an effective intervention with Latino immigrant families. In this case, the purpose of the intervention was to promote certain values and practices in the home that were intended to improve school readiness for preschoolers in the Countdown to Kindergarten program. Practicing the instructions and activities in the home strengthened the likelihood that those practices would be reinforced and adopted as part of the home routine, thereby complementing what children were doing in the playgroup.

Project Three: Pastores, Guatemala

The communication gap between home and school occurs not only for Latino immigrants like those in Somerville and East Boston in the USA but also for families in other countries. For the project in Pastores, Guatemala, the gap between home and school is largely social and economic, but we found that home visits and the methodology of the H-SCP have been effective for improving education for those children who were not reached by the public school system.

Pastores is a rural community of about 11,000, located 60 km to the southwest of Guatemala City. Agriculture is a primary activity, notably coffee and vegetable crops, and the town has a reputation in the region for its household fabrication of leather boots. Like most Guatemalan towns of its size, Pastores has a public elementary school. However, a significant number of children drop out early and some do not attend at all. Among the poorer families, many of the parents have no schooling themselves and given their economic needs and unfamiliarity with education, they tend not to require it for their children. Only some children consistently attend elementary school and graduate. Many attend for the first 2 or 3 years but when needs at home emerge or they are required to help in the field with agriculture, their parents take them out of school. Of those who finish elementary school, even fewer pursue high school education.

A team of educators and community workers who were concerned about low school performance took on the task of establishing a preschool program that would eventually lead to a kindergarten and to a six-grade school that would offer students high-quality education. The objective was to complement existing services by educating those children who tended not to be reached by the public elementary school. To reach those children and their families, the team realized that a different approach would be needed, and that approach relied heavily on establishing better communication between the home and school.

With this objective in mind, the *Cambiando Vidas* program, under the direction of Jannette Cuellar de Reyes, opened its first classroom for a group of 20 preschool children in 2007.[2] The school now has a total enrollment of 116 children attending from preschool to fourth grade and plans to add fifth and sixth grades during the next 2 years.

Cambiando Vidas was conceived from the start as an educational opportunity for children and parents to enable children to successfully complete elementary school. The students' participation in the program is promoted by conducting individual home visits to all the families with young children to explain the importance of early education in later school achievements and the benefits of their children participating in the program. All families who agreed to enroll their 4-year-old child at the school were visited before the beginning of the school year.

The purpose of these visits was to get to know the families well, to start familiarizing them with the school approach, and to discuss with parents the degree of involvement that would be expected from them by the school. Home–school communication and collaboration begins from day one; parents' commitment is required. Given the background of the families who participate, parents come to realize that in order to achieve excellent education for their children, they need to play a part in various ways that will improve their family life, promote strong educational values, and empower them to complete their elementary schooling.

The model of home–school educational services includes five major areas of activities that take place at school, and parents are actively engaged in all these activities as volunteers. Depending on their time availability and family responsibili-

[2] In English *Asociación Cambiando Vidas* (ACAVI) is "Changing Lives." ACAVI's school, *El Centro Educativo la Excelencia,* has received support from the Guatemalan government and several local and international donors to build the school facilities and cover salaries of teachers and staff and the expenses of extracurricular activities. Other founding members of *Cambiando Vidas* were Bertha Guadalupe Cuyún L., Mónica Angélica Gaytán, and Cecilia Martínez.

ties, parents rotate their involvement in school activities, having been provided the necessary training to work collaboratively with the school staff.

Children's School

The school adheres to the curriculum requirements of the Guatemalan Ministry of Education, and it integrates some elements of the Montessori and Waldorf approaches to education. An effort is made to have English-speaking instructors who conduct a part of the class each day in English to cover reading and writing, while exposing students to a more American didactic style which takes into account individual differences and promotes independent learning.

As the school has expanded upward over the years, they have been able to have the assistant teacher from one grade move up to become the head teacher of the next grade. This has provided an excellent continuity for the students and the families. In addition to continuing education on curriculum, teachers also regularly attend workshops offered by private schools in Guatemala City and by local and foreign professionals. These workshops deal with developmental issues in children's learning and the H-SCP approach to ensure efficient parent–teacher communication. All teachers are expected to become familiar with Pastores as a community and with the families of their students; they carry out home visits when appropriate. Additionally, families receive home visits from psychology interns who act as mediators to address issues related to individual children and to keep them motivated in the program.

Parental Education and the Mothers' Group

Regular parent group meetings are held monthly to furnish parents with information about aspects of children's growth and development. A curriculum is developed specifically to fulfill the goals of these sessions, and a staff member trained in psychology conducts the meetings. Topics include physical health, child rearing, discipline, temperament differences, supporting learning needs, and healthy eating. Mothers and fathers attend these parent education sessions. Additional workshops are also offered to parents on the use of computers and basic skills such as sewing and cooking healthy food.

In addition to regular educational meetings for parents, psychologists also conduct monthly support sessions attended by mothers only. These sessions provide mothers a forum to discuss personal family issues and to empower women in their marital relationships, encourage independent decision-making, and promote their self-esteem.

Nutrition and Preventive Health Services

Nutritional activities include offering breakfast to ensure that children do not attend class hungry, while taking the opportunity to involve parents in cooking and preparing meals so that they can learn about healthy food, nutrition, and managing their meal budgets. Nutrition also includes an inspired collaborative project in which parents and staff harvest and distribute vegetables and fruits donated by farmers in Pastores to all the families on a weekly basis. Besides offsetting needy families' food expenses, this aspect of the program enables community members to contribute to *Cambiando Vidas* in a meaningful way.

The academic curriculum for all classes includes a unit on nutrition, exercise, and health. Additionally, arrangements have been made with the public health clinics in Pastores for children to have regular checkups with the dentist, ophthalmologist, and pediatrician.

Every year the board evaluates the program; results are used to plan and improve activities in the program for the next school year. The accomplishments and contributions of this program are already significant for children, families, and the community, at large.

School attendance has been excellent on a daily basis as well as over the school years. Of the 20 children who started preschool in 2007, 17 are now completing fourth grade (the remaining 3 families having moved away from Pastores). Parental participation in all activities is remarkable. Parents consistently attend educational sessions, assume responsibility for routine school duties, and volunteer for additional tasks to support the school.

Students' academic achievement now surpasses grade-specific Guatemalan educational standards. Those students whose performance is below par are given additional help after school hours. Applications for enrollment now exceed the limit of 20 students per grade; a waiting list and first-come, first-served rules are applied to admit new families and siblings of students already attending the school.

Based on the school's reputation for academic progress, middle schools and high schools from elsewhere in Guatemala have offered openings with scholarships for some students when they finish sixth grade. Other schools in nearby communities have recognized the accomplishments of the program; during the last 2 years *Cambiando Vidas* has offered workshops and guided observation to kindergarten and elementary school teachers.

Ongoing subject content, training, and social support offered to the teachers has been a priority to sustain the quality of their teaching and the success of the academic component of the program. At the same time, we believe that it is the daily encouragement of their families behind the good school performances of the students. Unquestionably, this support comes from the deep and solid communication and collaboration that has been built between parents and teachers.

Conclusions

As early as 1946, Arnold Gesell, writing with Francis Ilg about successful school performance, emphasized the importance of the balance of responsibility between the parents, teachers, and students and the complexity of the relationship in the US schools (Gesell & Ilg, 1946). Gesell and Ilg probably were trying to explain this relationship as it was observed at that time for the majority of white students.

I have depicted that relationship as three overlapping circles to illustrate the importance of communication and understanding between the home, school, and the child. The three projects described here show how this triangular relationship grows in complexity, and also how it can be successfully managed and improved. The relationship is universal, although its particular expression will vary with the social setting and the times. The systemic nature of this relationship is seldom explicitly recognized and addressed, but it should be. What usually happens is that concerns emerge about the child's school performance; teachers manage as best they can, parents are uncertain about what is going on, and problems are not resolved effectively or on time. Over time, the gap between home and school persists, rather than being bridged by a long-lasting, supportive pattern of home–school communication.

The cases I have described of Latino immigrant children in Boston and children living in rural Guatemala illustrate the need for developing a common understanding of the relationship between home and school. The model of school adaptation developed for the H-SCP allows us to identify the relevant differences between home and school and to make those differences evident to the parents and teachers involved. Identifying those differences, then, was essential to agreeing on the appropriate ways to promote collaborations between parents and teachers to advance the students' school achievement.

Particular requirements to achieving school success were identified in each project, and accordingly different objectives were defined as outcomes for home intervention. For the immigrant children in Somerville, differences between parents and teachers were related to such issues as the importance of regular attendance, the need for a child to be referred for special evaluation, and the importance of children completing their homework on time. For the East Boston families, differences emerged in playgroup sessions when parents emphasized obedience and compliance over curiosity and autonomy in their toddlers' play. In Pastores, it began with finding ways for parents to understand the benefits of education.

In all cases, in order to achieve school success outcomes, parental involvement was needed and encouraged. The Somerville program brought parents and teachers together with the mediator's guidance to agree on a shared understanding and explicit goals for the child. The East Boston parents were shown how to promote their child's own learning behavior by conversing more with their toddlers, using an indirect style of interactions, and suggesting problem-solving strategies that promote intellectual autonomy. As for the parents in Pastores, assuming responsibility and involving themselves personally in the school was necessary and it was facilitated so that they could realize their own contribution to their child's school accomplishments and for the well-being of the their whole family.

Home visiting plays a crucial role in the methodology for improving home–school communication, and it was used in different ways in each of the three projects described here. For the purposes of learning about the home environment to support the child at school, observations conducted during home visits have shown to be an invaluable way to acquire information that would be impossible otherwise (Caldwell & Bradly, 2003). In Somerville, conversing with parents in their homes was essential to understanding their needs and perspectives for the design of the project itself. As the project continued, home visits enabled the mediators to bridge the gap between home and school so that they could guide parents and teachers to agreed-upon goals for the child.

In the East Boston project, the initial home visits served to establish a baseline understanding of mother–child interaction and the qualities of the home environment. Subsequently, the home was the venue for training intervention. That was important to ensure continuity of the patterns of interaction that were introduced during the sessions. For example, when the child had become accustomed to explorative play on the rug in the living room, continuing this behavior in the absence of the home visitor became natural. In Pastores, home visits were an important first step in reaching out to needy families and demonstrating respect and interest. Their acceptance was important in order to progress toward helping them understand the importance of education for their child and eventually assuming responsibilities in the school.

References

Baker, A., & Peterson, S. (2010). Participatory action research: An effective methodology for promoting community-based professional development. In S. Neuman & M. L. Kamil (Eds.), *Preparing teachers for the early childhood classroom*. Baltimore: Brookes.

Bradley, R. H. (2011). Immigration and acculturation, child care and schooling. In M. H. Bornstein, R. E. Tremblay, M. Boivin, & R. deV. Peters (Eds.), *Encyclopedia on early childhood development* (pp. 1–7). Montreal: Centre of Excellence for Early Childhood Development and Strategic Knowledge Cluster on Early Child Development.

Brizuela, B., & García-Sellers, M. J. (1998). School adaptation: A triangular process. *American Educational Research Journal, 36*(2), 345–370.

Brooks-Gunn, J., Berlin, L., & Fuligni, A. (2000). Early childhood intervention programs: What about the family? In J. P. Shonkoff & S. J. Meisels (Eds.), *Handbook of early childhood intervention*. Cambridge: Cambridge University Press.

Caldwell, B. M., & Bradley, R. H. (2003). *Home inventory administration manual* (comprehensive ed.). Little Rock: University of Arkansas for Medical Sciences and University of Arkansas at Little Rock.

Calzada, E., Fernandez, Y., & Cortes, D. (2010). Incorporating the cultural value of respeto into a framework of Latino parenting. *Cultural Diversity and Ethnic Minority Psychology, 16*(1), 77–86.

García-Sellers, M. J. (1997). *School adaptation of Hispanic immigrant children*. Poster symposium presented to the meeting of the Society for Research in Child Development, Washington, DC.

García-Sellers, M. J. (1998). *Preventing school failure: A model based approach for improving home–school communication*. Presented to the first international conference on child and adolescent mental health at the Chinese University of Hong Kong.

García, E., & Náñez, J. E., Sr. (2011). *Bilingualism and cognition: Informing research, pedagogy, and policy*. (pp. 57–77). Washington, DC: American Psychological Association.
García, E., & Ozturk, M. D. (2011). Education partnerships: From research to practice. *International Journal of the Humanities, 9*(4), 103–112.
Gesell, A., & Ilg, F. (1946). *The child from five to ten*. New York: Harper & Brothers.
Greene, J., & Winters, M. (2006). *Leaving boys behind: Public high school graduation rates*. Civic Reports No. 48. New York: Manhattan Institute for Policy Research Center for Civic Innovation.
Haskins, R., & Tienda, M. (2011). The future of immigrant children. *Future of Children, 21*(1), 1–7.
Jeynes, W. (2003). A meta-analysis: The effects of parental involvement on minority children's academic achievement. *Education and Urban Society, 35,* 202–218. doi:10.1177/0013124502239392.
Jeynes, W. (2005). A meta-analysis of the relation of parental involvement to urban elementary school student academic achievement. *Urban Education, 40,* 237–269. doi:10.1177/0042085905274540.
Jeynes, W. (2012). *Parental involvement and academic success*. New York: Routledge.
Kagan, J. (2006). Culture, values and the family. In L. Harrison & J. Kagan (Eds.), *Developing cultures: Essays on cultural change*. New York: Routledge.
Livas-Dlott, A., Fuller, B., Stein, G. L., Bridges, M., Mangual-Figueroa, A., & Mireles, L. (2010). Commands, competence, and cariño: Maternal socialization practices in Mexican-American families. *Developmental Psychology, 46*(3), 566–578.
Parra, M. L., & Garcia-Sellers, M. J. (2005). *Comunicación entre la escuela y la familia: Fortaleciendo las bases para éxito escolar*. (Editorial PAIDOS). Mexico: Paidós.
Pedraza, S. (1996). Origins and destinies: Immigration, race, and ethnicity in American history. In S. Pedraza & R. G. Rumbaut (Eds.), *Origins and destinies*. New York: Wadsworth.
Severns, M. (2011). Why ignoring the immigrant youth population is a mistake. http://earlyed.newamerica.net/blogposts/2011/ignoring_immigrant_children_the_labor_force_of_the_future-51484. Accessed 19 May 2011.
Soria, K. (2012). Book review: Higher education and first-generation students: Cultivating community, voice, and place for the new majority. *Urban Education, 47,* 689. doi:10.1177/0042085912440417.
Suárez-Orozco, M. (2000). Everything you ever wanted to know about assimilation but were afraid to ask. *Daedalus, 129*(4), 1–30.
Suárez-Orozco, M., & Páez, M. (2009). *Latinos: Remaking America* (2nd ed.). Cambridge: David Rockefeller Center for Latin American Studies at Harvard University and University of California Press.
Williams, T., & Sánchez, B. (2012) Parental involvement (and uninvolvement) at an inner-city high school. *Urban Education, 47,* 625–652. doi:10.1177/0042085912437794.

Martha Julia García-Sellers (USA): Professor, Tufts University, Child Development Department; Director, Home-School Connection Program (H-SCP) and the Family Values Project. She began her professional career in Guatemala as a psychologist in a multidisciplinary team carrying out applied research with malnourished children at the Institute of Nutrition of Central America and Panamá (INCAP), a unit of the Pan American Health Organization. Since completing her doctoral training in child development at Harvard University, she has devoted her efforts to the study of child–family assessment and preventive intervention of infants and preschool children. She is the founder and director of the Home-School Connection Program (H-SCP), a home visiting program strengthening communication among teachers, parents and children from immigrant families from Latin America living in the USA and in rural communities in Guatemala. At present, in collaboration with the Cultural Change Institute, she directs the Family Values Project for Hispanic and Brazilian immigrant families living in Boston, rural families living in Costa Rica, and Brazilian families in São Paulo.

Chapter 12
The Roving Caregivers Program: A Caribbean Model

Susan Branker Greene, Clive Murray, and Horis Lynch

The early childhood years have long been recognized by social scientists as the period during which children are in a position to acquire the social and cognitive skills that normally place them on a solid foundation toward building enduring positive relationships with parents, peers and favorable attitudes toward school and schooling (see Gilliam & Zigler, 2000; Marcon, 1999; Myers, 1992; Reynolds, 2000; Shonkoff & Phillips, 2000). Increasingly, the first 3 years of life have been recognized by governments and nongovernmental organizations around the world as an ideal time to provide early education. Programs from diverse philosophical backgrounds have been embraced as a beacon of hope for promoting better outcomes for children who live under difficult economic and social circumstances (see Roopnarine & Johnson, 2005).

Most early childhood programs in the developing world are center based and focus on prekindergarten age-children to prepare them academically for formal schooling (Snyder, Tan, & Hoffman, 2004). For a variety of reasons, some of which are rooted in economics, less attention has been paid to the threats to children's cognitive and social development during infancy and toddler years (0–3 years) when the acquisition of basic language and social skills are beginning to take shape and when children may be most vulnerable to environmental insults (Lamb, Bornstein, & Teti, 2002). Purportedly, there are sensitive periods during the initial few years of life when children are prone to learning specific developmental skills (Lombroso & Pruett, 2004), and some have pointed to the benefits of brain stimulation during this period (Shonkoff & Phillips, 2000).

S. B. Greene (✉)
Managing Director and Principal Consultant, Targeted Development Consulting Inc., Suite #1, 25 Cane Garden Park, St. Thomas, Barbados
e-mail: Smbranker@gmail.com

C. Murray · H. Lynch
Foundation for the Development of Caribbean Children, St. Michael, Barabado

L. Roggman, N. Cardia (eds.), *Home Visitation Programs*,
DOI 10.1007/978-3-319-17984-1_12

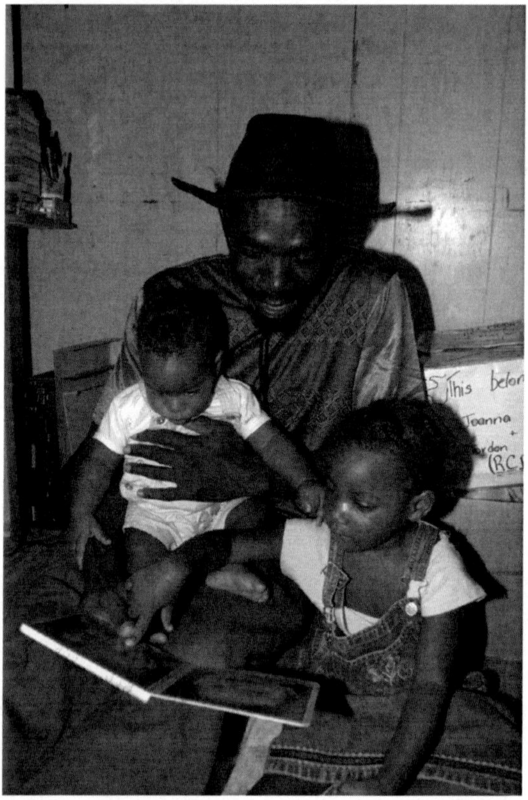

Roving Caregivers Program (RCP) parent interacting with his children. (Photo courtesy: Foundation for the Development of Caribbean Children (FDCC))

Early Childhood Development (ECD) in the Caribbean

A 1997 Caribbean Plan of Action (CPOA) for ECD revealed that the policy environment for early childhood programming was weak, particularly as it related to the provision of quality support services required for children between birth and 3 years old. The CPOA further noted that less than 30 % of children in this age cohort were accessing daycare provision and where there was such provision, a large percentage were privately owned and issues of quality and outcomes were of concern.

In addition, there were identified gaps in the provision of parenting support and therefore a required need for greater attention in this area. It revealed that there were few opportunities for parents to receive information on optimal parenting and much less child stimulation services. Another identified area of great concern was the fact that a large percentage of parents were young with low educational attainment and less than optimal parenting skills (Roopnarine & Gielen, 2005).

These unfortunate predicaments still continue to plague poor urban and rural families in the Caribbean today. Across the Caribbean region, 13 countries have reported formal policies being developed for early childhood care and education, with 10 of these still in draft awaiting approval. Ten of the eleven legal frameworks that have been developed for early childhood care and education are in draft awaiting approval (Charles, 2012). It is also significant to note the relative absence of institutional and legal frameworks that include early stimulation, developmental monitoring, and parental and family supports.

Among the English-speaking African Caribbean families, a significant number of families live at or below the poverty line. Poverty rates as a percentage of population range from as low as 5 % in Anguilla to 37.7 % in Grenada, with median rates being between 18.4 and 37.7 % (Charles & Williams, 2010). A majority of first-time births occur outside of marriage and during the teenage years. Too often the majority of child rearing and economic responsibility falls on the shoulders of young women who are often ill-prepared and unable to capably engage in effective parenting.

Mothers, especially those in the lower-income brackets, are not getting sufficient support in the increasingly challenging job of parenting. While middle- and upper-income parents are able to use their financial resources to ameliorate their situation (e.g., babysitters and special transportation arrangements), low-income women are unable to access similar support structures, and their children frequently remain unsupervised for extended periods (Reddock & Bobb-Smith, 2005, pp. 12–13). The levels of interaction and stimulation at home, particularly with young children, which impacts negatively on child development (Barrow & Ince, 2008).

The Roving Caregivers Program (RCP)—A Caribbean Model

The RCP is an informal ECD and parenting support program. Early stimulation for children and parenting education for parents form the core of the program. RCP addresses the developmental needs of the very young in disadvantaged conditions where children benefit from quality care and attention, development of basic skills, better health, and nutrition, and at the next level, better performance in preschool and future education.

Joyce Jarrett, a pioneer in ECD, created the RCP in 1993. The pivotal role of the RCP was to improve the childrearing beliefs and parenting practices of rural poor Jamaican parents, with the hope of reversing the developmental lags in cognitive and social skills that their young children show prior to entry into primary schools. Some of the developmental lags have been attributed to familial home environments that lack basic education and play materials and adequate doses of parental stimulation. By "coaching" parents in a personalized manner within the security of their own homes to improve the quality and quantity of cognitive and social stimulation with children between 0 and 3 years, it is argued that the RCP helps parents equip their children with the necessary intellectual and social acumen to prevent poor performance early in the schooling process. This program serves as an initial step in helping to dissolve the barriers between rural families and the larger community that may be attributed to geographical and social isolation—the very factors that may cause children to slip through social services cracks during the early infancy period.

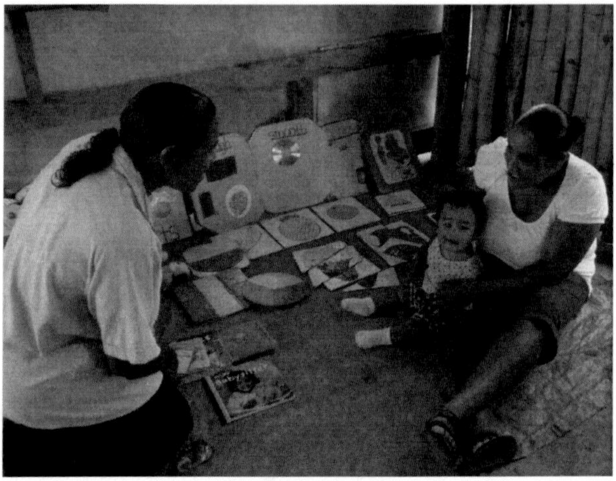

RCP Rover working with child and parent. (Photo courtesy: FDCC)

The RCP innovation starts with a conceptual advantage over traditional modes of care provision: It brings the service to the recipient; its methodology engages parents and caregivers actively in the service delivery; and it provides a vehicle for the conveyance of other related interventions (e.g., health, parenting). Like other home visiting programs, the RCP acknowledges the role of the parent/caregiver as the child's first teacher and lessens the financial burden on families to cover transportation and other costs that may act as deterrents to seeking or even contemplating seeking intervention services on their own.

In addition to the work that was already being done in Jamaica, the Bernard van Leer Foundation (BvLF) established the Caribbean Child Support Initiative (CCSI) from 2002 to 2011 to address issues relevant to poor parenting practices and inadequate cognitive stimulation of young children living under difficult social and economic circumstances. As an ECD and family support program, the CCSI was therefore aimed at strengthening the care environment for young children. Its mission, therefore, was to ensure that adequate resources are provided to enable young children to realize the immediate and long-term benefits of good quality ECD experiences.

As a consequence, the CCSI sought to replicate and introduce the BvLF-supported RCP to other countries in the region. The RCP was regarded as a proven concept—a robust, evaluated, tested outcome-led method for promoting effective child rearing practices. Quite importantly, it was established in the Caribbean for the

Caribbean and consequently was chosen for replication in the Eastern Caribbean. Five countries were part of the pilot replication experience. These included St. Lucia, St. Vincent and the Grenadines, Grenada, and Dominica for the pilot. A similar pilot was started in Belize in 2008.

CCSI's participation in the CPOA helped both to shape the wider policy context and to provide a grounded exemplar of a responsive model consistent with the aspirations of the regional framework. In addition, one outcome of the alliances that were forged with key agencies central to the child-care agenda in the region (i.e., United Nations Children's Fund (UNICEF), Caribbean Community and Common Market (CARICOM), and University of the West Indies (UWI)'s Caribbean Child Development Center) is that RCP was able to evolve in conformity with regional and international conventions.

A distinguishing feature of the CCSI was that its spheres of intervention were supportive and reinforced by the RCP as the primary arena of intervention. Research, for example, served to strengthen and refine the RCP methodology while also contributing to policy advocacy; training not only impacted on the RCP delivery capacity but also contributed to the establishment of standards which themselves were undergirded by research. The CCSI was mainstreamed through the establishment of the Foundation for the Development of Caribbean Children (FDCC), launched in June 2011 as an indigenous, regional response to the need for greater efforts and coordination to strengthen the care environment for young children in the Caribbean. Like the CCSI, the RCP, maintains its prominence as a flagship model for the FDCC. Figure 12.1 shows how the RCP model evolved.

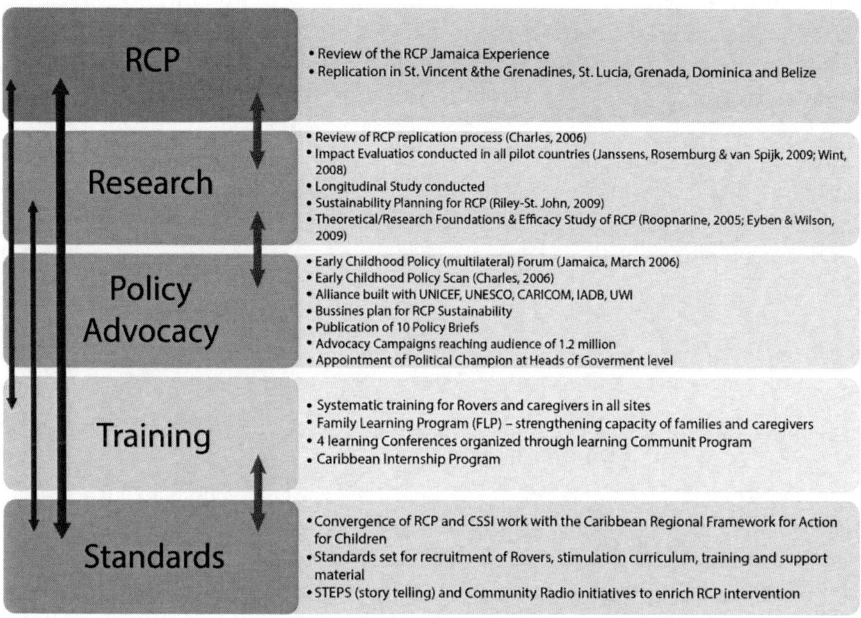

Fig. 12.1 Evolution of the Roving Caregivers Program (Jules, 2010)

Theoretical Foundations of the RCP

In 2005, the CCSI commissioned Professor Roopnarine Jaipaul of the University of Syracuse in the USA to examine the theoretical and research foundation and efficacy of the RCP model. He concluded that the RCP is not governed by a single set of theoretical principles. Rather it draws from theoretical discourses that focus on the intersection of classic childhood development theories, eco-cultural models that consider the developmental niche and micro-niche, and risk and resilience perspectives that embody prevention. He provided an examination of three main theoretical principles that govern the RCP as follows.

Childhood Development

The RCP espouses the importance of nurturing the spirit of the child. It relies on substantiated norms of social and cognitive skills and growth-promoting parenting behaviors proffered by cognitive development (Piaget, 1969), cognitive social learning (Bandura, 1986), attachment (Ainsworth & Bowlby, 1991; Bowlby, 1969), and other psychological theories. For instance, cognitive development theories stress the importance of sensor motor activities (e.g., play, grasping for objects, exploration, functional manipulation, and pretense) that are early building blocks to higher levels of development (Piaget, 1969); cognitive social learning theory underscores the role of observational learning (e.g., reproduction of an activity) and the development self-efficacy (Bandura, 1986); behavioral theories focus on dispensing positive feedback (e.g., encouragement) for the display of appropriate behaviors (Epstein, 2008; Graves, 2002); and attachment (Ainsworth & Bowlby, 1991) and psychodynamic theories (Erikson, 1950) help to define the emotional bonds between child and parent as fundamental in setting the stage for developing secure and trusting relationships with other individuals. Put simply, the RCP is eclectic in that it consults a range of child development and parenting theories in deciding which parent–child activity can be tailored to produce optimal levels of development in Caribbean children.

Cultural Relevance

It is hardly sufficient to speak of parenting practices and beliefs and childhood development in the context of attempts to intervene in people's lives without some attention to prevention. A three-phase approach is usually recommended when dealing with problems in childhood and adolescence: defining the problem, reviewing the relevant health and social science research to understand the etiology of the problem, and constructing a theoretical model for intervention based on identifiable protective factors that could be modified to make differences in children's and families' lives (Chambers & Gantham-McGregor, 1986). The RCP model has accomplished all of these goals by using intervention and health research conducted in the Caribbean to locate a point at which rural poor children begin to show development lags in cognitive functioning (Powell, 2004), identifying the inappropriate and inadequate parenting practices in the culture of the home environment (see Roopnarine & Evans, 2007) as malleable factors that can be modified, and implementing a home-stimulation approach to intervention that is culturally and developmentally sensitive.

The RCP strives to provide home visiting child stimulation to the rural poor with hopes of achieving some of the same long-term outcomes in maternal approaches to childrearing and school achievement in Caribbean families as those recorded in other intervention programs. Accordingly, the RCP aligns itself well with the deeply rooted home-based philosophical approach to educating young children by improving the parenting skills of primary and secondary caregivers (e.g., verbal stimulation, maternal interest in child growth and development, parental management strategies, and guided participation in different activities), and by targeting the infancy period as the time to intervene in children's lives.

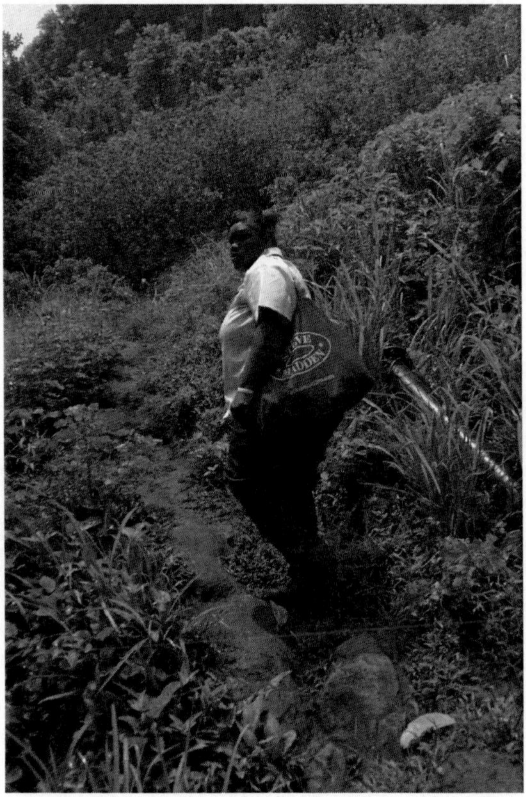

RCP Rover making her way to a home. (Photo courtesy: FDCC)

Prevention

Parenting beliefs and practices are braided into the RCP model of delivering services to rural Caribbean children and families. In the provision of home-based stimulation exercises, the RCP recognizes that harsh, controlling, and developmentally inappropriate parenting practices work against optimal childhood development. As a matter of fact, the RCP goals mesh well with a small body of studies that point to inadequate methods of child rearing among low-income Caribbean parents and the significant relationship between the quality of stimulation offered in the home and childhood development (Powell, Grantham-McGregor, & Walker, 1998). By virtue of its stand on these inappropriate/inadequate methods, the RCP is in a good position to enlist local community support to encourage changes in adults' internal working models of childrearing that are harsh and devoid of regular social and intellectual stimulation.

The RCP identifies key childhood developmental constructs to nurture (e.g., language development, psychomotor skills, and emotional stability), focuses on the development of good parenting skills, childhood safety and rights, and the nutritional status of children, all of which are essential to promoting successful parent–child relationships and the social and cognitive development during the early years of life.

RCP Major Working Principles

Additionally, in 2010, CCSI commissioned an examination of the RCP as a Caribbean Model by Dr. Didacus Jules (2010). He posited, based on his assessment of the model, that the following emerge as the situational preconditions that optimize the efficacy of the RCP model—indicators that point to optimal conditions for the RCP to make a significant difference: (1) absence of a continuum of service and support for ECD and education, (2) high-risk families and children who do not have access to ECD institutional structures (one reason the advocacy element is so important to forging new directions for RCP is that even the weak existing discourse conceptualizes the problem as a social deficit more than a rights issue), (3) policy environment that is weak in the countries that can most benefit from RCP so more strategic and aggressive policy interventions are needed, and (4) a strong regulatory regime that is necessary to guarantee standards of provision and thus acceptable outcomes.

Jules concluded that critical to the success of the RCP model are: the developmental aspects of the stimulation exercises, the mechanics of the program, and Rover qualifications and training. Stimulation activities are guided by solid data on the importance of parent–child emotional bonds, cognitive and language stimulation, and psychomotor and perceptual development during the infancy and toddler years. The activities are well conceived, based on developmentally and culturally appropriate practices (Bredekamp & Copple, 1997; Roopnarine & Metindogan, 2005), and integrate community input and parental socialization goals into stimulation routines. In addition, play and literacy materials that are made available to par-

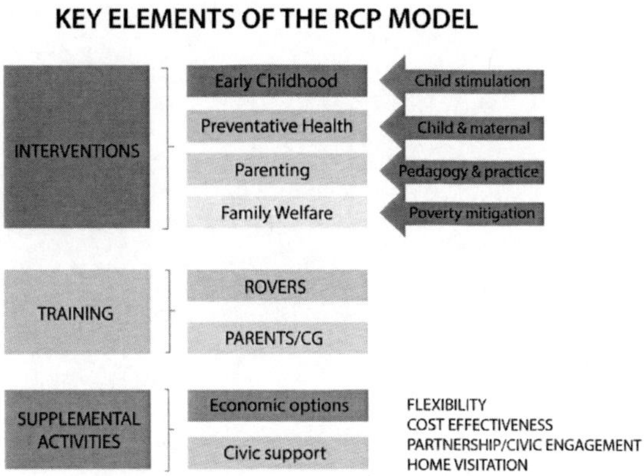

Fig. 12.2 Elements of the RCP as a Caribbean Model (Jules, 2010)

ents are constructed with culturally relevant information from the near environment and larger community.

The key elements that have evolved over time are identified in Fig. 12.2.

These elements have emerged from the ongoing critique of the interventions, the conclusions of evidence-based research, and the needs of the key constituencies. From that experience, the following could be distilled as the key working principles of the RCP: (1) Maintain a strong central focus primarily on the child and secondly on the immediate supporting familial and social apparatus surrounding the care, protection, and development of the child. (2) Prioritize rural, disadvantaged children and families. (3) Engage, train, and sensitize caregivers on child stimulation and development techniques, empowering parenting practices, and rights and responsibilities. (4) Involve community persons as Rovers, providing ongoing, systematic, and paraprofessional training to them. (5) Utilize a well-defined curriculum and activity sets that have proven effective in facilitating the cognitive and psychomotor development of the child. (6) Structure the program of visits and interventions to ensure regularity, and maximize the exposure of the children to stimulation. (7) Incorporate other social support networks (e.g., health and family literacy) in the outreach to family and community through the RCP.

The Role of the Rover

Additionally, attention must be paid to the role of the Rover who constitutes the primary facilitative agent in the interventions. The role of the Rover is to facilitate this evolving process in which there would be major spin-offs for both the child and the parent. It is vital therefore that in any future incarnations of the RCP, continuous attention be paid to capacity building of the Rover to ensure that this agent has the knowledge, skills, and competence required to effectively perform the role. In all of the project countries, much attention has been paid to this (Jules, 2010).

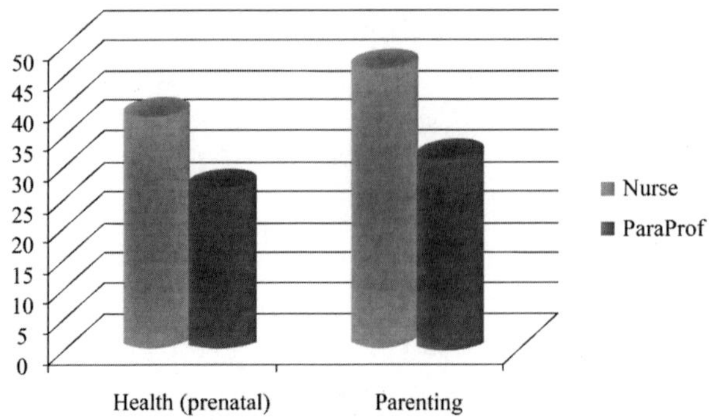

RCP Rovers (home visitors) in training. (Photo courtesy: FDCC)

An unintended consequence of the experience is the significant opportunity for national/community service for the young school leavers who served as Rovers. In 2008 alone, the 151 Rovers operating in four project countries received a total of 1363 hours of training. In one country, Rovers received paraprofessional training and were certified to National Council on Technical and Vocational Education and Training (NCTVET) Level 1. In that same year a total of 2550 children participated in the program in Dominica, Grenada, Jamaica, St. Lucia, and St. Vincent, and the Grenadines. Each of the 151 Rovers involved interacted with an average of 16 children. The Rovers held 137 community meetings and facilitated 2280 parent consultations.

RCP Impact Study

Although there is ample evidence on the benefits of ECD programs, the evidence for home-based as opposed to center-based interventions is still very limited, especially in the developing world. An experimental evaluation of the RCP in Jamaica in 2004 showed that RCP has a substantial impact on the cognitive development of young children after 1 year of enrollment. However, there was no evidence of impact in other Caribbean countries or on longer-term cognitive, nutritional, or socio-emotional development of young children.

In 2006, to help bridge this gap in knowledge, the BvLF commissioned a longitudinal quasi-experimental impact study of the RCP by the Amsterdam Institute for International Development (AIID) in St Lucia (Janssens & Rosemberg, 2013). One of the objectives of the impact study is to yield much-needed research evidence on the impact of a home visiting as opposed to a center-based approach to ECD interventions. The study, which was conducted over the period 2006–2014, was intended to measure the impact of the RCP on child development and parenting outcomes and show whether the program yields similar results in another setting that are sustained over time.

The key findings showed program outcomes as follows: (1) greater practical awareness of the value of good parenting practice in the formative years of childhood; (2) "significant changes in parenting practices, behavior, and parental social cognitions amongst parents from lower socioeconomic communities…(as well as) changes in the areas of hygiene, sanitation practices, nutrition, and where possible, the use of space"; (3) positive effects on the cognitive development of children between 6 and 18 months old, especially in fine motor skills and visual reception (an impact that diminished by the final round of the research); (4) enrollment at earlier ages that appeared to improve motor skills and language development; (5) substantially higher stimulating interactions occurring with RCP families; (6) reiteration of the importance of household poverty in "explaining an increasing gap in cognitive as well as socio-emotional development"; (7) confirmation of the negative impact of a "low educational level of the primary caregiver on cognitive child outcomes"; (8) confirmation that children born with a low birth weight, or with signs of stunting, show significantly slower development of their gross motor skills and receptive language development. RCP has had a significant and positive influence on the likelihood that parents in RCP communities engage in stimulating parent–child interactions with their children such as singing songs together. This propensity has increased substantially more than in non-RCP communities.

Several cursory analyses have suggested that the RCP program is more cost-effective than traditional forms of child-care provision. To bring authoritative definition to this point of view, the CCSI commissioned a cost analysis by the AIID. The report confirms the cost-effectiveness of the model (Van spijk, 2010) and provides the "final confirmation" needed to position the RCP as a viable and cost-effective model that can be adopted by governments and communities to expand the reach of provision.

Potential Application of RCP in Different Contexts

According to Jules (2010), it is not possible to speak about the potential application of the RCP in different contexts without reference to the "three-strand approach" developed by the CCSI and adopted by the FDCC. The strands are: (1) family and community intervention, (2) knowledge building and application, and (3) advocacy and communications for development. These strands overlap and operate in synergy to facilitate sustainable change, which shaped the evolution of the RCP.

Any future expansion of the RCP will continue to require some variant of the three strands. The RCP should remain the centerpiece of family and community interventions, and the nature of these interventions may vary according to the idiosyncrasies of the community and family environment. Equally so, the knowledge building strand—the continuous training, popularization of research, meetings, presentations, and other knowledge-building initiatives that may emerge—should contribute to knowledge sharing among primary target audiences including parents and other community members as well as policy-makers and actors in the private and public sectors.

Fig. 12.3 Process for applying RCP in different contexts

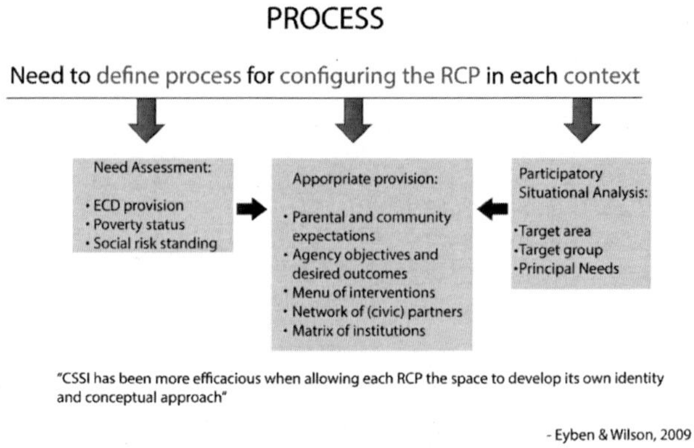

The advocacy and communications strand should serve as the impetus for sustained support. As the RCP initiative becomes adopted as an element of national child-care provision, the nature of advocacy would shift more toward ongoing public sensitization, and its content more toward public education on the rights of the child and better parenting. To successfully implement the RCP and other family and community intervention services, it is necessary to prepare the groundwork in each recipient country through advocacy and communications.

The framework represented by the three strands is, therefore, one that can be creatively appropriated in different institutional and other contexts. The three main steps of the process for future implementation of the RCP in any environment are identified as (1) pre-implementation needs identification, (2) configuration of the RCP in conformity to the needs identified, and (3) contextualizing the intervention.

Figure 12.3 explains how the RCP can be applied and configured for each context in a manner that ensures that it provides the best fit as a service delivery mode.

Partnership Opportunities for the RCP Model

The experience of the RCP replication has concretely demonstrated the potential of the RCP model to cost-effectively deliver a vital social service while incorporating multi-partner alliances. These relational roles are best conceptualized in Fig. 12.4.

Jules used Fig. 12.4 to demonstrate that the ECD Center (whether state or privately run) is an ideal community locus or base for the RCP. The ECD Center provides a logistical and operational base for the Rovers (and their supervisors), a training center for Rovers and community/family actors, and focal point for coordination with sectoral (especially governmental) agencies. Care support services can provide the underpinning of extension services and expertise through the RCP delivery mechanism, whereas the private sector and civic organizations can partner with government to provide support for the program. Indeed, it was argued that successful ECD, in any model, requires policy leadership by the state; multi-sectoral

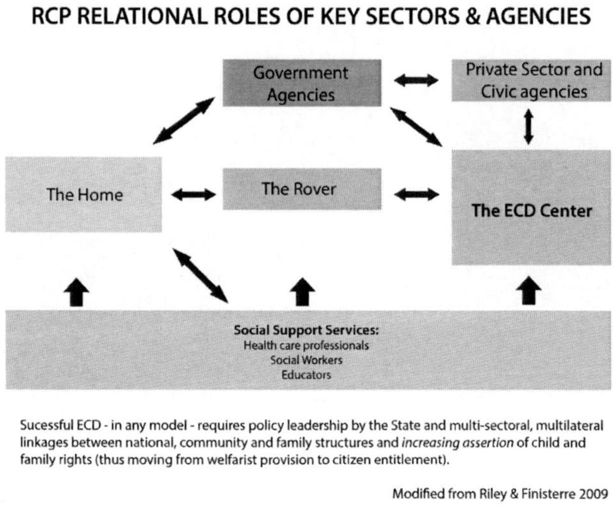

Fig. 12.4 Relational roles among RCP partners

and multi-lateral linkages between national, community, and family structures; and *increasing assertion* of child and family rights (thus moving from welfarist provision to citizen entitlement).

Conclusion

The RCP has demonstrated its ability to contribute to building human and social capital. Through this home- and community-based intervention, vulnerable children are also given the opportunity to escape from poverty and benefit from better career prospects and improved household and national prosperity. The program also helps parents to bring up their children with proper guidance and direction. The RCP has the potential to rebuild communities by creating social networks within disadvantaged communities as it offers parents a sense of inclusion in supporting the development of their children and lessens the inequality gap created by a lack of provision and access to quality ECD services.

The RCP is a proven sound and effective model for early intervention. The methodology is grounded within culturally relevant approaches for a Caribbean context and is based on broad theoretical underpinnings. It has demonstrated an impact in addressing the developmental needs of the very young in socially and economically disadvantaged conditions. The home visiting approach, as practiced through the RCP, allows for greater emphasis to be placed on the development of the child as well as on parent/caregiver participation in stimulation activities. Children therefore benefit from quality care and attention, development of basic skills, better health and nutrition, and at the next level, better performance in preschool and future education.

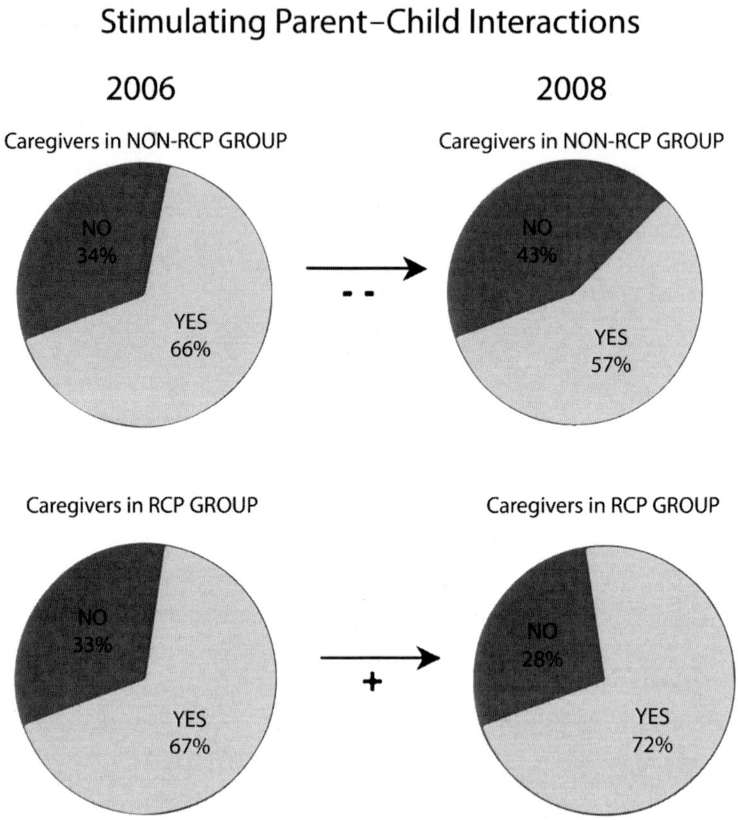

RCP child demonstrating mobility skills. (Photo courtesy: FDCC)

References

Ainsworth, M., & Bowlby, J. (1991). An ethological approach to personality development. *American Psychologist, 46,* 333–341.

Bandura, A. (1986). *Social foundations of thought and action: A social cognitive theory*. Englewood Cliffs: Prentice Hall.

Barrow, C., & Ince, M. (2008). *Early childhood in the Caribbean*. The Hague: Bernard van Leer Foundation.

Bowlby, J. (1969). *Attachment*. New York: Basic Books.

Bredekamp, S., & Copple, C. (Eds.). (1997). *Developmentally appropriate practice in early childhood programs* (revised ed.) Washington, DC: National Association for the Education of Young Children.

Chambers, C., & Grantham-McGregor, S. M. (1986). Patterns of development among young middle-class Jamaican children. *Journal of Child Psychology and Psychiatry, 27,* 117–123.

Charles, L. (2012) *Response opportunities and challenges for the Caribbean action agenda: An early childhood policy brief for The World Conference on Early Childhood Care and Education*. Kingston: United Nations Educational, Scientific and Cultural Organization (UNESCO).

Charles, L., & Williams, S. (2010). *Early childhood care and education in the Caribbean community: UNESCO Report prepared for The World Conference on Early Childhood Care and Education.* Moscow: United Nations Educational, Scientific and Cultural Organization (UNESCO).

Epstein, A. S. (2008). An early start on thinking. Educational Leadership, 65(5), 38.

Erikson, E. H. (1950). *Childhood and society*. New York: Norton.

Eybens, R., & Wilson, F. (2009). *The capacity to have an effect: An efficacy study of the Caribbean Child Support Initiative (CCSI).* Bridgetown, Barbados: CCSI.

Gilliam, W. S., & Zigler, E. F. (2000). A critical meta-analysis of all the evaluations of state-funded preschool from 1977 to 1998: Implications for policy, service delivery and program evaluation. *Early Childhood Research Quarterly, 15*(4), 441–473.

Graves, M. (2002). Working with a challenging child. Exceptional Children,17(1), 3–6.

Janssens, W., & Rosemberg, C. (2013). *The impact of a Caribbean home-visiting child development program on cognitive skills*. Amsterdam: Amsterdam Institute of International Development.

Janssens, W., Groot Bruinderink, M., & van der Gaag, J. (2011). *RCP impact evaluation St Lucia: Impact results 2009*. Amsterdam: Amsterdam Institute for International Development.

Jules, D. (2010). *Positioning the Roving Caregivers Programme as a Caribbean model.* Bridgetown: Caribbean Child Support Initiative.

Lamb, M. E., Bornstein, M. H., & Teti, D. M. (Eds.). (2002). *Development in infancy* (4th ed.). Mahwah: Lawrence Erlbaum Associates.

Lambroso, P. J., & Pruett, K. D. (2004). Critical periods in nervous systems development. In E. Zigler & S. J. Styfco (Eds.), *The Head Start debates* (pp. 435–447). Baltimore: Paul H. Brookes Publishing Company.

Lareau, A. (2003). *Unequal childhoods: Class, race, and family life*. Berkeley: University of California Press.

Marcon, R. A. (1999). Differential impact of preschool models on development and early learning of inner-city children. *Developmental Psychology, 35,* 358–375.

Myers, R. (1992). *The twelve who survive: Strengthening programmes of early childhood development in the third world.* London: Routledge.

Neisworth, J. T., & Buggey, T. J. (2005). Behaviour analysis and principles in early childhood education. In J. Roopnarine & J. E. Johnson (Eds.), *Approaches to early childhood education* (4th ed., pp. 196–210). Columbus: Merrill/Prentice Hall.

Piaget, J. (1969). *The language and thought of the child.* New York: World.

Powell, C. (2004). *An evaluation of the Roving Caregivers Program.* Unpublished manuscript. Mona: Tropical Medicine Unit, University of the West Indies.

Powell, C., Grantham-McGregor, S. M., & Walker, S. (1998). Early stimulation programmes in Jamaica. In *Recent advances in research on the effects of health and nutrition on the development of children living in poverty*. Washington, DC: Pan American Health Organization.

Reddock, R., & Bobb-Smith, Y. (2005). *Reconciling work and family: Issues and policies in Trinidad and Tobago: Working paper*. Geneva: International Labour Organization.

Reynolds, A. J. (2000). *Success in early intervention: The Chicago Child-Parent Centers.* Lincoln: University of Nebraska Press.

Riley-St. John, M., & Finisterre, F. (2009). *Study on regional replication of RCP*. Bridgetown: Caribbean Child Support Initiative.

Roopnarine, J. L. (2005). *The Roving Caregiver Program in Jamaica: Its theoretical and research foundations and efficacy*. The Hague: Benard van Leer Foundation.

Roopnarine, J. L., & Evans, M. E. (2007). Family structural organization, mother-child and father-child relationships and psychological outcomes in English speaking African Caribbean and Indo Caribbean families. In M. Sutherland (Ed.), *Psychology of development in the Caribbean.* Kingston: Ian Randle Publishers.

Roopnarine, J. L., & Gielen, U. (Eds.). (2005). *Families in global perspectives*. Boston: Allyn & Bacon.

Roopnarine, J. L., & Johnson, J. E. (Eds.). (2005). *Approaches to early childhood education* (4th ed.). Columbus: Merrill/Prentice Hall.
Roopnarine, J. L., & Metindogan, A. (2005). Early childhood education in cross-national perspective. In B. Spodek & O. Saracho (Eds.), *Handbook of research on the education of young children* (2nd ed.). Mahwah: Erlbaum.
Shonkoff, J., & Phillips, D. (2000). *From neurons to neighbourhoods: The science of early childhood development.* Washington, DC: National Academic Press.
Snyder, T.D., Tan, A.G., & Hoffman, C.M. (2004). *Digest of Education Statistics 2003,* (NCES 2005–025). U.S. Department of Education, National Center for Education Statistics. Washington, DC: Government Printing Office.
Van spijk, J. (2010). *Cost analysis of the Roving Caregivers Programme: A study on the costs and benefits of RCP in Dominica, Jamaica, Grenada, St Lucia and St Vincent and the Grenadines.* Amsterdam: Amsterdam Institute for International Development.

Susan Branker Greene (Barbados): A development and evaluation specialist consultant and former program director of the Bernard Van Leer Foundation's (BvLF) Caribbean Child Support Initiative (CCSI) Programme Management Unit (2001–2011) based in Barbados. She holds a Bachelor of Science degree in sociology and political science from the University of the West Indies, Cave Hill Campus, Barbados, and a Master of Science in international relations from the University of Southampton in the UK. She has over 15 years of multi-country and multi-sector program management and development evaluation experience with a strong track record of performance in the start-up and replication of nonformal, culturally relevant, and effective approaches to early childhood development and parenting support. She presented to regional and international audiences on the importance of quality, nonformal approaches to early childhood development, and family support service provision in the Caribbean context and is a strong advocate for mainstreaming such approaches into existing government systems and services.

Clive Murray (Barbados): Communication for development specialist with over 10 years of progressive work experience in the nonprofit sector in the Caribbean region. He has developed and managed initiatives in the areas of communication and advocacy for early childhood development, community development, donor management, and media relations. He holds a Master of Arts degree in social development and sustainable livelihoods from the University of Reading in the UK and a Bachelor of Arts in media and communication from the University of the West Indies (UWI) Mona; Kingston, Jamaica.

Horis Lynch (Barbados): Former research assistant with the Caribbean Child Support Initiative Programme Management Unit in Barbados. He holds a Bachelor of Science degree in political science and law from the University of the West Indies and is interested in social policy research and the effects of early childhood intervention on children's development from school entry to early adulthood. He studies family, school, and other social influences on children's educational success, and contextual factors that influence adolescent development, particularly for rural minorities.

Chapter 13
The Investment in Home Visit Programs in Rural Indigenous Communities as a Strategy to Grant a Good Start in Life for Young Children

J. Leonardo Yánez

Imagine you enter a rural house on a very distant community of the Amazonas, the Andes, or the semiarid areas of Brazil. In a corner, there are some toys and a few books with attractive pictures over a dry, clean, and soft piece of cloth or carpet. Older children and adults play and explore the materials with younger children. Sometimes, they even make new toys with objects that they can find around.

On a wall, a big poster keeps a visible record of the children's progress in height and weight. Other colorful posters remind the caregiver of important information related to the children: vaccinations, health control, recommended diet, and a schedule of activities that also marks the next time the home visitor will spend a time playing and talking to the mother, her family, and the baby.

The home visitor is a neighbor. She attends training and information sessions with a health agent from the capital city who comes 3–8 times in the year, on board of a ship of the municipality or, in some cases, the Armada (after all, they always watch over the safety of the most remote territories and peoples, and this is a strategic program).[1]

The agent provides the home visitor with materials, toys, information, and ideas to make her home visits to the parents and caretakers more enjoyable and productive. The home visitor advises the parents about playing and interacting with the child, and behaves as a role model for them.

[1] Actually, in Peru, the Armada has dedicated two fully furnished boats to bring a team that visits families with young children across the main rivers of the Amazonian territory of Loreto. The team includes health, education, protection, and other specialized staff that provide direct support to home visitors and other social agents in isolated communities. Ten more ships are under construction to scale the program.

J. L. Yánez (✉)
Bernard van Leer Foundation, The Hague, Netherlands
e-mail: leonardo.yanez@bvleerf.nl

L. Roggman, N. Cardia (eds.), *Home Visitation Programs*,
DOI 10.1007/978-3-319-17984-1_13

The home visitor monitors some basic indicators of child development and the environment of the child to feed that data into a digital device (e.g., tablet or mobile phone). The information is sent through an itinerant antenna to the health center that analyzes it in search for patterns of development or signs that would set off alarms.

The image described here is far from fictional. It portraits a range of diverse elements that can be observed in quality programs for rural families with young children that include a home visiting component. However, rarely can we see the combination of all of these elements in one single program. The local cultural and geographic context, the national policy, and the resources available to the program implementers define the prevalence of certain components over the others.

Nevertheless, this scenario illustrates some of the main issues that need to be taken into consideration when scaling up a home visiting program in isolated communities. The most apparent conclusion of this vision is that we seem to be clear about the content of a curriculum for this activity. The World Health Organization (WHO) and the United Nations Children's Fund (UNICEF) are promoting the Care for Child Development (CCD) package that, in my opinion, synthesizes our accumulated experience in early childhood development and health care. The package consists of "an evidence-based set of materials to help the health sector workers to support caregivers in improving the sensitivity, responsiveness and psychosocial stimulation of their children" (Christiansen et al., 2013, p. 23).

We are also stating that public awareness, which is needed to structure both the offer and the demand for home visitation services, is increasing. In the Americas, several leaders have made public commitments to invest more in children's early years. President Obama, President Rousseff, and President Humala have joined the leaders of Colombia and Chile in demanding priority to early learning and to pay special care to the most vulnerable. In every case, an estimate amount of the investment needed has been announced.

The origin of the investment is also open to opportunities. In some countries, it is expected that the public sector will make all of the investment, while in others the expectations are in favor of a greater commitment from the private sector. Finding the best mechanism to guarantee that every child has the same opportunity to access quality learning from the beginning of his or her life is the shared challenge.

We are also convinced that the quality of a service can only be sustained when the target population recognizes its benefits and gets organized to demand it. We all need to think of ways to raise awareness among the people, their leaders, local administrators, the private sector, and many other stakeholders who could be our interlocutors to the need to adapt high-quality home visiting programs for rural families with young children.

We are also aware that a program for early learning cannot be restricted to a single sector. An interdisciplinary approach to providing early care and development is necessary, if we are truly concerned about the best interests of the child. This aspect still poses some obstacles in a few countries in our region; however, examples of a multi-sector approach are gaining more terrain. The Brazilian programs Primeira Infância Melhor in Rio Grande do Sul and Mãe Coruja in Pernambuco are two excellent examples of inter-sectorial coordination and good governance. Both programs have built monitoring systems that provide accurate information to specialized teams that inform each relevant sector and lead the process of strategizing and decision-making. The initiative of the Peruvian Navy to join in an effort to ensure that every family with children from 0 to 3 years old in the Peruvian Amazon region has access to proper information, coaching, and support to foster their children's development is an outstanding example of the importance of including even quite different actors in such issues of priority in the early years of life.

A home visiting program is not just a program for young children; it is closely related to adult education and community development. The parents and caretakers are its main targets because they are the ones who spend most time with young children. Among the most relevant impacts of these programs are the increased quality of materials for playing with children and the enhancing of the environment where they grow up. A study of the scaling up of a home visiting program in rural communities in Colombia suggests that by helping adults, these changes are possible and sustainable (Attanacio et al., 2013). According to these researchers, "the overall aim of home visiting programs is to promote child development by improving parents' child-rearing beliefs and their ability to provide an enriching environment for their children" (p. 37).

Last but not least, technology is necessary to bridge the gap between political wish and practical feasibility to implement programs without sacrificing quality. The difficult access to certain populations in Africa, South Asia, and Latin America demands that we explore the use of communication and information technology to gain access to remote communities and give their children the right to a good start in life. A research study in progress, commissioned by the Bernard van Leer Foundation (BvLF), is yielding some promising results about the use of telephones to enhance the effectiveness of home visiting programs in some African countries (Ba & Bangura, 2013).

At the BvLF, we are convinced that everyone—from parents to policy-makers—has a role to play in supporting a child's growth. Our mission is to ensure that all children are able to reach their full potential by creating access to quality education and safe, healthy spaces for children to live, learn, and grow up. During more than 40 years, the BvLF has provided funding and technical support to innovative initiatives aimed at granting equal opportunities in education for children growing up in very challenging contexts. We have learned that often the children who fail or drop out of school come from very challenging environments: environments of poverty, isolation, or violence. Therefore, it is not fair to blame the failure on the child.

Children are born to learn, and learning is all about experiencing the world, expressing feelings, and being in constant transaction with the others. Learning is a social experience as much as it is an individual process of reorganization of the events that happen around us. Therefore, the best approaches to early learning include the family, the community, and the environment that surrounds the child and attracts her attention. In high-quality preschool centers this is well known. Planners know it too. We also know that learning starts before the child is born and that quality learning occurs when everyone in the community is involved and every aspect of the social, cultural, and economic life in a particular society is taken into account.

In the most humble and isolated community, there is accumulated knowledge and good practices of child rearing. Sometimes, competing information attempts against good traditional practice or certain cultural practice is unfavorable to a particular group of children (for instance girls). In those cases, the family needs access to trustable and opportune information. Such information must be available where they live. Every young child has the right to meaningful learning regardless of where and to whom they are born. Crèches and care centers are urban solutions, home visiting programs are the solution to quality learning in rural settlements and, sometimes, in certain urban slums.

To base professional staff in those communities is difficult, expensive, and often not possible. We have learned that it is also not necessary. There are better ways to attain quality, capitalizing on the existing capacities in the communities. Parents and caregivers are the best available human resource to create the environment for quality learning for children under 3 years of age. We should take advantage of this to scale-up fair opportunities to all children.

Understanding brain development and the complexity of child development requires specialized experts. Making it possible for a child to explore, play, learn, and enjoy the world requires loving and knowledgeable caregivers and a supportive community. Our big challenge is to help in creating the connection between sciences and care to ensure that every child has access to evidence-based high-quality care. This is why the BvLF is endorsing initiatives to scale-up home visiting programs starting with the most challenging regions. If this can be done there, there will be no doubts about doing it in areas that are more accessible.

There are plenty of good examples of the benefits of starting early and including everyone, in Brazil and also in other countries. In Brazil, Mãe Coruja, Primeira Infância Melhor (PIM), Asas da Floristania, and other amazing initiatives have shown the possibilities of bringing learning opportunities to where the children are going through home visiting programs that directly support parents and caregivers.

Each of these programs features a diverse range of adaptations responding to particular contexts and capacities. They all pack kits with relevant information about babies and toddlers for the parents; sometimes that information makes the difference between life and death. For instance, when staff of the Popular Centre for Culture and Development persuaded native parents in Maranhão about the danger of feeding feijoada (a meat stew popular in Brazil) to newborn babies, many lives were saved. In a place where infant mortality during the first 6 weeks of life is very high, providing useful information to the right person saved the lives of those babies without the direct intervention of experts. Knowing whom young mothers go to for advice is critical. We must identify the abilities and traits needed for a person to succeed as home visitors in rural communities.

Reducing domestic violence against children and mothers is a promising outcome of a good quality home visiting program. Innovative initiatives to interrupt violence, such as the program Ring-a-Bell, have shown that it is possible to change social norms regarding tolerance of violence. There are, however, still questions about how we can approach this issue in a way that does not backfire on those trying to interrupt violence. While early learning is critical during the first 3 years, experimenting or witnessing violence is a hindering factor to learning and brain development. A literature review commissioned to an important research center in Peru (Grupo de Análisis para el Desarrollo—GRADE, 2011) yields some interesting insights:

- Partner violence increases the risks of child abuse (Pinheiro, 2006).
- There is a 40 % overlap between violence against children and violence against mothers (Goddard & Bedi, 2010).
- Violence against mothers impacts on their children causing behavioral problem at home and at school: shyness, depression, post-traumatic stress, suicidal attitude, bad relationship with the mother, and risky behavior (Goddard & Bedi, 2010).
- There is a high association between community structure and violence at home: When there are more support networks, there is less isolation and less violence at home (Zielinski & Bradshaw, 2006).
- Violence against mothers is highly related to children's high prevalence of malnourishment, injuries, and respiratory and intestinal infections (Heaton & Forste, 2008).

GRADE's direct study in 36 communities in Peru confirmed the above-mentioned results in these communities. A regression analysis of primary data showed that violence against mothers was the best predictor of the prevalence of malnourishment, severe injuries, and infections among young children. They also found that violence against women was more frequent when children were younger (2011).

A rapid assessment, by the Peruvian Institute of Research, suggested that a family intervention in the highlands of Peru (Ayacucho) that included a home visiting program to provide advice and technology to poor families regarding child rearing practices, organizing their homes, and improving their livelihood, led to a remarkable reduction of accidents and child abuse in a very short period (Ames, 2014). An experimental study is underway to assess the quantitative and qualitative impact of this program in 12 communities in a neighboring region.

Despite the number of programs for young children in Latin America, it is quite difficult to find many cases that have counted on external and independent evaluation. We need to do more to change that. We do know the programs that have improved the early development of poor children in ways that help them succeed at school (Crece Contigo in Chile, Kusiwarma in Peru, Madres Guias in Honduras, Educa a tu Hijo in Cuba, and Hogares Comunitarios in Colombia, among many others). Program reports indicate good results; however, independent evaluations are still lacking, and rigorous evidence to support their use in policy-making is needed. For instance, in Pachacutec, an extremely poor urban slum of Lima, local teachers say that the children who were assisted by a local home visiting program (Kusiwarma) during the first 3 years of age, did better in school than those who were not. Even when no preschool is available, teachers report differences between children that received home visitation and those who did not at ages 0–3 years. Such programs are feasible in remote areas and have the potential to improve the lives of many of the world's poorest children. After more than 10 years of implementation of this program, it is just now that an experimental study is being designed to assess its results. We welcome studies of similar quality to that conducted by Attanacio et al. (2013) as a step in the right direction.

References

Ames, P. (2014). Improving home environments in the Andes to prevent violence against children. *Early Childhood Matters, 122*(June), 27–29. (Bernard van Leer Foundation)

Attanacio, O., Graham-MacGregor, S., Fernández, C., Fitzsimons, E., & Rubio-Codina, M. (2013). Enriching the home environment of low-income families in Colombia: A strategy to promote child development at scale. *Early Childhood Matters, 120*(June), 35–39. (Bernard van Leer Foundation)

Ba, H., & Bangura, L. (2013). Home visiting programmes: The evolving use of mobile phones. *Early Childhood Matters, 120*(June), 59–60. (Bernard van Leer Foundation)

Christiansen, C., Servili, C., Dua, T., & Daelmans, B. (2013). Health for learning: The Care for Child Development package. *Early Childhood Matters, 120*(June), 23–27. (Bernard van Leer Foundation)

Goddard, C., & Bedi, G. (2010). Intimate partner violence and child abuse: A child-centred perspective. *Child Abuse Review, 19*(1), 5–20.

GRADE (2011). *Baseline about violence, health and child care in Peru.* Commissioned by the Bernard van Leer Foundation. The Hague: Bernard van Leer Foundation.

Heaton, T. B., & Forste, R. (2008). Domestic violence, couple interaction and children's health in Latin America. *Journal of Family Violence, 23*(3), 183–193.

Pinheiro, P. S. (2006). *Rights of the child: Report of the independent expert for the United Nations study on violence against children.* New York: United Nations.

Zielinski, D. S., & Bradshaw, C. P. (2006). Ecological influences on the sequelae of child maltreatment: A review of the literature. *Child Maltreatment, 11*(1), 49–62.

J. Leonardo Yánez (Bernard van Leer Foundation/Netherlands): Senior program officer for Latin America at the Bernard van Leer Foundation. He worked in academia, NGOs, and government in Venezuela on primary and preschool care and education before joining the foundation in 2000, initially coordinating the "Effectiveness Initiative" before moving onto developing and managing programs in the Latin America region. He was national director of preschool education and general director of program coordination for social development in Venezuela and ex-chairman of the Primary and Preschool Education Department at the Andrés Bello University. He has contributed to the design, implementation, and evaluation of programs for early childhood care and development and worked as consultant for UNICEF, Social Science Research Centre, Book's Bank, National Institute for Child and Youth, and Ministries of Family and Social Development, Education and Planning, among others.

Index

L. Roggman, N. Cardia (eds.), *Home Visitation Programs*,
DOI 10.1007/978-3-319-17984-1

MIX
Papier aus verantwortungsvollen Quellen
Paper from responsible sources
FSC® C105338

Printed by Books on Demand, Germany